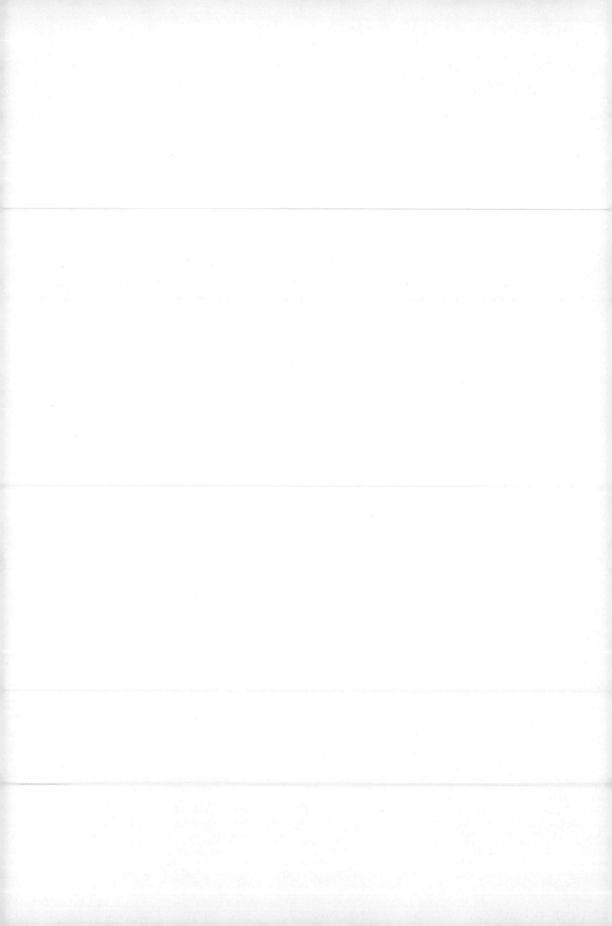

Head and Neck Cancer

Editors

PATRICIA A. HUDGINS
AMIT M. SAINDANE

NEUROIMAGING CLINICS OF NORTH AMERICA

www.neuroimaging.theclinics.com

Consulting Editor
SURESH K. MUKHERJI

February 2013 • Volume 23 • Number 1

ELSEVIER

1600 John F. Kennedy Boulevard ● Suite 1800 ● Philadelphia, Pennsylvania 19103-2899

http://www.theclinics.com

NEUROIMAGING CLINICS OF NORTH AMERICA Volume 23, Number 1
February 2013 ISSN 1052-5149, ISBN 13: 978-1-4557-7119-6

Editor: Pamela M. Hetherington
Developmental Editor: Donald Mumford

Neuroimaging Clinics of North America (ISSN 1052-5149) is published quarterly by Elsevier Inc., 360 Park Avenue South, New York, NY 10010-1710. Months of issue are February, May, August, and November. Business and editorial offices: 1600 John F. Kennedy Blvd., Suite 1800, Philadelphia, PA 19103-2899. Business and editorial offices: 6277 Sea Harbor Drive, Orlando, FL 32887-4800. Periodicals postage paid at New York, NY, and additional mailing offices. Subscription prices are USD 342 per year for US individuals, USD 471 per year for US institutions, USD 172 per year for US students and residents, USD 396 per year for Canadian individuals, USD 590 per year for Canadian institutions, USD 502 per year for international individuals, USD 590 per year for international institutions and USD 246 per year for Canadian and foreign students and residents. To receive student/resident rate, orders must be accompanied by name of affiliated institution, date of term, and the *signature* of program/residency coordinator on institution letterhead. Orders will be billed at individual rate until proof of status is received. Foreign air speed delivery is included in all *Clinics* subscription prices. All prices are subject to change without notice. POSTMASTER: Send address changes to *Neuroimaging Clinics of North America*, Elsevier Health Sciences Division, Subscription Customer Service, 3251 Riverport Lane, Maryland Heights, MO 63043. Telephone: 1-800-654-2452 (U.S. and Canada); 314-447-8871 (outside U.S. and Canada). Fax: 314-447-8029. E-mail: journalscustomerservice-usa@elsevier.com (for print support); journalsonlinesupport-usa@elsevier.com (for online support).

Reprints. For copies of 100 or more of articles in this publication, please contact the Commercial Reprints Department, Elsevier Inc., 360 Park Avenue South, New York, NY 10010-1710. Tel.: 212-633-3812; Fax: 212-462-1935; E-mail: reprints@elsevier.com.

Neuroimaging Clinics of North America is covered by *Excerpta Medica/EMBASE,* the RSNA Index of Imaging Literature, *MEDLINE/PubMed (Index Medicus),* MEDLINE/MEDLARS, SciSearch, Research Alert, and Neuroscience Citation Index.

Printed and bound by CPI Group (UK) Ltd, Croydon, CR0 4YY

Transferred to digital print 2012

PROGRAM OBJECTIVE:

The goal of *Neuroimaging Clinics of North America* is to keep practicing radiologists and radiology residents up to date with current clinical practice in radiology by providing timely articles reviewing the state of the art in patient care.

TARGET AUDIENCE

Practicing radiologists, radiology residents, and other healthcare professionals who utilize neuroimaging findings to provide patient care.

ACCREDITATION

The Elsevier Office of Continuing Medical Education (EOCME) is accredited by the Accreditation Council for Continuing Medical Education (ACCME) to provide continuing medical education for physicians.

The EOCME designates this journal-based CME activity for a maximum of 10 *AMA PRA Category 1 Credit*(s)™. Physicians should claim only the credit commensurate with the extent of their participation in the activity.

All other health care professionals completing continuing education credit for this activity will be issued a certificate of participation.

DISCLOSURE OF CONFLICTS OF INTEREST

The EOCME assesses conflict of interest with its instructors, faculty, planners, and other individuals who are in a position to control the content of CME activities. All relevant conflicts of interest that are identified are thoroughly vetted by EOCME for fair balance, scientific objectivity, and patient care recommendations. EOCME is committed to providing its learners with CME activities that promote improvements or quality in healthcare and not a specific proprietary business or a commercial interest.

The planning committee, staff, authors and editors listed below have identified no financial relationships or relationships to products or devices they or their spouse/life partner have with commercial interest related to the content of this CME activity:

Ashley H. Aiken, MD; Kriston L. Baugnon, MD; Jonathan J. Beitler, MD, MBA; Amy Y. Chen, MD; Nicole Congleton; Amanda Corey, MD; Elliott R. Friedman, MD; Patricia A. Hudgins, MD; Gamaliel Lorenzo, MD; Jill McNair; Nagaraj Paramasivam; Amit M. Saindane, MD; and Katelynn Steck.

The planning committee, staff, authors and editors listed below have identified financial relationships or relationships to products or devices they or their spouse/life partner have with commercial interest related to the content of this CME activity:

Christine M. Glastonbury, MBBS is a consultant/advisor and has received royalties/patents in Amirsys, Inc. Both herself and spouse own stock in Amirsys, Inc.
Suresh K. Mukherji, MD, FACR is a consultant or advisor for Philips.
Karen L. Salzman, MD is a consultant/advisor, owns stock, and has received royalties/patents from Amirsys, Inc.

UNAPPROVED / OFF-LABEL USE DISCLOSURE

The EOCME requires CME faculty to disclose to the participants:

1. When products or procedures being discussed are off-label, unlabelled, experimental, and/or investigational (not US Food and Drug Administration (FDA) approved; and
2. Any limitations on the information presented, such as data that are preliminary or that represent ongoing research, interim analyses, and/or unsupported opinions. Faculty may discuss information about pharmaceutical agents that is outside of DA-approved labelling. This information is intended solely for CME and is not intended to promote off-label use of these medications. If you have any questions, contact the medical affairs department of the manufacturer for the most recent prescribing information.

TO ENROLL

To enroll in the *Neuroimaging Clinics of North America* Continuing Medical Education program, call customer service at 1-800-654-2452 or sign up online at http://www.theclinics.com/home/cme. The CME program is available to subscribers for an additional annual fee of $212 USD.

METHOD OF PARTICIPATION

In order to claim credit, participants must complete the following:

1. Complete enrolment as indicated above.
2. Read the activity.
3. Complete the CME Test and Evaluation. Participants must achieve a score of 70% on the test. All CME Tests and Evaluations must be completed online.

CME INQUIRIES/SPECIAL NEEDS

For all CME inquiries or special needs, please contact elsevierCME@elsevier.com.

NEUROIMAGING CLINICS OF NORTH AMERICA

FORTHCOMING ISSUES

May 2013
Pediatric Demyelinating Disease
Manohar Shroff, MD, *Guest Editor*

August 2013
Modern Imaging of the Brain, Body and Spine
Lara Brandao, MD, *Guest Editor*

RECENT ISSUES

November 2012
Central Nervous System Infections
Gaurang V. Shah, MD, *Guest Editor*

August 2012
Socioeconomics of Neuroimaging
David M. Yousem, MD, MBA, *Guest Editor*

May 2012
Neuroradiology Applications of High-Field MR Imaging
Winfried A. Willinek, MD, *Guest Editor*

RELATED INTEREST

Magnetic Resonance Imaging Clinics, Vol. 20, No. 3, August 2012
Practical MR Imaging of the Head and Neck
Laurie A. Loevner, MD, *Guest Editor*

DOWNLOAD
Free App!

Review Articles
THE CLINICS

NOW AVAILABLE FOR YOUR iPhone and iPad

Contributors

CONSULTING EDITOR

SURESH K. MUKHERJI, MD, FACR
Department of Radiology, University of
Michigan Health System, Ann Arbor, Michigan

EDITORS

PATRICIA A. HUDGINS, MD, FACR
Director of Head and Neck Radiology;
Professor of Radiology and Imaging Sciences/
Otolaryngology, Head & Neck Section, Division
of Neuroradiology, Department of Radiology
and Imaging Sciences, Emory University
School of Medicine, Atlanta, Georgia

AMIT M. SAINDANE, MD
Director of Neuroradiology; Assistant
Professor of Radiology and Imaging
Sciences, Department of Radiology and
Imaging Sciences, Emory University School
of Medicine, Atlanta, Georgia

AUTHORS

ASHLEY H. AIKEN, MD
Assistant Professor of Radiology and Imaging
Sciences, Department of Radiology and
Imaging Sciences, Emory University, Atlanta,
Georgia

KRISTEN L. BAUGNON, MD
Assistant Professor of Radiology and Imaging
Sciences, Department of Radiology and
Imaging Sciences, Emory University School
of Medicine, Atlanta, Georgia

JONATHAN J. BEITLER, MD, MBA, FACR
Professor of Radiation Oncology, Department
of Radiation Oncology, Winship Cancer
Institute, Emory University School of Medicine,
Atlanta, Georgia

AMY Y. CHEN, MD
Professor of Otolaryngology-Head & Neck
Surgery, Department of Otolaryngology-Head
& Neck Surgery, Emory University School of
Medicine, Atlanta, Georgia

AMANDA COREY, MD
Assistant Professor, Department of Radiology
and Imaging Sciences, Emory University
School of Medicine, Atlanta, Georgia

ELLIOTT R. FRIEDMAN, MD
Assistant Professor of Radiology, Department
of Diagnostic and Interventional Imaging,
University of Texas Health Science Center at
Houston, Houston, Texas

CHRISTINE M. GLASTONBURY, MBBS
Professor of Clinical Radiology, Department of
Radiology and Biomedical Imaging, University
of California, San Francisco, San Francisco,
California

PATRICIA A. HUDGINS, MD, FACR
Professor of Radiology and Imaging Sciences/
Otolaryngology; Director of Head & Neck
Radiology, Head & Neck Section, Division of
Neuroradiology, Department of Radiology and
Imaging Sciences, Emory University School of
Medicine, Atlanta, Georgia

GAMALIEL LORENZO, MD
Department of Radiology and Imaging
Sciences, Emory University School of
Medicine, Atlanta, Georgia

AMIT M. SAINDANE, MD
Assistant Professor of Radiology and Imaging
Sciences, Director of Neuroradiology,

Department of Radiology and Imaging
Sciences, Emory University School of
Medicine, Atlanta, Georgia

KAREN L. SALZMAN, MD
Associate Professor of Radiology, Department
of Radiology, University of Utah, Salt Lake City,
Utah

Contents

> Cancer staging is how clinicians describe the state of the disease, predict prognosis, help determine best treatment, and interpret outcomes. Although several staging systems are available, the most widely used is the tumor node metastasis (TNM) system developed by the American Joint Committee on Cancer. Knowledge of normal anatomy and the myriad appearances of variations in anatomy is the basis of accurate tumor staging. Cross-sectional imaging is complementary to the clinical examination for accurate staging.

> Although nasopharyngeal carcinoma (NPC) is the most common primary malignancy of the nasopharynx, it is an uncommon malignancy in much of the Western world. Over the last several years, there have been important changes in the terminology used for histologic classification of NPC and important changes to the American Joint Committee on Cancer TNM staging of NPC. Accurate imaging assessment is critical for diagnose, to stage and plan radiation treatment, and for ongoing follow-up and surveillance. This article emphasizes important nasopharyngeal anatomy landmarks and the imaging appearances and pitfalls of NPC, its patterns of spread, and posttreatment appearances.

> Oral cavity cancer comprises nearly 30% of all malignant tumors of the head and neck. After a definitive diagnosis has been made, imaging is essential for staging the primary tumor by evaluating submucosal spread and invasion of adjacent structures, and to identify nodal or distant metastasis. Oral cavity anatomy is one of the most complex in the head and neck. Therefore, knowledge of anatomic subsites and spread patterns is critical for accurate staging. This article begins with a discussion of imaging techniques, and then presents a detailed review of normal anatomy followed by imaging's role in tumor staging highlighting potential pitfalls.

> The face of oropharyngeal squamous cell carcinoma (OPSCC) is changing. It has a dichotomous nature, with 1 subset of the disease associated with tobacco and

alcohol use and the other having proven association with human papilloma virus infection. Imaging plays an important role in the staging and surveillance of OPSCC, and a detailed knowledge of the anatomy and pitfalls is critical. This article will review the detailed anatomy of the oropharynx and epidemiology of OPSS, along with its staging, patterns of spread, and treatment.

To accurately interpret pretreatment and posttreatment imaging in patients with hypopharyngeal squamous cell carcinoma (SCC), one must understand the complex anatomy of this part of the aerodigestive system. Common patterns of spread must be recognized, andpitfalls in imaging must be understood. This article reviews the epidemiology, anatomy, staging, treatment, and pitfalls in imaging of hypopharyngeal SCC.

Laryngeal carcinoma is a devastating malignancy that severely affects patients' quality of life, with compromise of ability to talk, breathe, and swallow. Accurate tumor staging is imperative, because treatment plans focus on laryngeal conservation therapy whenever possible. Although the mucosal extent of tumor and vocal cord mobility is best assessed with endoscopic evaluation, cross-sectional imaging is essential for accurate T-staging, because only cross-sectional imaging can assess the submucosal extent of the tumor, cartilage invasion, and extralaryngeal spread. This article reviews topics crucial for interpreting imaging studies of patients with laryngeal squamous cell carcinoma.

The major salivary glands consist of the parotid, submandibular, and sublingual glands. Most neoplasms in other subsites in the head and neck are squamous cell carcinoma, but tumors of the salivary glands may be benign or malignant. Surgical treatment differs if the lesion is benign, and therefore preoperative fine needle aspiration is important in salivary neoplasms. The role of imaging is to attempt to determine histology, predict likelihood of a lesion being malignant, and report an imaging stage. This article reviews the various histologies, imaging features, and staging of major salivary gland neoplasms.

Thyroid cancer includes several neoplasms originating from the thyroid gland—from indolent and curable histologies of differentiated thyroid carcinoma to aggressive anaplastic thyroid carcinoma. Differentiation of thyroid nodules is problematic on CT and MR imaging unless there is evidence of extrathyroidal extension. Evaluation of regional lymph nodes is often performed clinically or with ultrasound. The retropharyngeal and mediastinal lymph nodes are better evaluated by CT and MR imaging. Nuclear scintigraphy is useful for staging and treatment of distant metastasis in differentiated thyroid carcinoma. PET may have a role in aggressive cancers. Accurate staging affects surgical management and subsequent therapy.

> Lymph nodes status is an important predictor of prognosis in head and neck squamous cell carcinoma, making accurate staging critical. The physical examination of the neck is highly inaccurate. CT, MR imaging, ultrasound (US), and positron emission tomography-CT (PET-CT) improve accuracy but have limitations. Size criteria, nodal shape and clustering, central necrosis, and findings of extracapsular spread and vascular encasement suggest metastatic involvement on CT and MR imaging. US features help differentiate benign from malignant nodes, aided by US-guided fine-needle aspiration for indeterminate cases. PET-CT is useful for staging the lymph nodes and detection of distant metastasis.

> Image-guided tissue sampling is becoming increasingly important for management of head and neck cancers. Ultrasound-guided fine-needle aspiration (UG-FNA) is safe, effective, and has many advantages compared with palpation-guided FNA and computed tomography-guided FNA. The technique of UG-FNA is highly operator and experience dependent; however, understanding the complex anatomy, disease processes, and patterns of nodal spread in the head and neck make this technique ideal for the neuroradiologist. Proper technique and recognition of pitfalls are critical to successful UG-FNA. Computed tomography–guided FNA is valuable for tissue sampling from deep lesions and for those without a sonographic window for UG-FNA.

Foreword

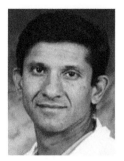

Suresh K. Mukherji, MD, FACR
Consulting Editor

We have entered the "Value-Added" era of medicine in which all physicians are being told to justify and document how we improve a patient's outcome. Head and neck oncologic imaging is clearly one of those areas where the value of imaging is indisputable. As mentioned in the preface, staging is the common language by which clinicians describe the state of the disease, predict prognosis, help determine the best treatment, and interpret outcomes. The importance of imaging and staging has evolved such that the 7th edition of the American Joint Committee on Cancer Staging Manuel fully integrates information obtained by imaging into clinical staging. In this edition, Drs Patricia Hudgins and Amit Saindane have taken a "value-added" approach. This is not a comprehensive review of head and neck anatomy but an issue showing how specific imaging findings affect staging and prognosis.

We are extremely fortunate to have such an outstanding group edit this edition. We are all aware of Dr Hudgin's extraordinary accomplishments and contributions to both Head and Neck and Neuroradiology. Dr Saindane is a "rising star," who is the Division Director of Neuroradiology at Emory. I cannot think of a more experienced and accomplished group to produce this edition and I would like to personally thank them and all the authors for their tremendous contributions. My hope is that other subspecialties will follow Drs Hudgins and Saindane's approach so that all of our health care colleagues will never doubt the "value-added" information provided by imaging.

Suresh K. Mukherji, MD, FACR
Department of Radiology
University of Michigan Health System
1500 East Medical Center
Ann Arbor, MI 48109-0030, USA

E-mail address:
mukherji@med.umich.edu

Neuroimag Clin N Am 23 (2013) xi
http://dx.doi.org/10.1016/j.nic.2012.09.002
1052-5149/13/$ – see front matter © 2013 Elsevier Inc. All rights reserved.

neuroimaging.theclinics.com

Preface

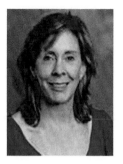 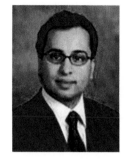

Patricia A. Hudgins, MD, FACR   Amit M. Saindane, MD
Guest Editors

Staging is the common language by which clinicians describe the state of the disease, predict prognosis, help determine best treatment, and interpret outcomes. The most widely used staging system is the tumor node metastasis (TNM) system developed by the American Joint Committee on Cancer (AJCC) in collaboration with the International Union for Cancer Control. The first AJCC staging manual was published in 1977, and the AJCC 7th edition published in 2010 (AJCC 7) is the current version. The manual is available as a 650-page book, a small handbook, and a CD-ROM. Head and Neck is the first anatomic area covered.

The TNM system categorizes each patient's disease based on location, size, and extent of the primary tumor (T), location, number, and extent of nodal metastases (N), and presence of distant metastases (M). Thus, the basis is anatomic. Factors that affect prognosis such as human papilloma virus 16 status, smoking or drinking history, and comorbidities are very important, but have not yet been incorporated into the staging system.

Despite the nearly universal use of the TNM staging system and the widespread availability of AJCC manuals in both written and electronic versions, in our experience diagnostic radiologists rarely include the anatomic stage of the primary tumor in the formal written imaging interpretation. That listing the stage in the dictation is the exception rather than the rule is puzzling. Because the AJCC staging system is anatomic, with the exception of mucosal or skin lesions, the best opportunity to accurately stage the patient is by interpretation of the modern imaging. Even endoscopic biopsies are limited in determining the deep extent of head and neck cancer. Why then, do even subspecialty trained radiologists hesitate to commit to an anatomic stage in each of their dictations?

Comprehensive review of head and neck anatomy is not the goal of this *Neuroimaging Clinics*. Instead, our goal is to show how the AJCC manual can be a guide to interpreting computed tomography (CT) or magnetic resonance (MR) imaging of the patient with head and neck cancer. Only with a thoughtful interpretation and dictation, clearly delineating the local extent of a primary head and neck tumor, can the radiologist offer a precise description of a tumor following guidelines of AJCC, giving value to the referring clinician, Tumor Board members, and the patient. Because of its detail, the AJCC staging manual is a wonderful guide for cross-sectional image interpretation and facilitates generating a useful, value-added CT or MR dictation for a patient with cancer of the head and neck. Using the AJCC manual guides the radiologist in making the most useful interpretations of the imaging.

Patricia A. Hudgins, MD, FACR
Department of Radiology and Imaging Sciences
Division of Neuroradiology, Head & Neck Section
Emory University School of Medicine
BG-27, 1364 Clifton Road, NE
Atlanta, GA 30322, USA

Amit M. Saindane, MD
Department of Radiology and Imaging Sciences
Emory University School of Medicine
BG-22, 1364 Clifton Road, NE
Atlanta, GA 30322, USA

E-mail addresses:
phudgin@emory.edu (P.A. Hudgins)
asainda@emory.edu (A.M. Saindane)

Neuroimag Clin N Am 23 (2013) xiii
http://dx.doi.org/10.1016/j.nic.2012.09.001
1052-5149/13/$ – see front matter © 2013 Elsevier Inc. All rights reserved.

neuroimaging.theclinics.com

Introduction to the Imaging and Staging of Cancer

Patricia A. Hudgins, MD[a],*, Jonathan J. Beitler, MD, MBA[b]

KEYWORDS

- Staging • Squamous cell carcinoma • American Joint Committee on Cancer • Ultrasound
- Computed tomography • Magnetic resonance imaging • Positron emission tomography
- Fine-needle aspiration

KEY POINTS

- Cancer staging is how clinicians describe the state of the disease, predict prognosis, help determine best treatment, and interpret outcomes.
- Although several staging systems are available, the most widely used is the tumor node metastasis (TNM) system developed by the American Joint Committee on Cancer.
- Knowledge of normal anatomy and the myriad appearances of variations in anatomy is the basis of accurate tumor staging.
- Cross-sectional imaging is complementary to the clinical examination for accurate staging.

THE TUMOR NODE METASTASIS STAGING SYSTEM

Cancer staging is the common language by which clinicians describe the state of the disease, predict prognosis, help determine best treatment, and interpret outcomes. Although there are several staging systems available, the most widely used is the tumor node metastasis (TNM) system developed by the American Joint Committee on Cancer (AJCC) in collaboration with the International Union for Cancer Control (UICC).[1] The first AJCC staging manual was published in 1977, and because the manual is revised every 6 to 8 years, the AJCC seventh edition published in 2010 (AJCC7) is the current version. The manual is available as a 650-page book, a small handbook, and on CD-ROM. The AJCC manual is organized by body part, and head and neck is the first anatomic area covered.

The TNM system categorizes each patient's disease based on location, size, and extent of the primary tumor (T), location, number and extent of nodal metastases (N), and presence of distant metastases (M). Thus, the basis is anatomic. Factors that affect prognosis such as human papillomavirus (HPV) 16 status, the smoking or drinking history, or comorbidities are important, but have not yet been incorporated into the staging system.

Tumors can be staged at various points through the treatment cycle. Specifically, clinical stage is at presentation before treatment, pathologic stage is after surgery, and posttherapy stage is after first course of nonoperative therapy, whether radiation, systemic, or both. The initial clinical stage remains the most significant factor to determine prognosis and additional therapy, and is the stage used in reporting survival statistics. The initial clinical stage often appears in every clinical and follow-up report. Thus, even years later and even if a patient is free of disease, clinical notes list the patient as a TNM stage.

[a] Department of Radiology and Imaging Sciences, Emory University School of Medicine, BG-27, 1364 Clifton Road, Northeast, Atlanta, GA 30322, USA
[b] Department of Radiation Oncology, Winship Cancer Institute, Emory University School of Medicine, 1701 Uppergate Drive, Atlanta, GA 30322, USA
* Corresponding author.
E-mail address: phudgin@emory.edu

Neuroimag Clin N Am 23 (2013) 1–7
http://dx.doi.org/10.1016/j.nic.2012.08.003
1052-5149/13/$ – see front matter © 2013 Elsevier Inc. All rights reserved.

Despite the nearly universal use of the TNM staging system and the widespread availability of AJCC manuals in both written and electronic versions, in our experience, diagnostic radiologists rarely include the anatomic stage of the primary tumor in the formal written imaging interpretation. That listing the stage in the dictation is the exception rather than the rule is puzzling. Because the AJCC staging system is anatomic, with the exception of mucosal or skin lesions, the best opportunity to accurately stage the patient is by interpretation of the modern imaging. Even endoscopic biopsies are limited in determining deep extent of head and neck cancer. Why, then, do even subspecialty-trained radiologists hesitate to commit to an anatomic stage in each of their dictations?

The answer, as with any significant medical question, is multifactorial, and likely is related to lack of knowledge regarding normal anatomy, patterns of tumor appearance and spread, and important locations of tumor extension that would change clinical staging. Normal head and neck anatomy is complicated, with small structures present in compact regions. The presence of some structures, such as cranial nerves, can be appreciated only by knowing normal anatomy, because they are so small as to evade visualization with current imaging equipment. Tumor resection and subsequent reconstruction to restore normal function and obtain adequate cosmetic result make follow-up imaging even more difficult.

In the past, the radiologist has had to rely on a frequently illegible blurb of a history on an imaging request form. With the advent of the electronic medical record, the radiologist has access to the clinical signs and symptoms to help their review of the imaging. For example, a history of pain along cranial nerve V2 distribution prompts a second look at that relevant anatomy.

Knowledge of normal anatomy and the myriad appearances of variations in anatomy is the basis of accurate tumor staging. Comprehensive review of head and neck anatomy is not the goal of this issue of *Clinics*. Instead, our goal is to show how the AJCC manual can be a guide to interpreting computed tomography (CT) or magnetic resonance (MR) imaging of the patient with head and neck cancer. Only with a thoughtful interpretation and dictation, clearly delineating the local extent of a primary head and neck tumor, can the radiologist offer a precise description of a tumor following guidelines of AJCC, giving value to the referring clinician, tumor board members, and the patient.

Consider the patient presenting with a mass in the tonsil. The referring clinician is likely aware of the mass, so a final dictation just confirming the mass is of little value. Frequently in our head and neck tumor board (HNTB), we see outside dictations that say "Impression: Large tonsillar mass, correlate clinically, tumor cannot be excluded." Questions that remain include size ("large" is vague and of little use when following the patient), whether there is extension to the base of tongue, soft palate, or pterygoids (all of which may affect whether the patient goes for surgery or the target volumes for the radiation oncologist) and does tumor approach, invade, or surround the internal carotid artery (a finding of tremendous prognostic significance that has direct bearing on the operability of the lesion, particularly in the era of transoral resections)? The interpretation offers little guidance for staging, and therefore no direction for treatment plan or prognosis for the patient. Is the patient a surgical candidate? Are radiation and chemotherapy more appropriate for treatment? Is the tumor curable? What is the prognosis? These pertinent questions arise in the HNTB, and the imaging interpretation is critical to answering the questions that the clinicians should be asking. In turn, a multidisciplinary HNTB significantly affects patient care, and the opportunity to actively participate in the HNTB should not be missed.[2]

Table 1 is current staging for cancer of the oropharynx from AJCC7. Because the tonsil is a subsite of the oropharynx, Table 1 should be used by the radiologist to offer a clinical stage based on imaging. Instead of reporting a large tumor, notice that gradations of size that affect tonsillar cancer stage are 2 cm or smaller (Fig. 1), more than 2 to less than 4 cm (Fig. 2), or greater than 4 cm. Report the actual tumor size as opposed to only the T stage.

Note that T1 and T2 are based exclusively on size. For T3 stage, size is important, greater than 4 cm, but presence of tumor on the epiglottis is important. More precisely, extension to the mucosal surface facing the oropharynx (the lingual surface) is another critical observation (Fig. 3). Therefore, both size and extension to the lingual epiglottic surface should be mentioned.

For all head and neck subsites, the T4 staging is now divided into "moderately advanced," or "very advanced" local disease. T4 tumors by definition have extended out of the boundaries of that subsite and involve surrounding sites. For staging a T4a oropharyngeal tumor, the radiologist must be able to identify the supraglottic larynx, extrinsic tongue muscles (the hyoglossus, styloglossus, genioglossus, and mylohyoid muscles), medial pterygoid muscle, hard palate, and mandible, because extension to 1 or more of those sites

Table 1 AJCC7 oropharynx primary site staging	
Primary Tumor (T)	
TX	Primary tumor cannot be assessed
T0	No evidence of primary tumor
Tis	Carcinoma in situ
T1	Tumor ≤2 cm in greatest dimension
T2	Tumor >2 cm but not >4 cm in greatest dimension
T3	Tumor >4 cm in greatest dimension or extension to the lingual surface of epiglottis
T4a	Moderately advanced local disease Tumor invades the larynx, extrinsic muscle of tongue, medial pterygoid, hard palate, or mandible[a]
T4b	Very advanced local disease. Tumor invades lateral pterygoid muscle, pterygoid plates, lateral nasopharynx, or skull base or encases carotid artery

[a] Mucosal extension to lingual surface of epiglottis from primary tumors of the base of the tongue and vallecula does not constitute invasion of larynx.

From Edge S, Byrd D, Compton C, et al. AJCC cancer staging manual. 7th edition. Chicago: Springer; 2010. p. 41–56; with permission.

infers the T4a stage (**Fig. 4**). T4b or "very advanced local disease" means that an oropharyngeal tumor has invaded the lateral pterygoid muscle or pterygoid plates, the lateral nasopharynx, skull base, or

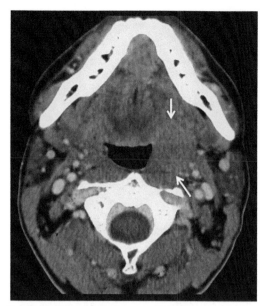

Fig. 2. Oropharyngeal SCC, tonsil subsite, stage T2 N0. Left tonsil mass (*arrows*) is greater than 2 cm, but less than 4 cm in maximum diameter.

is circumferential around the internal carotid artery.

Because of its detail, the AJCC staging manual is a wonderful guide for cross-sectional image interpretation, and facilitates generating a useful, value-added CT or MR dictation for a patient with cancer of the tonsil. Overall, using the AJCC

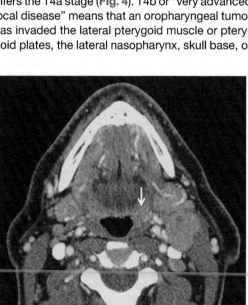

Fig. 1. Oropharyngeal SCC, tonsil subsite, stage T1 N2b. Small left tonsil mass (*arrow*) is less than 2 cm. Notice bulky left anterior and posterior IIA adenopathy. Patient was a nonsmoker and tumor was HPV-16 positive.

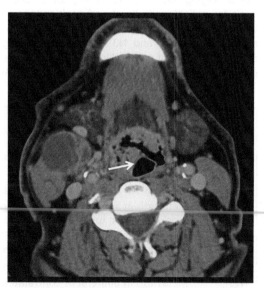

Fig. 3. Oropharyngeal SCC, tonsil subsite, stage T3 N2a. Right tonsil mass extends inferiorly to involve the lingual surface of the epiglottis (*arrow*). Bulky necrotic ipsilateral IIA nodal mass is also present.

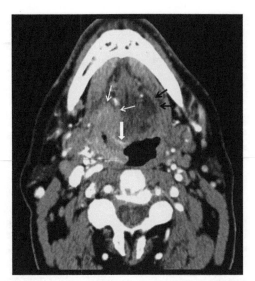

Fig. 4. Oropharyngeal SCC, tonsil subsite, stage T4a. Right oropharyngeal mass likely originated in tonsil, and has extended to base of tongue (*thick white arrow*) and to floor of mouth (*thin white arrows*), an oral cavity site. Note normal left hyoglossus muscle, an extrinsic tongue muscle (*black arrows*). Tumor has replaced right hyoglossus muscle. Based on involvement of hyoglossus muscle, tumor is staged as T4a or moderately advanced local disease.

manual guides the radiologist in making the most useful interpretations of the imaging.

NODAL STAGING

Nodal staging has a significant impact on prognosis for patients with head and neck cancer.[3–5] Designation of N0 denotes no metastatic adenopathy, and N1, N2, and N3 describe increasing number and size of nodes. Nodal staging can be pathologic, either by fine-needle aspiration (FNA) or surgical node dissection, or by imaging if there is unequivocal cross-sectional or metabolic [18F] fluorodeoxyglucose (FDG)-positron emission tomography (PET) evidence of disease. For example, a patient with a new neck mass may undergo FNA of the node, and the diagnosis of squamous cell carcinoma (SCC) may be made. A search for the primary tumor via conventional physical examination, imaging, and endoscopy follows. If multiple nodes are present on CT, MR imaging, or PET-CT, the nodal staging can be designated even if pathologic FNA is not performed on each node. It is crucial to evaluate the imaging carefully and accurately; treatment decisions are frequently made based on imaging.

The standard anatomic nodal description used universally by health care professionals should be routinely adopted by radiologists (**Table 2**).[6,7] This description of node location is used in the head and neck regardless of location of the primary cancer. Node groups that are not covered by the standard nodal system but may be involved with head and neck cancer are suboccipital, retropharyngeal, parapharyngeal, buccinator or facial nodes, preauricular, periparotid, or intraparotid.[1]

Cross-sectional imaging, although critical to nodal staging, carries poor sensitivity for detecting subclinical nodal metastases, especially micrometastases.[8] Microscopic nodal metastases cannot be detected by any current imaging modality. Size and central necrosis are criteria used routinely to detect macroscopic disease. Central nodal necrosis (in the absence of acute suppurative nodal infection) always denotes macroscopic metastatic disease. Nodal size is less sensitive for detecting metastasis, and less specific, because normal reactive nodes are variable in size. Choosing 8-mm to 10-mm short or long axis diameter as the size criteria for reporting

Table 2	
AJCC oropharynx and hypopharynx lymph node staging	
NX	Regional lymph nodes cannot be assessed
N0	No regional lymph node metastasis
N1	Metastasis in a single ipsilateral lymph node, ≤3 cm in greatest dimension
N2	Metastasis in a single ipsilateral lymph node, >3 cm but not >6 cm in greatest dimension; or in multiple ipsilateral lymph nodes, none >6 cm in greatest dimension; or in bilateral or contralateral lymph nodes, none >6 cm in greatest dimension
N2a	Metastasis in single ipsilateral lymph node >3 cm but not >6 cm in greatest dimension
N2b	Metastasis in multiple ipsilateral lymph nodes, none >6 cm in greatest dimension
N2c	Metastasis in bilateral or contralateral lymph nodes, none >6 cm in greatest dimension
N3	Metastasis in a lymph node >6 cm in greatest dimension

From Edge S, Byrd D, Compton C, et al. AJCC cancer staging manual. 7th edition. Chicago: Springer; 2010. p. 41–56; with permission.

a node as positive likely has high sensitivity, but low specificity, because many normal reactive nodes can be more than 10 mm in diameter. PET-CT has greatly improved nodal staging[9] but reactive nodes can be metabolically active on PET. A neck dissection has the best sensitivity for nodal staging, but nonsurgical management of neck disease is currently the mainstay for SCC of several subsites. The staging system takes into account the macroscopic staging of the neck, and the probability of subclinical disease should not lessen the radiologist's diligence in evaluating the neck. The radiologist should make every attempt to accurately stage the neck, using any imaging available as well as understanding the patterns of nodal metastasis.

Lymphatic drainage for head and neck cancer is frequently predictable, and nodal staging can be more precise when the radiologist is familiar with the drainage patterns for anatomic subsites.[8,10] In a patient with head and neck squamous cell carcinoma (HNSCC), metastases to nodes in levels II and III are common, whereas nodes in level V are less likely to harbor SCC metastases.

One change between the AJCC sixth edition and the current edition is that a descriptor has been added for extracapsular spread (ECS) of nodal disease, denoted as ECS+ or ECS−.[1] When describing a node that is likely pathologic, the radiologist should attempt to determine ECS. Clinically, ECS manifests as a neck mass that is fixed to overlying skin, surrounding muscle, or fibroadipose tissue, or has signs of cranial nerve extension. Radiographically, ECS can be presumed if the nodal margins are irregular or there is surrounding perinodal stranding and induration.[11,12] ECS of disease carries a poor outcome compared with intact nodal capsule.[13–15]

LIMITATIONS TO CROSS-SECTIONAL STAGING

Imaging is not perfect, and the best radiologist knows the limitations of each modality. In the head and neck, each separate subsite has imaging constraints that are specific for both location and modality. These constraints are discussed elsewhere in this issue. A common imaging limitation (tumor boundaries) deserves special mention.

Lesion size is a critical factor that is generally the major criterion that determines stage. The ability to define boundaries of a lesion with imaging is essential, and is related to several factors, including lesion size, vascularity and enhancement, and contrast between the mass and surrounding normal tissue. When mucosal lesions in the head and neck are small and superficial, with no deep invasion, even the best CT and MR imaging do not depict the mass. In that case, the formal interpretation could say, for example, "although there is a known lateral oral tongue mass, the contrast-enhanced CT is normal." Similarly, if there are no large or necrotic cervical lymph nodes in the locations routinely involved with a certain tumor subsite, the final impression should read "no significant cervical adenopathy, nodal disease is N0."

It should be obvious that accurate staging requires high-quality CT and MR imaging techniques. Careful attention to parameters that determine resolution and decrease artifacts, and intravenous contrast amount and timing, are necessary because they affect the accuracy of staging. Technologists should instruct the patient to remain still in the scanner, breathe normally during scan acquisition, and align the head and neck so that images are relatively straight, to optimize comparison of the normal and abnormal sides. In general, for both CT and MR imaging, slice thickness of 3 mm or less is necessary.[16] Thinner slices are important for coronal or sagittal reconstruction, because tumors of virtually every subsite have invasion patterns best appreciated in the nonaxial plane. For example, extension of a supraglottic mass across the laryngeal ventricle is best depicted in the coronal plane. Destruction of the extracranial surface of the sphenoid bone is often seen only in a nonaxial plane.

CT scan acquisition times are so fast that unless there is a built-in delay to obtain images, the CT may be optimized for CT angiography and not a soft tissue study. We have found a longer delay best for CT neck imaging because it allows for mucosal enhancement and showing tumor boundaries. The longer delay is best to detect nodal necrosis.

The current trend is to obtain PET-CT for initial staging of head and neck cancer, a practice that is supported in the literature.[17,18] Combined anatomic and physiologic imaging improves detection of the unknown primary and more accurately stages nodal disease than either technique alone. At our institution, all patients presenting with a new HNSCC undergo PET-CT for staging. One exception is a T1 glottic laryngeal carcinoma, which is accurately staged at endoscopy and has a low propensity for nodal metastases. For almost all other malignancies of the head and neck, the PET portion is interpreted by the nuclear medicine physicians, the contrast-enhanced CT by the head and neck radiologists, and 2 separate dictations are generated after the 2 groups consult with each other. If the findings on the PET and CT are concordant, that is mentioned in the final report. If the PET and CT are discordant (eg, if a metastatic node is detected on PET but has no malignant CT characteristics), a comment is made about which modality is more likely to be accurate or a method to resolve the difference is offered, typically an image-guided FNA.

AJCC7

Two important changes were made for staging head and neck cancer in the most recent edition. First, the terms "resectable" and "unresectable" were replaced with T4a "moderately advanced" and T4b "very advanced" when referring to the primary site. For virtually all the head and neck subsites, tumor encasing the internal or common carotid arteries upstages to T4b. For oral cavity cancer, extension to the masticator space, pterygoid plates, or skull base also describes T4b disease. For an oropharyngeal primary, tumor invading the lateral pterygoid muscles, pterygoid plates, lateral nasopharynx, or skull base describes T4b disease. For the larynx and hypopharynx, tumors invading the prevertebral space or fascia or extending to the mediastinum are T4b descriptors. T4 nasopharyngeal staging, which is not sub-divided into a or b, includes intracranial extension, cranial nerve involvement, hypopharyngeal or orbital extension, or invasion of the infratemporal fossa or masticator space.

Therefore, to incorporate the changes into practice, it is important for the interpreting radiologist to be familiar with the boundaries of each of the subsites, and to be able to identify the carotid artery, masticator space, the pterygoid plates, relevant muscles, the mediastinum, and the pre-vertebral space.

LIMITATIONS TO AJCC7 AND ANATOMIC STAGING

Because the revision cycle for staging is 6 to 8 years, scientific discoveries may occur that are not incorporated into the staging system. Thus, nonanatomic and biologic factors such as tumor type and grade, and HPV status, for example, are also considered when planning treatment. Anatomic characteristics remain the basis of staging, but additional factors are increasingly recognized as important when predicting prognosis. Although tumor stage, based on local and distant disease, has historically predicted survival, the molecular biology and status may play a more important role in determining prognosis and survival.[19] An HNTB, comprising specialists from all disciplines, therefore, is the single best way to assess each individual patient.

Pathologic characteristics of an individual tumor are not reflected in TNM staging. After biopsy or tumor resection, specifics of the tumor can be described: the degree of tumor differentiation (well, poor, or undifferentiated), presence of peri-neural invasion, and tumor vascularity, or micro-vascular density. Treatment recommendations from the HNTB therefore take more than just TNM stage into consideration.

There are important molecular factors that affect tumor development, and tumor resistance to radiotherapy and chemotherapy. The most important new development in head and neck cancer is the recognition of sexually transmitted HPV as a factor in HNSCC of the oropharynx. Base of tongue and tonsil cancers are associated with HPV-16 infections.[20,21] HPV-16 and HPV-18 have been recognized for many years as associated with cervical cancer, but the association with oropharyngeal cancer has been confirmed relatively recently. When there is HPV-16 infection, viral oncoproteins E6 and E7 inactivate p53 and pRb, both tumor suppressor proteins, disturbing cell cycle regulation.[22–24] Patients with HPV-16–associated oropharyngeal cancer, compared with tobacco-associated and alcohol-associated cancer, tend to be younger, and generally have a better prognosis. Proto-oncogenes that code for proteins promoting cellular proliferation, tumor suppressor genes that inhibit cellular proliferation, and a variety of growth factors that change the local microenvironment are all important in prognosis but are not routinely reflected in TNM staging.

HNSCC is therefore biologically heterogeneous, from patient to patient, and tumor environment in the same patient likely differs significantly on the molecular level within the primary lesion itself.

SUMMARY

It should be obvious that imaging-trained and subspecialty-trained radiologists, in combination with the physical examination and pathologic specimen, are essential to stage head and neck cancers (other than skin). The ear, nose, and throat surgeon or radiation oncologist can identify the primary site if there is a mucosal lesion, and can report palpable neck nodes. But these are crude measures of a head and neck tumor, and only cross-sectional imagers can determine the size or local extent of a tumor, and small necrotic or metabolically active nonpalpable lymph nodes. The exception is a T1 superficial mucosal tumor, best staged by direct visualization. When there is no deep invasion, CT or MR imaging may be normal, but even a normal study helps to confirm a T1 lesion.

The objectives of this issue of *Clinics* are to clearly describe the anatomic subsites of the head and neck, summarize the factors that can help stage a tumor in each of the subsites, and emphasize the anatomic structures that the radiologist must examine before assigning a stage. With AJCC7 as a guidebook, staging head and neck cancer is the subspecialty-trained radiologist's responsibility.

REFERENCES

1. Edge SB, Byrd DR, Compton CC, et al, editors. American Joint Committee on Cancer: Cancer Staging Manual. 7th edition. New York: Springer; 2010.

2. Wheless SA, McKinney KA, Zanation AM. A prospective study of the clinical impact of a multidisciplinary head and neck tumor board. Otolaryngol Head Neck Surg 2010;143:650–4.

3. Van den Brekel MW, Stel HV, Castelijns JA, et al. Cervical lymph node metastasis: assessment of radiologic criteria. Radiology 1990;177(2):379–84.

4. Spiro RH. The management of neck nodes in head and neck cancer: a surgeon's view. Bull N Y Acad Med 1985;61:629–37.

5. Van den Brekel MW, Bartelink H, Snow GB. The value of staging of neck nodes in patients treated with radiotherapy. Radiother Oncol 1994;32:193–6.

6. Som PM, Curtin HD, Mancuso AA. The new imaging-based classification for describing the location of lymph nodes in the neck with particular regard to cervical lymph nodes in relation to cancer of the larynx. ORL J Otorhinolaryngol Relat Spec 2000; 62:186–98.

7. Robbins KT, Clayman G, Levine PA, et al, American Head and Neck Society; American Academic of Otolaryngology–Head and Neck Surgery. Neck dissection classification update: revisions proposed by the American Head and Neck Society and the American Academy of Otolaryngology–Head and Neck Surgery. Arch Otolaryngol Head Neck Surg 2002;128(7):751–8.

8. Som P, Brandwein-Gensler MS. Lymph nodes of the neck. In: Som PM, Curtin HD, editors. Head and neck imaging. 5th edition. St Louis (MO): Mosby Elsevier; 2011.

9. Liao XB, Mao YP, Liu LZ, et al. How does magnetic resonance imaging influence staging according to AJCC staging system for nasopharyngeal carcinoma compared with computed tomography? Int J Radiat Oncol Biol Phys 2008;72(5):1368–77.

10. Shah JP. Patterns of cervical lymph node metastasis from squamous carcinomas of the upper aerodigestive tract. Am J Surg 1990;160(4):405–9.

11. Yousem DM, Som PM, Hackney DB, et al. Central nodal necrosis and extracapsular neoplastic spread in cervical lymph nodes: MR imaging versus CT. Radiology 1992;182:753–9.

12. Gor DM, Langer JE, Loevner LA. Imaging of cervical lymph nodes in head and neck cancer: the basics. Radiol Clin North Am 2006;44(1):101–10.

13. Larsen SR, Johansen J, Sorensen JA, et al. The prognostic significance of histological features in oral squamous cell carcinoma. J Oral Pathol Med 2009;38(8):657–62.

14. Woolgar JA, Rogers SN, Lowe D, et al. Cervical lymph node metastasis in oral cancer: the importance of even microscopic extracapsular spread. Oral Oncol 2003;39:130–7.

15. Woolgar JA. The topography of cervical lymph node metastases revisited: the histological findings in 526 sides of neck dissection from 439 previously untreated patients. Int J Oral Maxillofac Surg 2007; 36(3):219–25.

16. Lell MM, Gmelin C, Panknin C, et al. Thin-slice MDCT of the neck: impact on cancer staging. Am J Roentgenol 2008;190(3):785–9.

17. Branstetter BF, Blodgett TM, Zimmer LA, et al. Head and neck malignancy: is PET/CT more accurate than PET or CT alone? Radiology 2005;235:580–6.

18. Jeong HS, Baek CH, Son YI, et al. Use of integrated ^{18}F-FDG PET/CT to improve the accuracy of initial cervical nodal evaluation in patients with head and neck squamous cell carcinoma. Head Neck 2007; 29:203–10.

19. Ang K, Harris J, Wheeler R, et al. Human papillomavirus and survival of patients with oropharyngeal cancer. N Engl J Med 2010;363:24–35.

20. D'Souza G, Kreimer AR, Viscidi R, et al. Case-control study of human papillomavirus and oropharyngeal cancer. N Engl J Med 2007;356:1944–56.

21. Syrjanen S. Human papillomaviruses in head and neck carcinomas. N Engl J Med 2007;356:1993–5.

22. Mork J, Lie AK, Glattre E, et al. Human papillomavirus infection as a risk factor for squamous-cell carcinoma of the head and neck. N Engl J Med 2001;344:1125–31.

23. Leemans CR, Braakhuis BJM, Brakenhoff RH. The molecular biology of head and neck cancer. Nat Rev Cancer 2011;11:9–22.

24. Brandwein-Gensler M, Smith RV. Prognostic indicators in head and neck oncology including the new 7th edition of the AJCC staging system. Head Neck Pathol 2010;4:53–61.

Pitfalls in the Staging of Cancer of Nasopharyngeal Carcinoma

Christine M. Glastonbury, MBBS[a],*, Karen L. Salzman, MD[b]

KEYWORDS

• Staging • Nasopharyngeal carcinoma • Nasopharynx • Epstein-Barr virus

KEY POINTS

• Although nasopharyngeal carcinoma (NPC) is the most common primary malignancy of the naso-pharynx, it is an uncommon malignancy in much of the Western world.
• Over the last several years, there have been important changes in the terminology used for the histologic classification of NPC and important changes to the American Joint Committee on Cancer TNM staging of NPC.
• Accurate imaging assessment is critical for diagnose, to stage and plan the radiation treatment, and for ongoing follow-up and surveillance.
• This article emphasizes important nasopharyngeal anatomy landmarks and the imaging appearances and pitfalls of nasopharyngeal carcinoma, its patterns of spread, and posttreatment appearances.

INTRODUCTION

Although nasopharyngeal carcinoma (NPC) is the most common primary malignancy of the naso-pharynx, it is an uncommon malignancy in much of the Western world where it has an incidence of less than 10 per 1 000 000. Over the last several years, there have been important changes in the terminology used for the histologic classification of NPC and important changes to the American Joint Committee on Cancer (AJCC) TNM staging of NPC. Imaging already plays a central role in the evaluation of nasopharyngeal disease because this region may be difficult to examine clinically. With NPC, our clinical colleagues depend on accurate radiologic assessment to diagnose, stage, and plan the radiation treatment and for ongoing follow-up and surveillance. This article empha-sizes important nasopharyngeal anatomy land-marks and the imaging appearances and pitfalls of NPC and its patterns of spread and posttreatment appearances. The updated histology and new AJCC TNM staging are presented, emphasizing key changes that are of relevance to the radiologist.

NASOPHARYNGEAL ANATOMY

The nasopharynx is the most superior portion of the tubular pharynx, located immediately caudal to the central skull base. The inferior limit of the nasopharynx is the soft palate, and it is at this level that the pharynx is deemed oropharynx. The posterior and lateral walls of the nasopharynx are in continuity with the posterior and lateral oropha-ryngeal walls, respectively. On axial imaging, the nasopharynx is located posterior to the nasal cavity, with which it communicates through the choanae (Figs. 1 and 2). The pharyngobasilar fascia of the superior constrictor muscle, which forms the wall of the nasopharynx, attaches the pharynx to the undersurface of the clivus.[1] There

a Department of Radiology and Biomedical Imaging, University of California, San Francisco, Box 0628, Room L358, 505 Parnassus Avenue, San Francisco, CA 94143-0628, USA; b Department of Radiology, University of Utah, 30 North 1900 East #1A071, Salt Lake City, UT 84132-2140, USA
* Corresponding author.
E-mail address: christine.glastonbury@ucsf.edu

Neuroimag Clin N Am 23 (2013) 9–25
http://dx.doi.org/10.1016/j.nic.2012.08.006

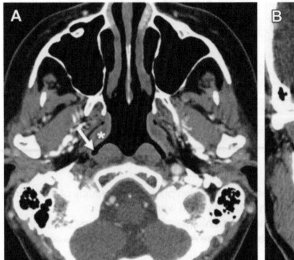
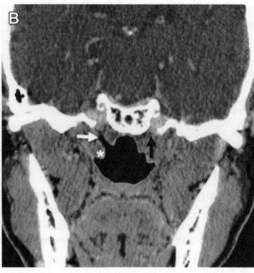

Fig. 1. Axial (A) and coronal (B) contrast-enhanced computed tomography images through the nasopharynx illustrating normal anatomic landmarks. The nasopharynx is posterior to the nasal cavity. The posterior wall in this adult has an undulating contour from the prevertebral longus capitis muscles, and the adenoidal tissue is almost completely atrophic. The lateral pharyngeal recess or fossa of Rosenmüller (arrow) is delineated by the lateral margin of these muscles. Note that in the axial plane the recess is posterior to the torus tubarius (asterisk), whereas the recess (white arrow) is superior to the torus tubarius (asterisk) in the coronal plane. The coronal plane best emphasizes the intimate relation of the nasopharynx to the central skull base and the foramen lacerum (black arrow).

is a small lateral hiatus or opening in this skull base attachment, known as the foramen of Morgagni, through which the eustachian (pharyngotympanic) tube and levator veli palatini muscle pass.[2] The levator veli palatini and the tensor veli palatini muscles are identifiable on magnetic resonance (MR) scans in the lateral wall of the nasopharynx and are responsible for opening the eustachian tube and for tensing and elevating the palate to prevent oronasal reflux (see Fig. 2). The eustachian tube communicates with the middle ear, allowing both middle ear aeration and drainage; its

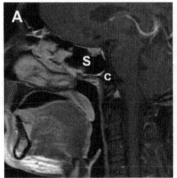
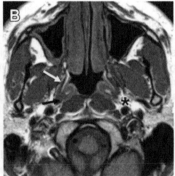
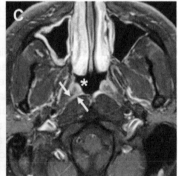

Fig. 2. Sagittal fat-saturated postcontrast T1-weighted (A), axial T1-weighted (B), and axial fat-saturated postcontrast T1-weighted (C) images of the nasopharynx illustrating normal anatomy. (A) The sagittal projection demonstrates the normal adult contour of the nasopharynx. Note the sloping roof or vault, formed by the clivus (c) and sphenoid sinus (s). There is little adenoidal tissue in this adult patient. (B) Axial T1-weighed image shows the tensor veli palatine muscle (white arrow) in the lateral wall, innervated by a branch of the mandibular division of the trigeminal nerve. The levator veli palatini muscle (black arrow) is innervated by the pharyngeal plexus. Bright parapharyngeal fat (asterisk) is evident lateral to the nasopharynx. (C) Postcontrast imaging shows normal enhancement of the mucosa of the torus tubarius (asterisk) and of the mucosa lining the lateral recess (arrows). The prevertebral muscles are distinct from this mucosal enhancement.

opening in the superolateral aspect of the naso-pharyngeal wall is marked by the torus tubarius, an elevation of the wall of the nasopharynx formed by the eustachian tube cartilage. The foramen of Morgagni is an essential anatomic structure but is also a potential weak spot in the head and neck through which nasopharyngeal neoplasms or infections may spread directly to the skull base or laterally to the parapharyngeal fat.

The lateral pharyngeal recess (often known by its eponym, the fossa of Rosenmüller) is superolat-eral to the torus tubarius and the opening of the eustachian tube. On axial images, the lateral pharyngeal recess is located posterior to the torus tubarius and it is superior to the torus tubarius on coronal images (see Fig. 1). It is within the lateral recess (fossa of Rosenmüller) that most nasopha-ryngeal carcinomas arise.

The midline posterior nasopharyngeal wall con-necting the two lateral recesses is superficial to the prevertebral longus capitis and longus colli muscles that attach to the basiocciput and upper cervical vertebrae. The posterior nasopharyngeal wall, as well as the roof or vault in younger patients, is the location of the nasopharyngeal tonsillar tissue or adenoids. Adenoidal hypertrophy in response to infection may mimic neoplastic enlargement or a nasopharyngeal mass. However, reactive hypertrophy is never associated with inva-sion of the prevertebral muscles, and these struc-tures are clearly delineated on MR imaging.

The overall shape of the nasopharyngeal cavity varies depending on the bulk of the prevertebral muscles and the adenoids. In older patients, the nasopharynx may appear enlarged but shallow with loss of muscle bulk and atrophy of the adenoids, whereas the nasopharyngeal cavity may be entirely obliterated in children by large adenoids.

EPIDEMIOLOGY OF NPC

There have been many changes to the terminology used for the classification of NPC. Currently, the World Health Organization (WHO) divides NPC into a histologic classification of 4 types, with epidemiology reflecting the different pathologic types (Table 1).[3-6] Broadly defined, NPC is defined as keratinizing (previously termed type I or squamous cell carcinoma), nonkeratinizing (NK), and basaloid squamous cell carcinoma

Table 1 Comparison of different histologic types of NPC			
WHO Classification	Previous Terminologies	Epidemiology	Prognosis
Keratinizing	Type I, squamous cell carcinoma	~25% NPC cases Rare <40 y of age Men greater than women Weak EBV association Environmental risk factors	20%–40% 5-y survival
Nonkeratinizing		Overall ~75% NPC cases Most common fifth to seventh decades 70% men, 30% women Strong EBV association Genetic & environmental risk factors	
Differentiated	Type II, transitional carcinoma	~15% NPC cases	~75% 5-y survival
Undifferentiated	Type III, lymphoepithelial carcinoma	~60% NPC cases May occur in children	~75% 5-y survival
BSCC		Rare Sixth to seventh decades, mean age = 55 y Men greater than women Associated with excessive alcohol and tobacco use	Seems to be less aggressive than BSCC in other sites but overall poor prognosis

Abbreviations: BSCC, basaloid squamous cell carcinoma; EBV, Epstein-Barr virus.

(BSCC). NK NPC is further subdivided into differentiated (previously termed type II or transitional carcinoma) and undifferentiated (previously termed type III or lymphoepithelioma).

NK NPC is the most common form, with undifferentiated NK being approximately 4 times as common as the differentiated form. The subtypes of NK NPC share the same proposed epidemiologic and etiologic factors. Both are strongly associated with Epstein-Barr virus (EBV) infection, are most commonly found in Asian (particularly Chinese) men, and are most often found in patients from 40 to 80 years of age. Although pediatric NPC is relatively rare, undifferentiated NK NPC is the most common form.[7–9] The incidence rate of NPC at less than 20 years of age is higher for African Americans than for American Asians.[10] NK NPC is highly radiosensitive, which results in reasonably good 5-year survival statistics of approximately 75%.[4,7,11]

Keratinizing NPC was previously termed NPC type I and is the histologic type found in approximately a quarter of NPC cases.[5] It is graded as poorly, moderately, or well differentiated, with well differentiated being the least commonly occurring. Keratinizing NPC is not typically associated with EBV but is associated with cigarette smoking; prior radiation; and occupational exposures, such as to chemical fumes, smoke, and formaldehyde. Five-year survival is significantly lower for keratinizing NPC (20%–40%) and this is largely because of poor local control. The US statistics for relative survival at 5 years from diagnosis overall for all nasopharyngeal carcinomas varies from 47% to 78% depending on the tumor stage at presentation of stage IV to stage I, respectively.[11]

Another common malignancy to involve the nasopharynx is lymphoma arising in or secondarily affecting the adenoid tissue. Diffuse large B-cell lymphoma is the most common type to affect the Waldeyer ring and is weakly associated with EBV infection. Lymphoma mimics NPC on imaging and can be a diagnostic dilemma for the radiologist. However, lymphoma is more commonly midline in origin; when invading the skull base, it tends to expand the clivus rather than just infiltrate the marrow.

Other uncommon malignancies that involve the nasopharyngeal mucosa include adenoid cystic carcinoma (ACC) and small cell undifferentiated neuroendocrine carcinoma (SCNEC). There is a rare nasopharyngeal papillary adenocarcinoma (NPPA) that most often presents as an exophytic obstructing nasopharyngeal mass. This slow-growing low-grade neoplasm does not typically metastasize and is cured by complete excision. There are no known viral or environmental etiologic factors for ACC, SCNEC, or NPPA.[12]

AJCC SEVENTH EDITION STAGING

The seventh edition of the AJCC, published in January 2010, brought important changes to the way in which NPC is staged and these were largely simplifications of the prior system.[3,13] With regard to staging the primary tumor site (T stage), it has been determined that tumors extending to the oropharynx or nasal cavity (previously staged as T2a) did not have a worse prognosis than tumors confined to the nasopharynx (T1) and so are now staged as T1 (Box 1, Fig. 3).[3,13] Parapharyngeal space extension, which is posterolaterally spread through the pharyngobasilar fascia to the parapharyngeal fat, denotes T2 stage (Fig. 4). T3 and T4 designations remain unchanged from the prior AJCC staging system (Figs. 5 and 6).

Additional changes were made to the regional lymph node status staging (N stage), which clarified the status of retropharyngeal nodes. It was unclear before the seventh edition how to stage retropharyngeal nodal metastasis in the absence of jugular chain adenopathy. Some institutions would determine this to be N1 disease, whereas others would determine it to be N0. It has now been clarified that unilateral or bilateral retropharyngeal nodal metastases, less than or equal to 6 cm in greatest dimension, are now considered N1 disease (see Box 1, Fig. 6). No other changes were made to the nodal staging system in the current edition. The most difficult designation for radiologists remains the determination of N3b, that is, the presence of supraclavicular adenopathy. This stage is a clinical stage, determined by the anatomic boundaries of the triangle of Ho; but in the authors' practice, a low level IV or VB node, or any node on the same slice as the clavicle on cross-sectional imaging, should be specifically described as a potential supraclavicular node because it may upstage the nodal status to N3b, stage IVB (see Box 1, Fig. 7, Table 2).[3] The M designation remains unchanged as M0 for no distant metastasis and M1 for the presence of metastasis. MX is commonly used when metastatic disease status is unknown.

When looking at the overall anatomic stage/prognostic groups (stage 0–IV), the only changes made were to reflect the removal of the separate designations, T2a and T2b, again resulting in the simplification of NPC staging (Table 3).

Box 1
AJCC seventh edition nasopharynx staging

Primary tumor (T)

TX: Primary tumor cannot be assessed

T0: No evidence of primary tumor

Tis: Carcinoma in situ

T1: Tumor confined to the nasopharynx or extends to oropharynx and/or nasal cavity without parapharyngeal extension

T2: Tumor extends to parapharyngeal fat

T3: Tumor involves bone of skull base and/or paranasal sinuses

T4: Intracranial extension and/or involvement of cranial nerves, orbit, hypopharynx, and/or extension to the infratemporal fossa or masticator space

Regional lymph nodes (N)

NX: Regional lymph nodes cannot be assessed

N0: No regional lymph node metastasis

N1: Unilateral nodes 6 cm or less in greatest dimension and/or unilateral or bilateral retropharyngeal nodes 6 cm or less in greatest dimension

N2: Bilateral nodes 6 cm or less in greatest dimension

N3: Metastasis in a lymph node more than 6 cm in greatest dimension or extension to supraclavicular fossa

N3a: Nodes 6 cm or more in dimension

N3b: Nodal metastasis in supraclavicular fossa

Distant Metastasis (M)

M0: No distant metastasis

M1: Distant metastasis

From Edge SB, Byrd DR, Compton CC, et al, editors. AJCC cancer staging handbook. Seventh edition. New York: Springer-Verlag; 2010. p. 63–79; with permission.

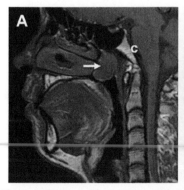
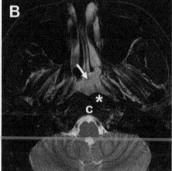
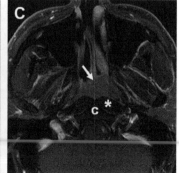

Fig. 3. A 29-year-old Asian man with 4 months of recurrent sneezing and trace epistaxis and a nasopharyngeal mass evident on ear, nose and throat examination. Sagittal T1-weighted (*A*), axial fat-saturated T2-weighted (*B*), and axial fat-saturated postcontrast T1-weighted (*C*) MR images demonstrate an asymmetric exophytic mass (*arrow*) that likely arose from the left fossa of Rosenmüller. There is no evidence of infiltration of the prevertebral muscles (*asterisk*) or parapharyngeal fat, and the clivus (c) has preserved signal intensity. There was no adenopathy in the neck on MR imaging and the whole-body positron emission tomography–computed tomography was negative. This NPC is T1N0M0 (stage I), EBV positive, and undifferentiated. It was treated with radiation alone.

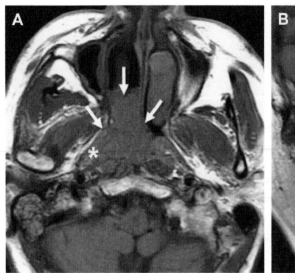
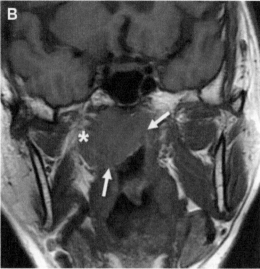

Fig. 4. Axial (*A*) and coronal (*B*) T1-weighted MR images in a 60-year-old man with nasal congestion of several months duration. The images demonstrate an asymmetric nasopharyngeal mass (*arrows*) that extends anteriorly through the right choana to the posterior right nasal cavity. There is lateral extension of the mass to the right parapharyngeal fat (*asterisk*), indicating T2 disease. The mass infiltrates the right prevertebral muscle but does not invade the skull base. This undifferentiated NPC was staged as T2N1 (stage II disease) and treated with chemoradiation.

TRENDS IN NPC TREATMENT AFFECTING STAGING

NPC, particularly nonkeratinizing NPC, is typically a very radiosensitive tumor. Additionally, given its approximation to the skull base and pattern of spread, it is generally not amenable to surgical resection. For this reason, radiation has been the primary mode of therapy and is often augmented with systemic chemotherapy. Keratinizing NPC is

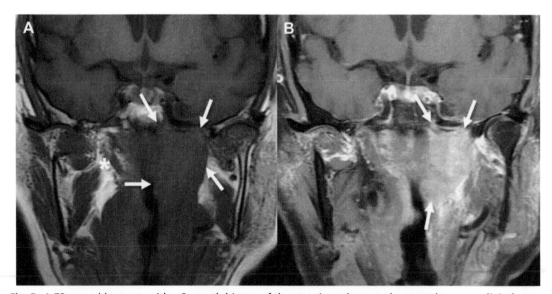

Fig. 5. A 73-year-old woman with a 2-month history of throat pain and a nasopharyngeal mass on clinical examination. Coronal T1-weighted (*A*) and coronal fat-saturated postcontrast T1-weighted (*B*) MR images show a left nasopharyngeal mass (*arrows*) that extends almost down to the oropharynx. Superiorly, the mass infiltrates the skull base around foramen lacerum with subtle but real loss of the normally T1 hyperintense fatty skull base marrow. Postcontrast imaging shows enhancement of the mass and of the skull base involvement without clear intracranial extension that would have designated this as T4 tumor. The WHO II NPC tumor was staged as T3 N1, which is stage III disease. The patient is currently undergoing treatment with chemoradiation.

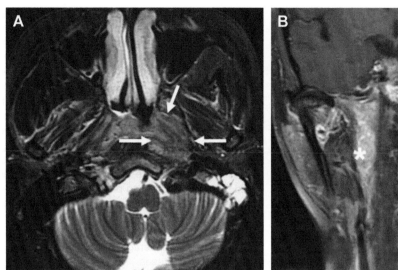
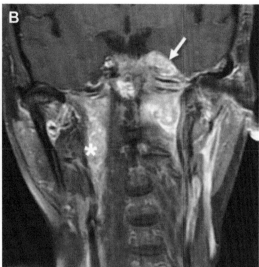

Fig. 6. Axial fat-saturated T2-weighted (*A*) and coronal fat-saturated postcontrast T1-weighted (*B*) MR images in a 44-year-old Asian woman with left-sided hearing loss and a nasopharyngeal mass on clinical examination. Axial imaging (*A*) shows an endophytic mass centered in the left fossa of Rosenmüller (*arrows*) that infiltrates the left prevertebral muscle and the lateral nasopharyngeal wall. Note T2 hyperintense secretions in the left mastoid air cells from the obstructed eustachian tube. Coronal imaging (*B*) shows that although this is not a large primary mass, it has extended cranially through the left foramen lacerum and skull base so that it is involving the left cavernous sinus (*arrow*) and the Meckel cave. Intracranial extension indicates this is T4 disease. Although there was no palpable neck adenopathy, there is a pathologically enlarged retropharyngeal node (*asterisk*) indicating N1 disease. This NPC is staged as T4, N1, or stage IVA.

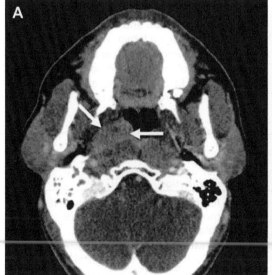
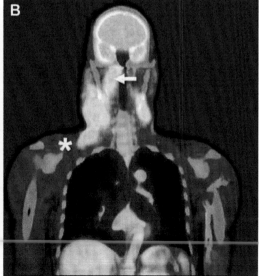

Fig. 7. Axial contrast-enhanced computed tomography (CT) (*A*) performed as part of a positron emission tomography (PET)-CT and coronal fused PET-CT (*B*) in a 49-year-old construction worker from China with a 3-year history of enlarging right neck mass and new left mass. The axial image shows minimal enhancement of a right nasopharyngeal mass that seems to invade the parapharyngeal fat. The fused PET-CT reveals intense uptake in the primary undifferentiated NPC (*arrows*) and intense uptake in bilateral neck nodes. Note the low location of the right adenopathy (*asterisk*) indicating supraclavicular nodal involvement. This NPC was staged as T2N3b, which is stage IVB, and the patient was treated with chemoradiation.

Table 2
Final tumor stage using the AJCC staging system for nasopharyngeal carcinoma, seventh edition

Stage 0	Tis	N0	M0
Stage I	T1	N0	M0
Stage II	T1/T2	N1	M0
	T2	N0	M0
Stage III	T1/T2	N2	M0
	T3	N0/N1/N2	M0
Stage IVA	T4	N0/N1/N2	M0
Stage IVB	Any T	N3	M0
Stage IVC	Any T	Any N	M1

From Edge SB, Byrd DR, Compton CC, et al, editors. AJCC cancer staging handbook. Seventh edition. New York: Springer-Verlag; 2010. p. 63–79; with permission.

also treated with chemoradiation, whereas BSCC of the nasopharynx may be treated initially with surgical resection if possible.

External beam radiation therapy (EBRT) with opposed lateral fields has been the traditional form of radiation therapy for NPC. This therapy has many limitations because it is difficult to maximally irradiate the tumor while sparing vital adjacent tissues, such as the temporal lobes and brainstem.[14] Other tissues, such as the parotid glands, are almost impossible to spare with this traditional radiation therapy technique. Radiation parotitis results in xerostomia, which is the most common cause of significant morbidity in this group of patients and can be irreversible with a high dose (>40–50 Gy) to most of the gland. Intensity modulated radiation therapy (IMRT) is a form of 3-dimensional conformal radiotherapy

that allows high-dose radiation delivery to specific tissues and, therefore, improves tumor coverage. At the same time, the irradiated area is carefully contoured so as to spare normal adjacent tissues and, thus, reduce radiation-associated toxicity.[14,15] In many institutions, IMRT is replacing EBRT as the treatment of choice for NPC. This change to treatment has not so much affected staging as affected treatment planning and now requires more detailed understanding on the part of the radiation oncologist of the anatomic structures of the skull base and deep face. The head and neck radiologist can play an important role in treatment planning in concert with the radiation oncologist and specifically checking or redelineating the gross total volume (GTV) contours to ensure correct coverage of the primary tumor and nodal metastases.

T1N0M0 disease is typically treated with radiation alone. The current standard of care for treatment of NPC when there is evidence of T2-T4 or N1-N3 disease is concurrent chemoradiation followed by adjuvant chemotherapy or induction chemotherapy followed by chemoradiation.[16] Accurate TNM staging is, thus, important for treatment planning.

PATTERNS OF NPC DISEASE SPREAD

It is important to understand the potential patterns of tumor spread with any head and neck malignancy to anticipate and detect subtle findings that might upstage a tumor and potentially change therapy. NPC tends to behave with a fairly predictable pattern of local and nodal spread, although there seems to be much variability from patient to patient in the relationship of the T stage of the

Table 3
Pitfalls in staging of NPC

Pitfall	Recommendation
Failure to recognize parapharyngeal fat involvement, understaging as T1 instead of T2	Look for loss of normal fat density and precontrast T1 fat signal from the parapharyngeal fat
Indeterminate skull base invasion on CT	Perform MR imaging with close attention to precontrast coronal and sagittal T1-weighted images
Failure to recognize perineural and intracranial extension	Closely evaluate the skull base foramina on precontrast T1-weighted and postcontrast, fat-saturated, T1-weighted MR images
Underevaluating for distant metastatic disease	Recommend PET-CT to evaluate for distant metastases when N2 or N3 disease is present

Abbreviation: PET-CT, positron emission tomography–computed tomography.

primary tumor and the presence, size, and extent of nodal metastases (Fig. 8).

Because NPC most often arises in the fossa of Rosenmüller, small tumors can present with obstruction of the adjacent opening of the eustachian tube and stasis of secretions in the middle ear (serous otitis). Obstruction of middle ear drainage is not ubiquitous with NPC but is common. Unilateral serous otitis or the observation of unilateral middle ear/mastoid fluid on adult head imaging necessitates evaluation of the nasopharynx for a primary nasopharyngeal mass.

From this early stage as a small T1 tumor, NPC may enlarge in an exophytic fashion to fill the nasopharynx and may extend anteriorly into the nasal cavity through the choanae or inferiorly to the oropharynx. Any of these patterns of growth are considered T1 using the AJCC TNM staging system.[3] This growth is radiographically very similar to both benign lymphoid hypertrophy and

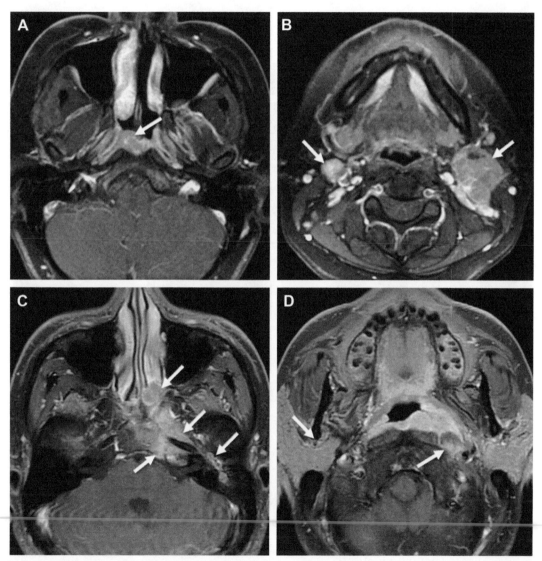

Fig. 8. Variability of N staging in relation to tumor T staging. Axial fat-saturated postcontrast T1-weighted MR images from patient 1 (A, B), a 25-year-old woman who presented with N2 neck adenopathy (arrows in B) found to be caused by a small (T1) exophytic primary right NPC (arrow in A). Note in particular the very large, heterogeneous left level II node. By comparison, axial fat-saturated postcontrast T1-weighted MR images from patient 2 (C, D), a 43-year-old man with a locally infiltrative left NPC (arrows in C) that spread superiorly through the skull base to involve multiple cranial nerves (T4). This patient had only one retropharyngeal node (arrows in D) evident on imaging, N1.

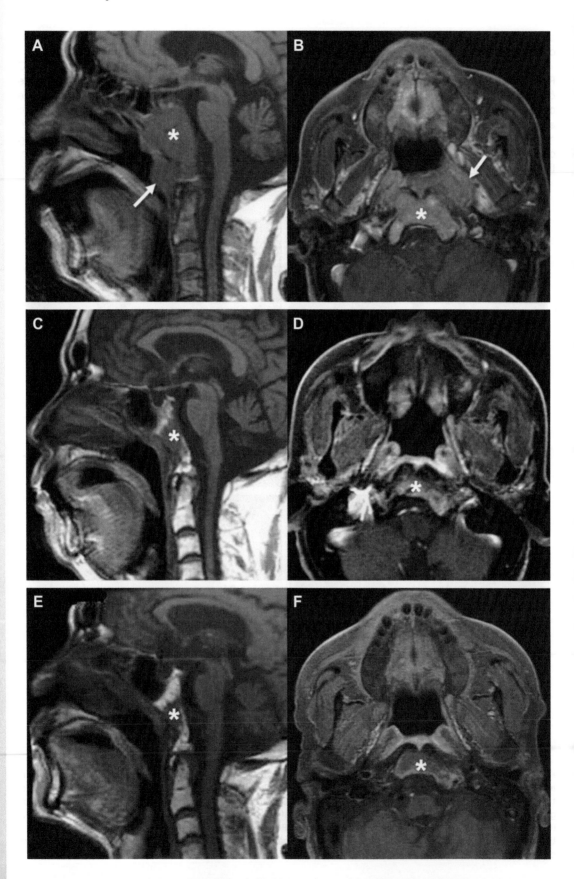

lymphoma involving the nasopharyngeal adenoids. Lymphoid hypertrophy can usually be distinguished from NPC by the striated appearance of normal lymphoid crypts on T2-weighted or postcontrast T1-weighted imaging, whereas NPC shows more homogenous mild enhancement.[17] NPC tends to be more asymmetric than lymphoma because it most often arises from the lateral aspect of the nasopharynx and not the midline tonsillar tissue.[18] Both NPC and lymphoma, but not lymphoid hypertrophy, may infiltrate posteriorly into the prevertebral muscles through the deep layer of deep cervical fascia. This infiltration does not change the staging for NPC but should heighten concern for invasion of the skull base and for metastatic nodal disease through retropharyngeal lymphatics.

Invasion of bone of the skull base can be imperceptible on computed tomography (CT) but denotes T3 stage. It is, thus, preferable that MR imaging be used for NPC staging.[3,19,20] In the authors' experience, the T1-weighted images in 3 planes, but particularly the coronal and sagittal plane, are excellent for evaluation of the normally hyperintense (fat signal) skull base marrow. When tumor abuts the skull base, loss of the fat signal indicates bone infiltration. Once this is determined, it is important to consider more extensive intracranial disease spread through the skull base foramina along cranial nerves or along the internal carotid artery. This disease spread is also best seen with MR imaging and designates T4 tumor.

NPC may also spread laterally from the nasopharynx through the pharyngobasilar fascia or through the foramen of Morgagni to the parapharyngeal fat with or without skull base invasion. Parapharyngeal fat involvement, which is well seen on either CT or MR imaging owing to the fat's low CT density and high T1 signal intensity on MR imaging, denotes T2 tumor. Further lateral spread through the superficial layer of the deep cervical fascia into the masticator space, however, upstages the tumor to T4 and is an independent prognostic factor for overall survival and local relapse-free survival.[21] Because the masticator muscles are supplied by the mandibular division

of the trigeminal nerve and are located inferior to the greater sphenoid wing, it is important to look for involvement of the foramen ovale for intracranial spread once masticator space involvement is determined. This involvement will not change tumor staging because intracranial spread is also T4, but it is important for radiation planning.

Nasopharyngeal tumors commonly spread to the retropharyngeal lymph nodes (RPN) first and then the upper jugular (level II) and spinal accessory (level V) nodal groups. RPN metastasis is now designated as N1 disease whether unilateral or bilateral. Nodal involvement follows an orderly spread down the neck to levels III and then level IV and supraclavicular nodes.[22–25] Metastatic nodal disease is often bilateral.[26] N0 disease is distinctly uncommon, and probably in the range of 4%, when staging is performed with MR imaging, which is more sensitive for detection of retropharyngeal adenopathy.

NPC has a strong tendency for systemic metastases to the bone, chest, and/or liver, with up to 5% of patients having distant metastasis at presentation. M1 tumor staging determines stage IVC disease.[7,27] Up to 30% of patients will have distant recurrence after radiation therapy.[15,28] National Comprehensive Cancer Network (NCCN) practice guidelines recommend positron emission tomography–computed tomography (PET-CT) to evaluate for distant metastases when N2 or N3 disease is present.[16]

PITFALLS IN NPC STAGING

For many institutions and practices, the greatest change to a treatment plan occurs when a tumor is designated as T2 (or more), and not T1, because chemotherapy is added to the treatment regimen. The presence of T2 disease portends a greater likelihood of distant treatment failure (ie, recurrence with metastatic disease). Thus if a T1 tumor is suspected clinically it is very important for the radiologist to look carefully for imaging features that may upstage the tumor

Fig. 9. A 66-year-old man diagnosed with T4N1 NPC (moderate to poorly differentiated nonkeratinizing) demonstrating expected changes to the skull base with treatment. All images are sagittal T1-weighted and axial fat-saturated postcontrast T1-weighted MR images. (A, B) These images were, at the time of diagnosis, demonstrating a large mass (arrow) centered in the left fossa of Rosenmüller and infiltrating the skull base (asterisk). Bilateral, left-greater-than-right cavernous sinus infiltration was also present. (C, D) These images were obtained 7 months later on completion of chemoradiation, showing almost complete resolution of the left nasopharyngeal mass. Note that the skull base shows ongoing low signal intensity (asterisk) with some enhancement, although loss of fullness of this infiltrative tumor. Surveillance images (E, F) were obtained 6 years later and show no evidence of a recurrent mass but residual loss of fat signal in the clivus (asterisk), which has minimal enhancement. The patient was asymptomatic and had a normal PET study. He remains well 30 months later.

such as parapharyngeal fat involvement (T2) and skull base involvement (T3).

The use of IMRT mandates that the radiation oncologist have a more precise knowledge of the local extent of disease to ensure that the tumor is encompassed in the radiation GTV. MR imaging is clearly the best imaging modality for evaluating intracranial and skull base involvement, which can be underestimated or completely occult on CT.[17,19,20] In addition, MR imaging, with its improved soft tissue contrast as compared with CT, makes the detection of abnormal RLN easier. In the authors' practice, the most common staging errors seen are understaging of the primary or lymph nodes when CT or, less often, positron emission tomography (PET)-CT is used without MR imaging. As described previously, fluorodeoxyglucose (FDG)-PET is of the most value when there is concern for distant metastatic disease at presentation (N2-N3 disease) or at the time of recurrence when distant metastases are more commonly found.[27,29,30]

PITFALLS IN NPC SURVEILLANCE AND APPEARANCE OF RECURRENCE

The NCCN guidelines recommend a baseline scan to be obtained within 6 months of completion of chemoradiation and only in those patients with T3-4 and/or N2-3. Further imaging is only recommended "as indicated based on signs/symptoms."[16] In the authors' practice, a baseline imaging scan is obtained at 2 to 3 months because it is perceived to be valuable for detecting subclinical residual adenopathy and also serves as a baseline to detect future more subtle recurrences.[31] Because the original tumor should have been staged with MR imaging, this modality is typically also used to establish a post-treatment baseline. The baseline scan should show significant decrease in size of the presenting primary mass, and it is not uncommon to find residual soft tissue that may represent granulation tissue and fibrosis (Fig. 9). If the pretreatment study showed infiltration of the parapharyngeal space, the pterygopalatine fossa, orbits, or the skull base, abnormal signal intensity may persist. The initial scan may also show significant posttreatment edema of the pharyngeal mucosa. There should be no residual enlarged lymph nodes, however; if these are found on the new baseline scan, a neck dissection is typically performed.[16] There is no defined surveillance protocol following successfully treated NPC. If further imaging studies are obtained after the baseline evaluation, any nasopharyngeal, deep face, or skull base soft tissue MR imaging signal abnormality should remain stable over this period or show further reduction in volume. The nasopharynx tends to lose its normal contours and develop a fibrosed appearance on MR imaging with effacement of the lateral pharyngeal recess primary site. This atrophic nasopharyngeal appearance also stabilizes over time, and any progression of soft tissue as compared with the baseline study must be considered recurrence until proven otherwise. Any new enlarged nodes must also be viewed with suspicion and fine-needle aspiration or biopsy is recommended.

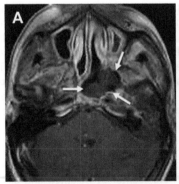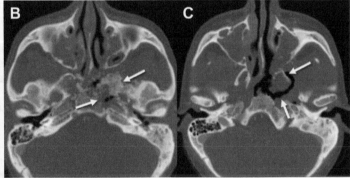

Fig. 10. Skull base osteoradionecrosis complicating treatment of a 40-year-old man treated 9 years ago with radiation for NPC. He was subsequently treated with radiation 6 years ago for local recurrence. Patient now presents with severe headaches, blurry vision, diplopia, and malodor. (A) Axial, fat-saturated, postcontrast, T1-weighted MR images show no solid enhancement to indicate local recurrence but an unusual appearance in the skull base with a rounded area of nonenhancement (arrows). (B, C) Axial contrast-enhanced CT images show the clivus and sphenoid left greater wing (arrows) to have ill-defined heterogeneous texture with air extending up to the skull base. PET showed no uptake, and operative biopsy showed necrotic amorphous material with degenerative changes.

The red marrow of the irradiated skull base becomes replaced with yellow (fatty) marrow and so appears hyperintense on T1-weighted images. If skull base invasion was present before chemoradiation, the treated tumor here tends to become scar tissue. This scar tissue is of variable signal intensity on MR imaging but tends to be hypointense on T1-weighted images, hyperintense on T2-weighted images, and may continue to enhance (see **Fig. 9**). Any increase in bulk of abnormal signal in the skull base on MR imaging after baseline imaging may represent recurrent disease. Osteoradionecrosis with or without osteomyelitis can be extremely difficult to differentiate from recurrent tumor, although frank bone destruction without a soft-tissue mass is most

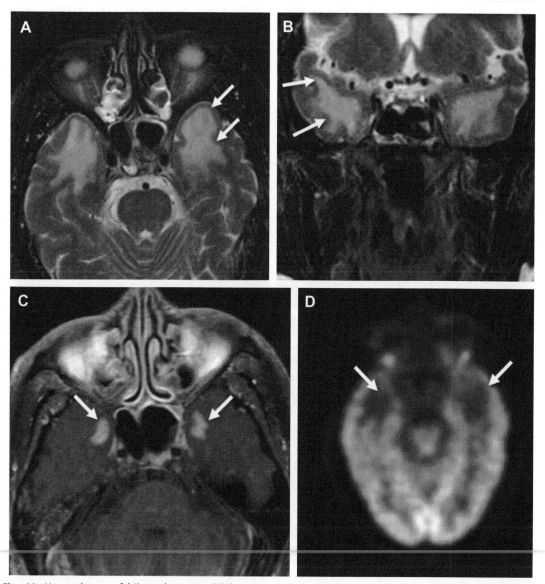

Fig. 11. Unusual case of bilateral temporal lobe necrosis in a 59-year-old man with T3N1 NPC treated with external beam radiation 8 years before and lost to follow-up. The patient returns for follow-up for nasopharyngeal wall pain from ulceration but is otherwise asymptomatic. Axial (*A*) and coronal (*B*) fat-saturated T2-weighted MR images demonstrate hyperintensity of the white matter of both temporal lobes (*arrows*). Both lobes appear expanded indicating edema rather than gliosis. Axial, fat-saturated, postcontrast, T1-weighted MR image (*C*) reveals focal enhancement of the medial aspects of the temporal lobes (*arrows*). The characteristic location with history is key for this diagnosis, although bilateral necrosis is very unusual. Axial FDG-PET image (*D*) demonstrates relative reduced uptake in both temporal lobes (*arrows*) as is typically seen with necrosis.

suggestive of osteoradionecrosis (**Fig. 10**).[32] CT classically shows bony cortical disruption with loss of marrow trabeculations. When a bulky soft tissue mass is seen in conjunction with bone destruction, a biopsy should be performed to exclude tumor recurrence.[33,34]

Trismus is seen in up to 35% of patients treated with traditional radiation therapy and is thought to be caused by sclerosis in the pterygoid muscles and temporomandibular joint.[32,35] MR imaging is recommended for patients with prior treated NPC and new trismus to look for evidence of perineural tumor or a recurrent mass and distinguish this from radiation-induced muscle inflammation. In some patients, extensive abnormal T2 signal and muscle atrophy is evident on MR imaging, and evidence of a clear field effect should differentiate radiation myopathy from denervation of the masticator muscles from perineural tumor involving the third division of the trigeminal nerve.[31]

One of the most serious side effects from traditional EBRT is temporal lobe necrosis, which

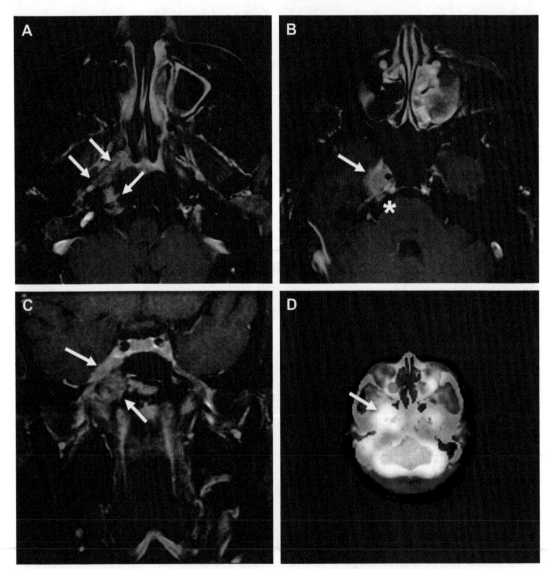

Fig. 12. Patient with local recurrence with intracranial extension. Axial (*A, B*) and coronal (*C*) fat-saturated, post-contrast, T1-weighted MR images in a 39-year-old man treated 6 years before with chemoradiation for T3N1 disease. The patient returns with facial pain, which is caused by an infiltrating mass in the right skull base that extends through foramen ovale to Meckel cave (*arrows*). Subtle perineural tumor is also seen along the cisternal segment of the trigeminal nerve (*asterisk*). Axial fused PET-CT (*D*) in the same patient reveals intense uptake at the right skull base corresponding to this local recurrence (*arrow*). This area can be difficult to evaluate on PET because of the intense, normal FDG uptake by the brain.

peaks at approximately 12 to15 months after treatment but can occur after more than 5 years. It is seen in up to 40% of patients treated with EBRT for NPC but seems to be markedly decreased with the use of targeted IMRT.[33] Temporal lobe necrosis appears as white matter edema with T2 and fluid-attenuated inversion recovery hyperintensity and variable focal enhancement in the anteromedial temporal lobe. It typically follows a waxing and waning time course; if the edema or symptoms are severe, then it is typically treated with steroids. Temporal lobe necrosis is well described but is infrequently mistaken for metastatic brain disease. Brain metastases from NPC are uncommon and the characteristic location of this abnormality coupled with the absence of other brain lesions is key for the correct imaging diagnosis (Fig. 11).

In those long-term survivors of NPC, for which there are expected to be many, the possibility of a radiation-induced neoplasm must also be considered when reviewing follow-up examinations. Radiation-induced sarcomas of the deep face and sinuses have been reported 5 to 10 years after completion of treatment and generally have a poor prognosis.[36] Squamous cell carcinoma, particularly of the external auditory canal, may also be a late complication of traditional EBRT radiation for NPC, seen 10 to 15 years after treatment.[33]

Most NPC recurrences occur within the first 2 years after treatment and can be manifest as local or systemic; 10% to 20% of patients with local or systemic recurrence may be curable with additional treatment.[7] Any enlarging posttreatment soft tissue mass or any new deep face or intracranial enhancement is concerning for recurrent disease (Fig. 12). At the authors' institution, those patients with a suspicious MR scan typically also undergo PET-CT. Additionally, for those patients with a suspicious clinical examination, both PET-CT and MR imaging are performed to restage patients before confirmatory biopsy. MR imaging has excellent sensitivity for the detection of small recurrences and can even detect primary lesions that are endoscopically not evident.[37] Current literature shows that MR imaging trends toward higher accuracy than PET-CT in detecting local residual and/or recurrent disease. However, the combined use of MR imaging and PET-CT is more accurate for tumor restaging than either modality independently.[38]

FUTURE DIRECTIONS AND ADVANCED IMAGING

Diffusion-weighted imaging has been performed to look at primary nasopharyngeal tumors; however, it is limited by extensive artifact at the skull base. Overlapping apparent diffusion coefficient values do not permit differentiation of NPC from other tumors, such as lymphoma.[39] Diffusion may yet prove to be useful for the detection of early local recurrence and differentiation from posttreatment changes.

Early MR spectroscopic data suggest that both primary and metastatic NPC (>1 cm^3) have abnormally elevated choline (creatine ratios compared with normal muscles).[40] MR spectroscopy shows potential as an additive tool for detecting residual disease after treatment and for differentiating recurrent tumor from treated disease. This may also have a future application for predicting tumoral behavior and monitoring treatment or, with technical advances that minimize the sample volume, it may be possible to detect small nodal metastases.

REFERENCES

1. Berkowitz KB. Pharynx Chapter 35. In: Standring S, editor. Gray's anatomy. London, UK: Elsevier; 2005. p. 619–22.
2. Harnsberger HR. Pharyngeal mucosal space. In: Diagnostic and surgical imaging anatomy: brain, head & neck and spine, vol. 11. Salt Lake City, Utah: Amirsys; 2006. p. 148–59.
3. American Joint Committee on Cancer. Pharynx. In: Edge SB, Byrd DR, Compton CC, et al, editors. AJCC cancer staging handbook. 7th edition. New York: Springer-Verlag; 2010. p. 63–79.
4. Wenig BM. Nasopharyngeal carcinoma, nonkeratinizing types. In: Thompson LD, Wenig BM, editors. Diagnostic pathology: head and neck, vol. 2. Salt Lake City, Utah: Amirsys; 2011. p. 24–31.
5. Wenig BM. Nasopharyngeal carcinoma, keratinizing type. In: Thompson LD, Wenig BM, editors. Diagnostic pathology: head and neck, vol. 2. Salt Lake City, Utah: Amirsys; 2011. p. 32–3.
6. Wenig BM. Nasopharyngeal carcinoma, basaloid squamous cell carcinoma. In: Thompson LD, Wenig BM, editors. Diagnostic pathology: head and neck, vol. 2. Salt Lake City, Utah: Amirsys; 2011. p. 34–7.
7. Vokes EE, Liebowitz DN, Weichselbaum RR. Nasopharyngeal carcinoma. Lancet 1997;350:1087–91.
8. Stambuk HE, Patel SG, Mosier KM, et al. Nasopharyngeal carcinoma: recognizing the radiographic features in children. AJNR Am J Neuroradiol 2005; 26:1575–9.
9. Chia KS, Lee HP. Epidemiology. In: Chong VF, Tsao SY, editors. Nasopharyngeal carcinoma. Hong Kong (China): Armour Publishing; 1997. p. 1–5.
10. Richey LM, Olshan AF, George J, et al. Incidence and survival rates for young blacks with nasopharyngeal carcinoma in the United States.

Arch Otolaryngol Head Neck Surg 2006;132: 1035–40.

11. Piccirillo JF, Costas I, Reichman ME. Chapter 2. Cancers of the head and neck. In: SEER survival monograph: cancer survival among adults: US SEER Program, 1988-2001, patient and tumor characteristics. Washington, DC: National Cancer Institute; 2007. p. 7–22.

12. Wenig BM. Nasopharyngeal papillary adenocarcinoma. In: Thompson LD, Wenig BM, editors. Diagnostic pathology: head and neck, vol. 2. Salt Lake City, Utah: Amirsys; 2011. p. 38–9.

13. American Joint Committee on Cancer. Pharynx. In: Greene FL, Page DL, Fleming ID, et al, editors. AJCC cancer staging handbook. 6th edition. New York: Springer-Verlag; 2002. p. 47–60.

14. Lee N, Xia P, Quivey J, et al. Intensity-modulated radiotherapy in the treatment of nasopharyngeal carcinoma: an update of the UCSF experience. Int J Radiat Oncol Biol Phys 2002;53:12–22.

15. Lee AW, Law SC, Foo W, et al. Retrospective analysis of patients with nasopharyngeal carcinoma treated during 1976-1985: survival after local recurrence. Int J Radiat Oncol Biol Phys 1993;26:773–82.

16. Pfister DG, et al. Cancers of the nasopharynx. In: Head and neck cancers. NCCN clinical practice guidelines in oncology. v.2.2011. National Comprehensive Cancer Network (NCCN). Available at: http://www.nccn.org/professionals/physician_gls/f_guidelines.asp. Accessed January 12, 2012.

17. King AD, Vlantis AC, Tsang RK, et al. Magnetic resonance imaging for the detection of nasopharyngeal carcinoma. AJNR Am J Neuroradiol 2006; 27:1288–91.

18. Chin SC, Fatterpekar G, Chen CY, et al. MR imaging of diverse manifestations of nasopharyngeal carcinomas. AJR Am J Roentgenol 2003;180(6):1715–22.

19. Chung NN, Ting LL, Hsu WC, et al. Impact of magnetic resonance imaging versus CT on nasopharyngeal carcinoma: primary tumor target delineation for radiotherapy. Head Neck 2004;26:241–6.

20. Liao XB, Mao YP, Liu LZ, et al. How does magnetic resonance imaging influence staging according to AJCC staging system for nasopharyngeal carcinoma compared with computed tomography? Int J Radiat Oncol Biol Phys 2008;72(5):1368–77.

21. Tang LL, Li WF, Chen L, et al. Prognostic value and staging categories of anatomic masticator space involvement in nasopharyngeal carcinoma: a study of 924 cases with MR imaging. Radiology 2010; 257(1):151–7.

22. Ng WT, Lee AW, Kan WK, et al. N-staging by magnetic resonance imaging for patients with nasopharyngeal carcinoma: pattern of nodal involvement by radiological levels. Radiother Oncol 2007;82:70–5.

23. Ng SH, Chang JT, Chan SC, et al. Nodal metastases of nasopharyngeal carcinoma: patterns of disease on MRI and FDG PET. Eur J Nucl Med Mol Imaging 2004;31:1073–80.

24. Ma J, Liu L, Tang L, et al. Retropharyngeal lymph node metastasis in nasopharyngeal carcinoma: prognostic value and staging categories. Clin Cancer Res 2007;13:1445–52.

25. Liu LZ, Zhang GY, Xie CM, et al. Magnetic resonance imaging of retropharyngeal lymph node metastasis in nasopharyngeal carcinoma: patterns of spread. Int J Radiat Oncol Biol Phys 2006;66:721–30.

26. King AD, Ahuja AT, Leung SF, et al. Neck node metastases from nasopharyngeal carcinoma: MR imaging of patterns of disease. Head Neck 2000; 22:275–81.

27. Teo PM, Kwan WH, Lee WY, et al. Prognosticators determining survival subsequent to distant metastasis from nasopharyngeal carcinoma. Cancer 1996;77:2423–31.

28. Vikram B, Mishra UB, Strong EW, et al. Patterns of failure in carcinoma of the nasopharynx: failure at distant sites. Head Neck Surg 1986;8:276–9.

29. Yen TC, Chang JT, Ng SH, et al. The value of 18F-FDG PET in the detection of stage M0 carcinoma of the nasopharynx. J Nucl Med 2005;46: 405–10.

30. Chang JT, Chan SC, Yen TC, et al. Nasopharyngeal carcinoma staging by (18)F-fluorodeoxyglucose positron emission tomography. Int J Radiat Oncol Biol Phys 2005;62:501–7.

31. Glastonbury CM. Nasopharyngeal carcinoma: the role of magnetic resonance imaging in diagnosis, staging, treatment, and follow-up. Top Magn Reson Imaging 2007;18(4):225–35.

32. King AD, Ahuja AT, Yeung DK, et al. Delayed complications of radiotherapy treatment for nasopharyngeal carcinoma: imaging findings. Clin Radiol 2007;62:195–203.

33. Ng SH, Liu HM, Ko SF, et al. Posttreatment imaging of the nasopharynx. Eur J Radiol 2002;44(2):82–95.

34. Glastonbury CM, Parker EE, Hoang JK. The postradiation neck: evaluating response to treatment and recognizing complications. AJR Am J Roentgenol 2010;195(2):W164–71.

35. Spano JP, Busson P, Atlan D, et al. Nasopharyngeal carcinomas: an update. Eur J Cancer 2003;39: 2121–35.

36. Amemiya K, Shibuya H, Yoshimura R, et al. The risk of radiation-induced cancer in patients with squamous cell carcinoma of the head and neck and its results of treatment. Br J Radiol 2005;78(935): 1028–33.

37. King AD, Vlantis AC, Bhatia KS, et al. Primary nasopharyngeal carcinoma: diagnostic accuracy of MR imaging versus that of endoscopy and endoscopic biopsy. Radiology 2011;258(2):531–7.

38. Comoretto M, Balestreri L, Borsatti E, et al. Detection and restaging of residual and/or recurrent

nasopharyngeal carcinoma after chemotherapy and radiation therapy: comparison of MR imaging and FDG PET/CT. Radiology 2008;249(1):203–11.

39. Fong D, Bhatia KS, Yeung D, et al. Diagnostic accuracy of diffusion-weighted MR imaging for nasopharyngeal carcinoma, head and neck lymphoma and squamous cell carcinoma at the primary site. Oral Oncol 2010;46(8):603–6.

40. King AD, Yeung DK, Ahuja AT, et al. In vivo proton MR spectroscopy of primary and nodal nasopharyngeal carcinoma. AJNR Am J Neuroradiol 2004;25: 484–90.

Pitfalls in the Staging of Cancer of Oral Cavity Cancer

Ashley H. Aiken, MD

KEYWORDS

- Squamous cell carcinoma • Oral cavity • Retromolar trigone • Floor of mouth

KEY POINTS

- Staging OC tumors requires knowledge of OC anatomy, the OC subsites, and tumor spread patterns.
- Radiologists should always assess for features that would upstage to a T4a disease, including invasion of the extrinsic tongue muscles or mandible, and features that upstage to potentially unresectable T4b disease, including involvement of the masticator space, skull base, and encasement of the internal carotid artery.
- This article reviews the detailed imaging anatomy of the OC, and epidemiology, staging, and surveillance for OCSCC.

INTRODUCTION AND EPIDEMIOLOGY

Oral cavity (OC) cancer comprises nearly 30% of all malignant tumors of the head and neck. A total of 90% of cases are squamous cell carcinoma (SCC). The remaining 10% represent minor salivary gland neoplasms, melanoma, lymphoma, and rare varieties of squamous cell and odontogenic tumors.[1] Oral cavity cancer is the sixth leading cause of cancer-related mortality in the world.[2] Although it only accounts for a small percentage (0.6%–5%) of cancers in Western societies, it represents nearly 45% of cancers in certain countries, such as India, secondary to risk factors, such as betel nut chewing. Oral cavity cancer occurs most commonly in middle aged and elderly individuals. However, recent evidence suggests an increased incidence in younger individuals (<40 years) from 3% in 1973 to 6% in 1993.[3] The primary causative risk factors in North America include alcohol and tobacco, which are independent and synergistic. Human papillomavirus is strongly associated with oropharyngeal cancers, but only a minority of OC cancers.[4] Oral cancer is often diagnosed at a late stage contributing to the low 5-year survival rates, hovering at 50 60% overall and as low as 22% for late stage.[5,6]

The OC is the most anterior subdivision of the aerodigestive tract with a wide variety of tissue types for such a small region. The posterior OC is separated from the oropharynx (OP) by an imaginary ring drawn across the circumvallate papillae, anterior tonsillar pillars, and junction of the hard and soft palate. This is a critical distinction because carcinomas in the OC versus OP differ in presentation, treatment, and prognosis. However, it is not uncommon for OC tumors to spread to the OP and vice versa. The remaining boundaries of the OC include the lips anteriorly; the cheeks laterally; the hard palate and superior alveolar ridge superiorly; and the inferior alveolar ridge and mylohyoid muscle inferiorly (**Figs. 1** and **2**). The oral mucosal space refers to the nonkeratinized stratified squamous epithelium lining the entire OC including the buccal (cheek), gingival (gums), palatal, and lingual surfaces.[7] These are the potential sites for SCC. In addition, subepithelial collections of minor salivary glands are found throughout the OC, most commonly along the inner surface of the lip, buccal

Department of Radiology and Imaging Sciences, Emory University, BG-21, 1364 Clifton Road, Northeast, Atlanta, GA 30322, USA
E-mail address: ashley.aiken@emoryhealthcare.org

Neuroimag Clin N Am 23 (2013) 27–45
http://dx.doi.org/10.1016/j.nic.2012.08.004
1052-5149/13/$ – see front matter © 2013 Elsevier Inc. All rights reserved.

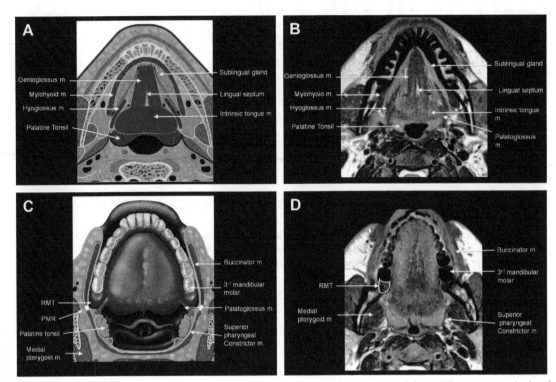

Fig. 1. Normal OC anatomy: axial at the level of the floor of mouth and oral tongue. (*A*) Axial illustration at the level of the floor of mouth demonstrating the extrinsic tongue muscles and sublingual space. (*B*) Axial T2-weighted image at the level of the floor of mouth. (*C*) Axial illustration at the level of the oral tongue demonstrating the oral tongue and retromolar trigone (RMT). PMR, pterygomandibular raphe (facial band connecting the buccinator and superior constrictor muscles). (*D*) Axial T2-weighted image at the level of the oral tongue. (*Courtesy of* Eric Jablonowski.)

mucosa, and hard palate. These are potential sites for minor salivary gland neoplasms, such as adenoid cystic and mucoepidermoid carcinomas.

The OC is readily accessible, so oral cancer screening and initial evaluation should be accomplished by clinical examination. Changes in the mucosa are easily identified and evaluated. After a definitive diagnosis has been made, imaging is essential for staging the primary tumor by evaluating submucosal spread and invasion of adjacent structures, and to identify nodal or distant metastasis. OC anatomy is one of the most complex in the head and neck; therefore, knowledge of anatomic subsites and spread patterns is critical for accurate staging. This article begins with a discussion of imaging techniques, and then presents a detailed review of normal anatomy followed by imaging's role in tumor staging highlighting potential pitfalls (**Table 1**).

IMAGING PROTOCOLS

The choice of imaging modality is often determined by the clinical question and treatment options.

Computed tomography (CT) is generally the workhorse modality for OC cancer. It can be acquired within minutes limiting motion artifact, and can easily be reformatted in coronal and sagittal planes. CT is also preferred to evaluate for early cortical bone involvement.[8] MR imaging may complement CT of the OC because it offers advantages in delineating soft tissue anatomy, especially where accurate tumor extent is critical for surgical planning and negative margins. MR imaging may also be preferable in patients with excessive dental amalgam artifact obscuring the primary tumor and tumor extent. The overall accuracy of CT versus MR imaging for T staging is comparable.[9] However, many subsites, especially the hard palate, can be understaged with CT and therefore MR imaging is invaluable for accurately defining margins and evaluating for perineural extension.[10] CT is more affected by artifact caused by dental metals, whereas MR imaging is more affected by artifact caused by movements of the patient. Most studies that have compared the accuracy of CT and MR imaging for the assessment of the neck have also found no difference.[11] Although

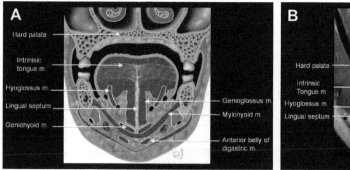

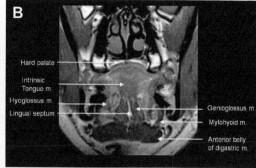

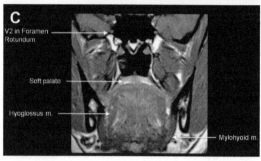

Fig. 2. Normal OC anatomy: coronal at the level of the hard and soft palate. (*A*) Coronal illustration through the hard palate. Note the mylohyoid muscle forming the inferior and lateral borders of the OC, the close relationship to the mandible, and the extrinsic tongue muscles (hyoglossus and genioglossus). (*B, C*) Coronal T1-weighted image through the hard palate and soft palate, respectively. (*Courtesy of* Eric Jablonowski.)

positron emission tomography (PET) and PET-CT have the potential to increase sensitivity for nodal disease, some authors have found that the diagnostic accuracy for OC nodal metastasis did not improve significantly compared with CT or MR imaging alone.[12–14]

Although protocols vary based on institution, my CT protocol includes 1.25-mm helical images after injection of intravenous contrast, reconstructed at 2.5 mm from the orbits through the thoracic inlet, with routine use of sagittal and coronal reformations. I also obtain a second set of images through

Table 1	
Pitfalls in staging of OC SCC	
Pitfall	**Advice**
Upstage to T4a: Misinterpreting odontogenic disease as mandible invasion	Thin section bone CT with multiplanar reformats
Upstage to T4a: Misinterpreting atrophic edentulous mandible as tumor invasion/ destruction	Thin section bone CT with multiplanar reformats
Upstage to T4a: Not recognizing extrinsic tongue muscle involvement significance rather than intrinsic	Know anatomy of hyoglossus and genioglossus MR imaging may help in difficult cases
Hard palate primary: Understaging with CT	Recommend MR imaging for all cases being considered for resection to delineate tumor spread
PET-CT too early after surgery or biopsy	Wait at least 8 wk
Upstaging to T4b: Overcalling involvement of masticator space	Tumor may bulge rather than invade medial pterygoid muscle. Most surgeons will still attempt resection for medial pterygoid involvement

the OC with delayed mucosal enhancement and butterfly angled images to decrease dental amalgam artifact (Fig. 3).

An ideal MR imaging protocol includes axial, sagittal, and coronal images obtained with a dedicated neck coil and section thickness of 4 mm or less.[15] Optimal field of view is 16 to 18 cm on T1- and 18 to 20 cm on T2-weighted images allowing for improved signal-to-noise ratio.[16] Three planes of precontrast T1-weighted imaging are desirable to delineate normal anatomy and obliteration of fat and muscle planes. Postgadolinium T1-weighted fat-saturated sequences are especially useful for delineating enhancing tumor margins from intrinsically high signal intensity fat, and in the evaluation for perineural tumor.[16,17] However, fat suppression can result in artifacts with signal loss and distortion.[18] In this case, I prefer to add postgadolinium sequences without fat saturation.

STAGING

The American Joint Committee on Cancer (AJCC) staging for lip and OC can be found in Table 2. This TNM staging system is only used for epithelial tumors including SCC and minor salivary gland carcinoma. T1, T2, and T3 lesions of the OC are distinguished based on 2-cm increments in size. Patterns of invasion are used to upstage to a T4a or T4b lesion. The primary considerations to upstage to T4a disease include bone invasion (mandible or maxilla) or involvement of the extrinsic tongue muscles. It is critical, therefore, that the radiologist be able to routinely identify

the extrinsic tongue muscles. The sixth edition of the *AJCC Cancer Staging Manual* modified OC staging by the addition of T4b, which denoted unresectable disease. Since that time, the seventh edition of the AJCC has replaced the "resectable" versus "unresectable" terminology for T4a and T4b respectively to "moderately advanced" and "very advanced" disease. T4b still refers to tumor invasion of the masticator space, pterygoid plates, or skull base and tumor encasement of the internal carotid artery. The criteria for nodal staging of OC are identical to the criteria for other sites in the pharynx and larynx, with the exception of nasopharynx.

Additional Prognostic Indicators and Trends in Treatment Important for Staging

Tumor thickness and depth of invasion are important prognostic factors and surgical planning tools in OC cancer that are not included in the T staging of the AJCC. Tumor thickness and depth of invasion have been associated with local recurrence and survival for cancer of the oral tongue.[19] The exact depth of invasion that predicts nodal disease is not clear, but several studies have suggested that tumor thickness greater than 4 mm increases the chance of cervical metastasis.[20] Elective neck dissection for early T1-T2 N0 disease continues to be investigated. Clinically and radiographically occult nodal disease found only at surgery increases the risk of recurrence and decreases 5-year survival from 82% to 53%.[21] Furthermore, Kligerman and colleagues[22] showed that

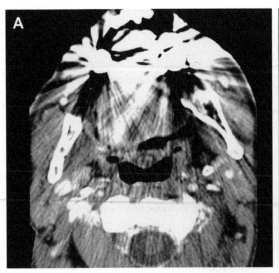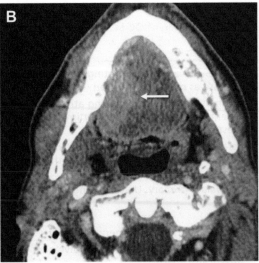

Fig. 3. SCC of the right oral tongue: usefulness of reangled images. (*A*) Axial contrast-enhanced (CE) CT through the oral cavity is nondiagnostic because of dental amalgam and extensive streak artifact. (*B*) Delayed and reangled axial CE CT image shows a large enhancing right oral tongue mass (*arrow*), effacing the right sublingual space.

Table 2
AJCC 7 lip and oral cavity staging

	Primary Tumor (T)
TX	Primary tumor cannot be assessed
T0	No evidence of primary tumor
Tis	Carcinoma *in situ*
T1	Tumor 2 cm or less in greatest dimension
T2	Tumor more than 2 cm but not more than 4 cm in greatest dimension
T3	Tumor more than 4 cm in greatest dimension
T4a	Moderately advanced local disease (lip) Tumor invades through cortical bone, inferior alveolar nerve, floor of mouth, or skin of face, i.e., chin or nose (oral cavity) Tumor invades adjacent structures only (e.g., through cortical bone, [mandible or maxilla] into deep [extrinsic] muscle of tongue [genioglossus, hyoglossus, palatoglossus, and styloglossus], maxillary sinus, skin of face)
T4b	T4b Very advanced local disease Tumor invades masticator space, pterygoid plates, or skull base and/or encases internal carotid artery Note: Superficial erosion alone of bone/tooth socket by gingival primary is not sufficient to classify a tumor as T4
	Regional Lymph Nodes (N)
NX	Regional lymph nodes cannot be assessed
N0	No regional lymph node metastasis
N1	Metastasis in a single ipsilateral lymph node, 3 cm or less in greatest dimension
N2	Metastasis in a single ipsilateral lymph node, more than 3 cm but not more than 6 cm in greatest dimension; or in multiple ipsilateral lymph nodes, none more than 6 cm in greatest dimension; or in bilateral or contralateral lymph nodes, none more than 6 cm in greatest dimension
N2a	Metastasis in single ipsilateral lymph node more than 3 cm but not more than 6 cm in greatest dimension
N2b	Metastasis in multiple ipsilateral lymph nodes, none more than 6 cm in greatest dimension
N2c	Metastasis in bilateral or contralateral lymph nodes, none more than 6 cm in greatest dimension
N3	Metastasis in a lymph node more than 6 cm in greatest dimension
	Distant Metastasis (M)
M0	No distant metastasis
M1	Distant metastasis

From Edge S, Byrd D, Compton C, et al. AJCC Cancer Staging Manual. 7th edition. Chicago (IL): Springer; 2010. p. 41–56; with permission.

a prophylactic neck dissection in patients with low-volume primary and N0 neck reduced recurrence rate from 33% to 12%, compared with those in whom the neck was treated with watchful waiting. Some authors advocate a prophylactic neck dissection for all OC cancers, regardless of depth of invasion.[14] Others recommend a staging supraomohyoid neck dissection for all patients with T2 disease at the primary site, and T1 disease with greater than 4 mm depth of invasion. Because 70% to 80% of neck dissection specimens are negative for regional metastatic disease, recently some authors advocate a sentinel node biopsy.[21,23]

Perineural invasion and lymphocytic response are additional histopathologic parameters that are not accounted for in the current AJCC staging system.[12] Extracapsular spread (ECS) may have a significant impact on the prognosis of patients with regional disease, with up to 50% reduction in survival.[24] On imaging, ill-defined margins of the lymph node and stranding are the biggest clues to ECS (**Fig. 4**). Patients with ECS are commonly treated with adjuvant radiation and chemotherapy.

Superficial carcinomas of the OC can be treated with excellent cure rates with either radiation or

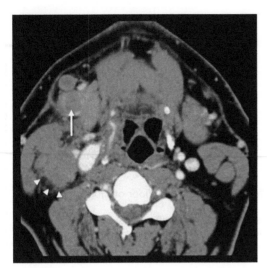

Fig. 4. SCC of the floor of mouth with lymph node metastasis. Axial CE CT shows multiple level IB and IIA nodes that are pathologically enlarged. The IB nodes show central necrosis (*arrow*). The IIA nodes have extensive surrounding stranding (*arrowheads*) suggesting extracapsular spread. This pattern of nodal drainage suggests an OC primary.

surgery. However, because surgical cure can be achieved rapidly with minimal morbidity, it is often preferred.[12] Advanced disease is often managed with multimodality therapy. Surgery with or without reconstruction coupled with preoperative or postoperative radiation therapy is often used. Most centers perform surgery followed by postoperative radiation because of the higher rate of postoperative complications with preoperative radiation treatment.[12] Although primary surgical management has been advocated for most advanced OC cancer, recent evidence suggests that primary chemoradiotherapy may be effective for selected T4 patients, especially in cases of "functional irresectability," such as patients requiring total glossectomy.[25]

T STAGE

Primary SCCs in the OC are usually infiltrative mucosal lesions with variable enhancement on CT and MR imaging. Larger tumors may have central necrosis. On MR imaging, the precontrast T1-weighted sequence is often particularly helpful to show the T1 hypointense tumor, especially to contrast the signal intensity of the fibrofatty oral tongue. These tumors are minimally T2 hyperintense and variably enhancing postgadolinium.

Conversely, minor salivary gland tumors are submucosal and often more well circumscribed. The most common minor salivary neoplasms are adenoid cystic and mucoepidermoid carcinomas.

Adenocarcinoma is less common. On MR imaging, these tumors are T1 isointense to muscle, mildly T2 hyperintense, and avidly enhancing.

IMAGING ANATOMY AND PATTERNS OF SPREAD BY SUBSITE

OC cancers are classified into the following subsites: (1) lip, (2) buccal mucosa, (3) upper and lower gingiva, (4) retromolar trigone (RMT), (5) hard palate, (6) oral tongue, and (7) floor of mouth (FOM) (**Fig. 5**).

Lip Carcinoma

Keratinizing squamous epithelium covers the outer lips, whereas the inner surface and gingiva are covered by nonkeratinizing stratified squamous epithelium. The motor branch of cranial nerve (CN) VII innervates the lips. The primary lymphatic drainage is to submental (level IA) and submandibular (level IB) nodes.

The lip is the most common site of SCC in the OC, representing roughly 40% of cases.[26] Carcinomas of the lip usually arise from the vermillion border and may spread laterally to adjacent skin or deeply to the orbicularis oris muscle. If the tumor invades skin or bone, it becomes upstaged to a T4a.

Buccal Mucosa and Gingiva

The gingiva or "gums" refers to the mucosal covering of the lingual (medial) and buccal (lateral) surfaces of the alveolar mandible and maxilla. The junction between the gingival and the buccal mucosa lining the cheek is called the gingivobuccal sulcus.

Buccal carcinomas often originate along the lateral margins of the buccal mucosa lining the

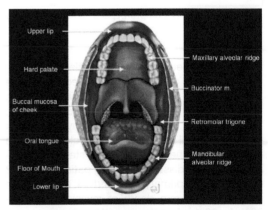

Fig. 5. Graphic drawing illustrating the mucosal subsites for oral cavity SCC. (*Courtesy of* Eric Jablonowski.)

cheeks. Some authors find it helpful to have patients puff their cheeks outward to reveal more subtle mucosal lesions (**Fig. 6**). I do not routinely use this technique, because it is primarily the clinician's role to identify mucosal extent. Imaging is critical to identify submucosal tumor, bone involvement, perineural extension, or extension to the masticator space. A common route of spread is lateral extension along the buccinator muscle to the RMT and ptergomandibular raphe. Buccal tumors that invade the buccinator muscle and have nodal disease or other poor prognostic indicators should undergo postoperative radiation. Therefore, it is important that the radiologist identifies involvement of the buccinator muscle and RMT, because involvement of the RMT provides numerous paths of tumor spread and makes surgical management more difficult (**Fig. 7**). More than half of buccal tumors present as deeply invasive tumors that may track along the parotid duct (**Fig. 8**), masseter muscle, or into the palate. Involvement of the parotid duct requires the surgeon to trace the duct retrograde to ensure negative margins. These lesions also spread along the submucosal surface and may eventually involve the skin.

Tumors of the gingiva along the maxillary or mandibular alveolar ridges account for less than 10% of OC carcinomas.[16,27] Because of the proximity to cortical bone, it is critical to assess for bone invasion and perineural extension, particularly along the inferior alveolar nerve for SCCs of the lower alveolar ridge (**Fig. 9**).

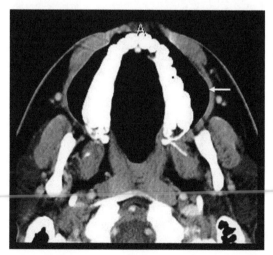

Fig. 6. Puffed cheek technique. Axial CE CT shows a patient "puffing" their cheeks, which may demonstrate the mucosal buccal space with better detail. Note the margins of the buccinator muscle are also better defined (*arrow*).

Retromolar Trigone

The RMT refers to the small triangular-shaped mucosa overlying the area just posterior to the last mandibular molar. The RMT is an important subsite of the OC because it represents a crossroads for tumor spread to and from the OC, OP, buccal space, FOM, and masticator space. The RMT refers to the small triangular-shaped mucosa overlying the area just posterior to the last mandibular molar. The pterygomandibular raphe lies just beneath the mucosa of the RMT and provides attachment for the buccinator and superior pharyngeal constrictor muscles (**Fig. 10**). This fibrous band connects the posterior mylohyoid line of the mandible to the hamulus of the medial pterygoid plate, and thereby it serves as a route of tumor spread superiorly from the RMT to the pterygoid process or posterior maxillary alveolus (**Fig. 11**). Tumors of the RMT are in close proximity to the mandible and maxilla, and therefore have a high propensity to invade bone.

Hard Palate

The hard palate is a thin horizontal bone formed by the palatine processes of the maxillae and the horizontal plates of the palatine bones (see **Fig. 2**). It spans the arch formed by the alveolar ridges and upper teeth. Posteriorly, the hard palate is contiguous with the soft palate, which is a subsite of the OP. It forms the superior margin of the OC and inferior margin of the nasal cavity. The greater palatine foramen is located medial to the posterior third molar within the lateral border of the bony palate.[28] The greater palatine nerve runs through this foramen and is a potential source of perineural spread of tumor along branches of CN V2 into the ptergopalatine fossa.[29] The incisive canal houses the nasopalatine nerves and arteries, and is found within the hard palate, just posterior to the incisor teeth.

Unlike other areas of the OC where SCC predominates, the palate is rich in minor salivary glands. OC minor salivary gland tumors are most commonly found at the junction of the hard and soft palate. Preoperative imaging is a key to assess invasion of the maxillary sinus, palatal bone, and nasal cavity. Important features to identify on CT are erosion of the hard palate and widening of the greater palatine foramen, suggesting perineural spread (**Fig. 12**). MR imaging is critical to define the extent of these infiltrating tumors and to assess for perineural spread, because these tumors have a propensity to spread along the greater and lesser palatine nerves into the ptergopalatine fossa, allowing intracranial access along V2 through foramen rotundum or the vidian nerve in the vidian

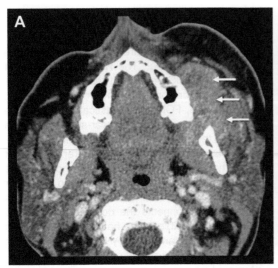
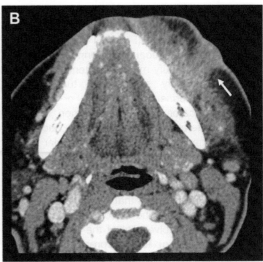

Fig. 7. SCC of the left buccal mucosa, T4a. (*A*) Axial CE CT shows large left buccal mass (*arrows*) extending to maxillary RMT. (*B*) Axial CE CT (inferior to *A*) shows inferior and lateral extension to involve the skin (*arrow*). Involvement of the skin critical to note, because the tumor is upstaged to T4a.

canal. Achieving negative margins at surgery is essential to a good outcome. Minor salivary gland tumors of the hard palate rarely metastasize to the neck, so that a neck dissection is rarely warranted in the absence of gross disease.

Oral Tongue

The oral tongue denotes the anterior two-thirds of the tongue separated from the base of tongue (OP) by a line across the circumvallate papilla. The tongue is composed of intrinsic and extrinsic muscle fibers. The four interdigitating intrinsic tongue muscles include the superior and inferior longitudinal, transverse, and oblique muscles. The extrinsic tongue muscles originate from bony or soft tissue attachments outside the tongue and have distal fibers that interdigitate with the intrinsic tongue muscles. They are the genioglossus, stylogossus, hyoglossus, and palatoglossus

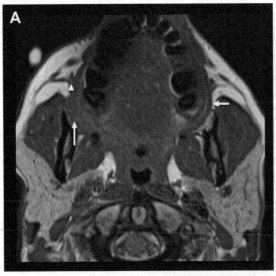
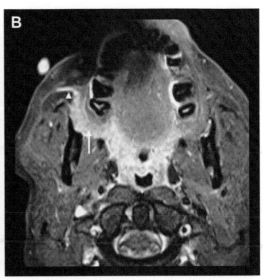

Fig. 8. Right buccal mucosa adenoid cystic carcinoma. (*A*) Axial T1-weighted image shows a right buccal mass (*arrow on right*), extending to the RMT and invading the buccinator muscle (*arrow on left* shows normal buccinator muscle) and extending to distal parotid duct (*arrowhead*). (*B*) Postcontrast fat-saturated axial T1-weighted image results in increased conspicuity of the mass (*arrow*) and parotid duct involvement (*arrowhead*). Note this example of limitation of fat saturation with increased artifact from dental amalgam.

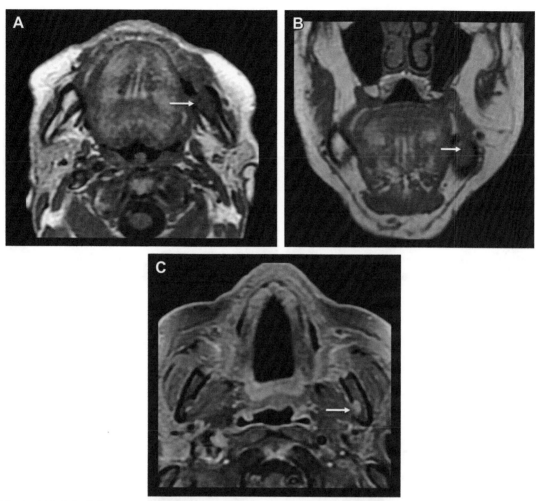

Fig. 9. SCC of the left posterior alveolar ridge, T4a. (*A*) Axial T1-weighted image shows an isointense mass with cortical and medullary cavity invasion of the mandible (*arrow*). Notice the interruption of the T1 hypointense line of the cortex, but also replacement of normal T1 hyperintense marrow signal intensity. (*B*) Coronal T1-weighted image also shows involvement and near complete replacement of normal marrow signal in the mandible (*arrow*). Cortical involvement was confirmed on a CT (not shown). Bone involvement upstages to a T4a. (*C*) Postcontrast fat-saturated T1-weighted image shows perineural spread along the inferior alveolar nerve (*arrow*). It is important to assess foramen ovale for intracranial extension.

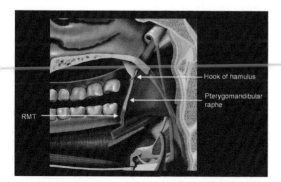

Fig. 10. Normal anatomy of pterygomandibular raphe.

muscles and originate from the genial tubercle of the inner mandible, anterior styloid process, cornua of the hyoid bone, and soft palate, respectively (see **Fig. 1**). The extrinsic tongue muscles are crucial to evaluate because involvement upstages OC carcinomas to at least a T4a.

The intrinsic and extrinsic tongue muscles are innervated by the hypoglossal nerve (CN XII), which emerges from nasopharyngeal carotid space and runs in the sublingual space with the lingual artery between the hyoglossus and mylohyoid muscles. The palatoglossus also receives supply from the vagus nerve (CN X) and the pharyngeal plexus. The sensory supply to the anterior two thirds of the tongue is by the lingual nerve, a branch of the trigeminal nerve (CN V)

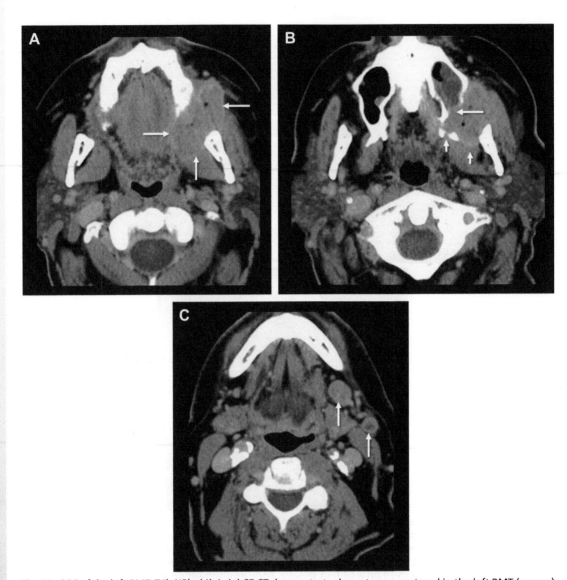

Fig. 11. SCC of the left RMT, T4b N2b. (*A*) Axial CE CT demonstrates large tumor centered in the left RMT (*arrows*). (*B*) Axial CE CT (cranial to *A*) shows obvious invasion of the posterior maxilla involving the maxillary sinus (*long arrow*) from tumor growing superiorly along the pterygomandibular raphe. Tumor is therefore upstaged to T4a. Also note tumor extension to medial pterygoid plate and masticator space (*short arrows*), resulting in overall T4b stage. (*C*) Axial CE CT shows metastatic level I and II nodes (*arrows*). Some have central low density, a very specific sign for metastasis.

and taste fibers from the chorda tympani nerve, a branch of the facial nerve (CN VII). The primary lymphatic drainage is by the superficial mucosa and deep collecting system, which both drain into anterior submandibular nodes (level IB). The superficial lymphatics are directed to level IB and IIA nodes, whereas the deeper lymphatics of the oral tongue have pathways to both sides of the neck. For this reason, tumor depth of 4 to 5 mm or greater has increased risk of bilateral lymphadenopathy.[12]

Nearly all tongue carcinomas occur along the lateral margin or undersurface. Prognosis and treatment depends on depth of invasion. Although superficial tumors are not easily seen on CT or MR imaging, it is not the radiologist's role to diagnosis mucosal lesions. It is critical that the radiologist assess the extrinsic tongue muscles as discussed previously to upstage to T4a. Assessment of involvement of the midline lingual septum is critical to determine whether the patient requires a hemiglossectomy or total glossectomy. Advanced

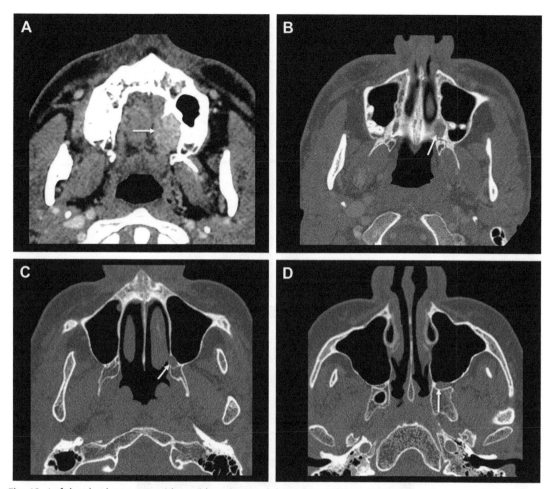

Fig. 12. Left hard palate mucoepidermoid carcinoma. (*A*) Axial CE CT shows 2-cm enhancing mass with fairly well-circumscribed borders (*arrow*) in the left hard palate. Well-circumscribed borders are common in minor salivary gland malignancies, making it difficult to differentiate them from benign minor salivary gland tumors. (*B, C*) bone window from axial CE CT images (at the level of the hard palate [*B*] and just above) show asymmetric widening of the left greater palatine foramen (*arrow*), compatible with perineural tumor extension. (*D*) Bone window from axial CE CT images shows extension of abnormal widening to the left pterygopalatine fossa (*arrow*). An MR image is needed to assess for proximal intracranial extension to determine if this tumor was resectable.

tumors have defined routes of infiltration. Anterior third tumors tend to invade the FOM (**Fig. 13**). Middle-third lesions invade the musculature of the tongue and subsequently the FOM (**Fig. 14**). Posterior-third tumors grow into the anterior tonsillar pillar, tongue base, and glossotonsillar sulcus.[8] Involvement of the tongue base is critical to note, because it may necessitate a total laryngectomy to prevent aspiration.[30]

Up to 35% of patients have nodal metastasis on presentation (see **Fig. 13**). Even in the clinically N0 neck, 30% have occult metastasis.[8] The first nodal drainage group is level IB or submandibular, then level IIA or high jugular chain. Most authors suggest that greater than 4 mm depth (some advocate 5 mm) is associated with an increased risk of cervical nodal metastasis and therefore recommend

elective treatment of the clinically N0 neck.[20] Multiple studies have demonstrated the impact of tumor size on overall survival, thus the importance of the T factor on the AJCC chart. Overall survival decreases from 90% for tumors less than 2 cm to 60% to 63% for tumors greater than 2 cm.[31]

Floor of Mouth

The mylohyoid muscle forms the inferior border of FOM and divides the sublingual space from the submandibular space. It arises from the mylohyoid line of the mandible and inserts into the hyoid bone. This U-shaped sling is best visualized in the coronal plane (see **Fig. 2**). The mylohyoid muscle is innervated by the mylohyoid nerve, a branch of the inferior alveolar nerve (CN V3). Primary FOM

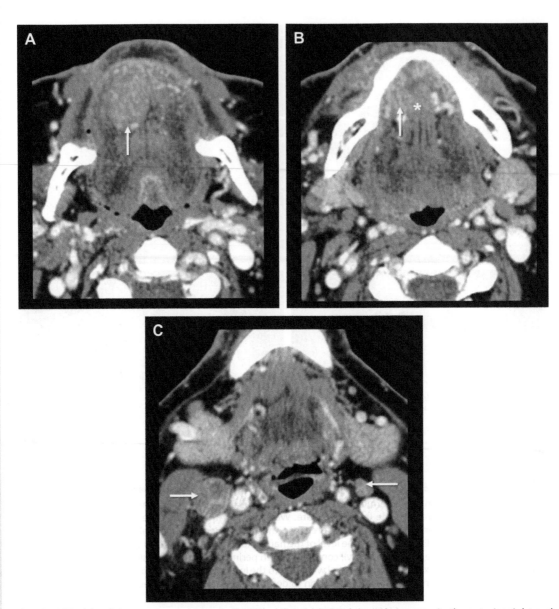

Fig. 13. SCC of the right anterior oral tongue, T4aN2c. (*A*) Axial CE CT shows a large mass in the anterior right oral tongue (*arrow*). (*B*) Axial CE CT (slightly inferior to *A*) shows extension to the floor of mouth (*arrow*), with efface-ment of sublingual space fat and involvement of genioglossus muscle (*asterisk*). The genioglossus muscle is an extrinsic tongue muscle and involvement upstages to T4a. (*C*) Axial CE CT shows abnormal bilateral level IIA nodes (*arrows*). Both have areas of low density consistent with necrosis, a morphologic abnormality with high speci-ficity, even though the left level IIA node is not abnormal by size criteria. The right level IIA node has surrounding fat stranding suggesting ECS. This is compatible with N2C disease.

carcinomas arise along the mucosal surface, including the crescent-shaped mucosa overlying the mylohyoid, sublingual space, and undersurface of the anterior two-thirds of the tongue.[28] FOM carcinomas tend to arise within 2 cm of the anterior midline and spread laterally to the adjacent mandible or ipsalateral or contralateral neurovas-cular bundle (Fig. 15). The neurovascular bundle, including the lingual artery and hypoglossal nerve, traverses the sublingual space. Ipsilateral tumor involvement necessitates sacrifice, but the remain-ing contralateral supply preserves viable tongue function. However, if tumor extends to the contra-lateral neurovascular bundle, this necessitates sacrifice of both bundles and total glossectomy. Nonsurgical management is often considered in these cases. Because the FOM is rich in neurovas-cular structures, frequent metastases occur to the

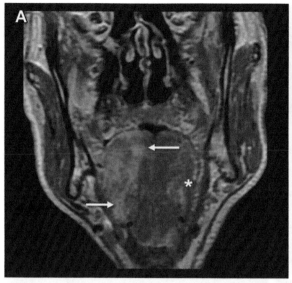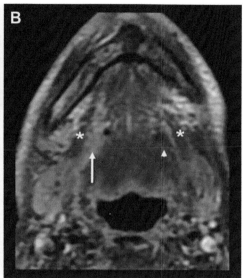

Fig. 14. SCC right oral tongue, T4a. (*A*) Coronal postcontrast T1-weighted image (fat saturation was not used secondary to excessive dental artifact) shows a large right oral tongue mass (*arrows*) extending to midline and inferiorly to involve the hyoglossus muscle. Note the normal left hyoglossus muscle (*asterisk*). (*B*) Axial postcontrast fat-saturated T1-weighted image shows the enhancing mass invading the right hyoglossus muscle (*arrow*). Note normal left hyoglossus muscle (*arrowhead*). Involvement of the hyoglossus (extrinsic tongue muscle) upstages to a T4a. The more lateral right and left mylohyoid muscles can also be seen (*asterisks*), but seem to have normal signal.

level I and II nodal groups. MR imaging provides better delineation of tumor extent in the FOM or toward the tongue base, but CT may be complementary to evaluate bone involvement.

Mandibular Invasion (T4a)

The presence of osseous involvement upstages OC carcinomas to at least stage T4a. Such subsites as the FOM, RMT, and the lower alveolus can invade the mandible directly. CT and MR imaging may be complementary for evaluation of mandibular involvement. In the RMT, one study suggests that CT is specific with a high positive predictive value (90%), but limited sensitivity (50%).[32] Other authors report high diagnostic accuracy for predicting mandibular invasion with thin-section CT Dentascan (sensitivity 95% and specificity 79%).[33] MR imaging offers superior evaluation of the medullary cavity, but may overestimate marrow involvement, secondary to adjacent odontogenic disease or edema. Although MR imaging may have good sensitivity, pitfalls result in low specificity.[34] The radiologist should closely examine the mandible for signs of invasion, including T1 hypointensity replacing normal fatty marrow, loss of low signal intensity cortex, and contrast-enhancement within the bone or along the inferior alveolar nerve. However, one potential

pitfall on MR imaging occurs in the setting of odontogenic disease, which can cause false-positive marrow replacement and even enhancement. Another pitfall on CT occurs in the evaluation of the edentulous patient, who may have a demineralized or even heterogeneous appearance of the mandible at baseline, making evaluation for subtle cortical invasion more difficult. Reformations in the oblique sagittal and coronal plane are often useful in these cases (**Fig. 16**).

Tumors invading the mandible can be managed with a marginal or segmental resection. Tumor invasion of only the periosteum without gross cortical invasion or involvement of the medullary cavity can be managed with a marginal mandibulectomy, which provides an adequate resection while maintaining the integrity of the bone. Tumors with gross cortical erosion or invasion of the medullary cavity require a segmental resection, meaning resection of the entire involved segment of mandible.[12] MR imaging may be complementary to CT to assess for medullary involvement. The segmental resection necessitates a more complex reconstruction, requiring vascularized bone and soft tissue, often a fibular free flap. In many cases, the most accurate measure of bony invasion is determined at the time of surgery. Unless there is frank invasion of the bony cortex on imaging or examination, wide excision and

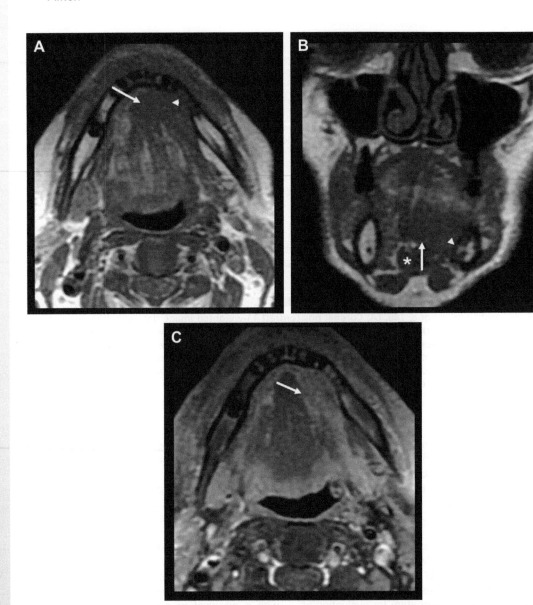

Fig. 15. SCC of the left floor of mouth, T4a. (*A*) Axial T1-weighted image shows a left anterior floor of mouth mass with medial extension to invade the anterior genioglossus (*arrow*) and lateral extension to invade the mandible (*arrowhead*). Both the genioglossus (extrinsic tongue muscle) and mandible invasion upstage to T4a. (*B*) Coronal T1-weighted image shows interruption of the mandible cortex (*arrowhead*) and medial extension to genioglossus muscle (*arrow*). The normal right geniohyoid muscle (*asterisk*) is seen just inferiorly. (*C*) Axial postcontrast fat-saturated T1-weighted image shows the borders of the mass and interface with midline genioglossus musculature (*arrow*).

periosteal stripping followed by frozen section examination at the time of surgery is often the most reliable measure of bone invasion.[12] If there is no cortical invasion, wide excision with periosteal stripping may suffice.

T4 DISEASE

The primary role of imaging in assessing the primary tumor is determination of T4a or T4b disease. The presence or absence of the following criteria should be reported for all OC tumors.

Extrinsic Muscle Invasion (T4a)

Invasion of the extrinsic tongue muscles should be assessed for all OC and OP primary tumors, because of the importance in upstaging to a T4a. Extrinsic tongue muscles include only the genioglossus, hyoglossus, styoglossus, and palatoglossus.

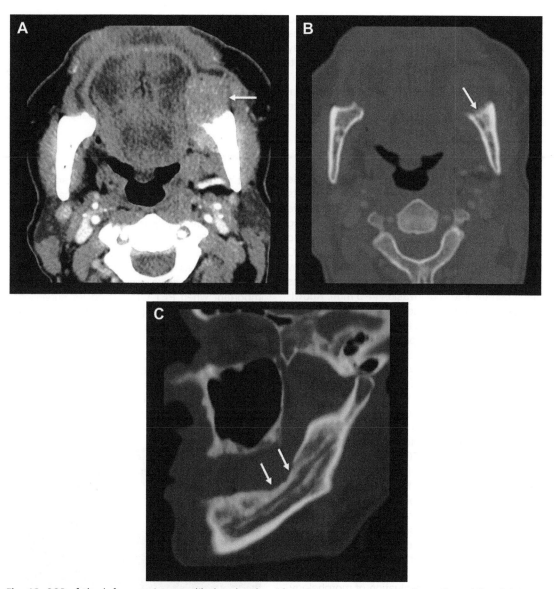

Fig. 16. SCC of the left posterior mandibular alveolar ridge, T4a: importance of reformations. (*A*) Axial CE CT shows a large mass along the posterior left mandibular alveolar ridge (*arrow*). (*B*) Axial CE CT in bone window demonstrates subtle cortical irregularity along the anterior mandibular angle/ramus junction (*arrow*). (*C*) Reformatted sagittal image confirms the focal cortical erosion (*arrows*).

The genioglossus and hyoglossus are most often involved and easily visualized on imaging to upstage to T4a. The hyoglossus muscle can be found just medial and parallel to the mylohyoid; it divides the sublingual space into medial and lateral portions (see **Figs.** 1 and 2). The paired genioglossus muscles can be found on either side of the lingual septum, just below the intrinsic tongue muscles (see **Figs.** 1 and 2). One potential pitfall is not understanding the anatomy or "speaking the same language" as the surgeons. The mylohyoid and geniohyoid are not extrinsic tongue muscles and their involvement does not upstage, but involvement is useful to report to surgeons.

Very Advanced Disease (T4b)

Tumor invasion of the masticator space, pterygoid plates, skull base, or encasement of internal carotid artery upstages to T4b (see **Fig.** 11). Resection may still be attempted for T4b disease, based upon masticator space invasion, but invasion of the skull base or internal carotid artery often deems a patient unresectable. Therefore, it is critical to assess these structures for every OC tumor and clearly outline their involvement. However, it is important not to "overcall" because this may preclude surgery in a potentially resectable patient. For example, large tumors often seem to "bulge" into the masticator space and displace the medial pterygoid muscle, but this often does not translate into true invasion at surgery.

N STAGE

The N status of the cervical lymph nodes is the most important predictor of outcome in patients with SCC of the OC.[10] Most studies that have compared the accuracy of CT and MR imaging for assessment of lymph nodes have found no difference.[11,35–37] For lymph node staging of OC carcinoma it is important to remember that many surgeons perform prophylactic neck dissections for certain thickness of invasion (4–5 mm). Knowledge of the surgeons' practice at a particular institution dictates when careful discrimination of nodes is most critical to plan surgery and when it is not. Ultrasound-guided fine-needle aspiration of a suspicious node may be helpful for the clinically N0 neck, if this would affect surgical management. Level I and II lymph nodes are often the first involved. In the untreated neck, metastases to levels IV or V are rare in the absence of known metastasis at levels I to III. Among different subsites, the RMT and FOM show the strongest predilection for lymphatic involvement, with nearly 50% patients presenting the metastatic nodes.[26] Oral tongue SCCs present with regional lymph node metastasis in up to 40% cases, whereas primaries in the lip, buccal mucosa, and hard palate are less likely to have nodal involvement.[38] The imaging assessment of cervical lymphadenopathy is complex and includes not only determination of size, but also evaluation of morphology, borders, density, and number. A commonly used size criterion is no more than a maximal long axis diameter of 15 mm for levels I and II and no more than a maximal longitudinal diameter of 10 mm for all other levels.[39] If minimal diameter is used, then the threshold of 11 mm for level II nodes and 10 mm for all other levels has been used.

Regardless of the size, central low density is indicative of central necrosis and a metastatic node. Other highly suspicious features include rounded morphology with loss of the fatty hilum, heterogenous enhancement, clustering, and ill-defined margins. Ill-defined margins and soft tissue stranding indicate ECS. A more detailed discussion of lymph node drainage and metastatic lymphadenopathy is found elsewhere in this issue.

M STAGE

Distant metastasis from the OC is rare at presentation, so there is no cost-effective role for PET-CT in most patients with oral SCC. However, for more locally advanced cases PET-CT can be helpful to assess lymph nodes status, distant metastasis, or a second primary tumor, especially in the chest.

SURVEILLANCE

Most recurrences occur at the local site, so this should be the focus of surveillance imaging. Recurrence can be challenging to assess on imaging because of posttreatment changes, such as edema, fibrosis, and distortion of anatomy after surgical manipulation. It is standard to wait at least 10 to 12 weeks after surgery before imaging to reduce false-positive results. This is especially important when PET-CT is used for surveillance after surgical resection (or for staging after biopsy), because it is a common pitfall to see avid fluoro-deoxyglucose uptake in areas of postsurgical inflammation (Fig. 17). The role of PET-CT has been assessed in other head and neck tumors, such as laryngeal and hypopharyngeal, but has not been established in OC SCC surveillance.[40] Nevertheless, it is not uncommon for surgeons to

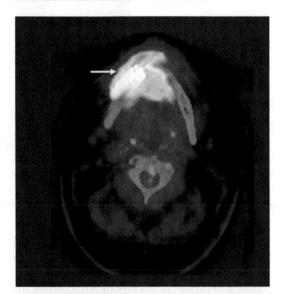

Fig. 17. Pitfall in PET-CT at the OC primary site. Axial fused PET-CT demonstrates intense fluorodeoxyglucose uptake 4 weeks after resection of floor of mouth. SCC (arrow). The patient had negative margins on pathology and a negative clinical examination. The increased fluorodeoxyglucose activity is caused by postoperative inflammation and is a common, expected postoperative appearance in this time frame. This examination was performed for lymph node staging.

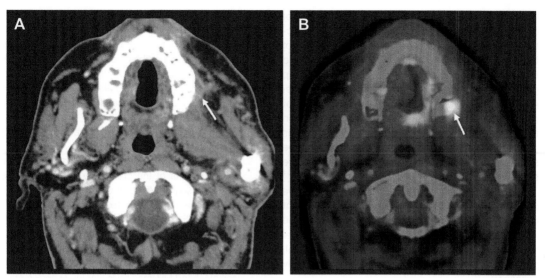

Fig. 18. Role of combined PET-CT to find early left RMT recurrence. (*A*) Axial CE CT showing postoperative changes after segmental mandibulectomy for an RMT primary. There is some effacement of buccal fat and mild prominence of soft tissue posterolateral to the maxillary alveolus (*arrow*); however, the findings are subtle and fairly nonspecific on this first postoperative baseline study. (*B*) The fused PET-CT image clearly identifies a focal area of increased uptake in this region (*arrow*). This was a pathologically proved recurrence. PET can add sensitivity to the CE CT, but it is important to be aware of false-positives.

use PET-CT surveillance after treatment for advanced OC tumors. In this setting, a diagnostic CT neck with contrast is performed and fused with PET images, interpreted by nuclear medicine and head and neck radiologists, and can be a powerful tool to detect recurrences in the complicated postoperative neck (**Fig. 18**).

Patients with advanced OC SCC treated with composite (removal of bone and soft tissue) resection and flap reconstruction present a particular challenge to the radiologist. The radial forearm flap is a fasciocutaneous flap commonly used to reconstruct the OC. The free fibula composite flap is often used to reconstruct after mandible

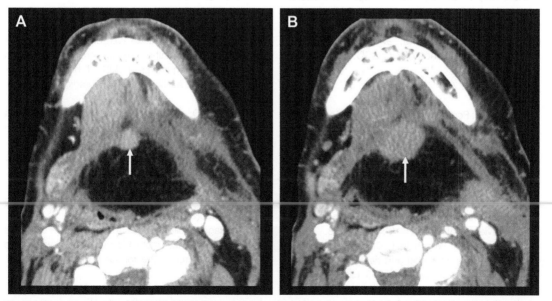

Fig. 19. Flap recurrence. (*A*) Axial CE CT shows a minimally enhancing 1-cm nodular density (*arrow*) along anterior aspect of the fatty portion of the flap at the interface between the flap and native floor of mouth structures. (*B*) Axial CE CT 2 months later shows interval increase in size of the mass (*arrow*).

resection. The radiologist should be aware of complications, such as seroma, hematoma, infection, fistulas, and recurrent tumor. Knowledge of the surgical procedure, type of flap used, and familiarity of the expected appearance of a flap greatly aid in interpreting the image. Therefore, reading operative reports is very useful. Tumor recurrence is commonly along the flap margins in the primary tumor bed. Focal nodular masses along the flap in the recipient bed, progressive soft tissue thickening, and local invasion are the strongest indicators of recurrent tumor (**Fig. 19**).[41]

Recurrence in the lymph nodes should also be assessed. Lymphatic metastasis after treatment can be unpredictable because of alterations in the normal lymphatic pathways, so even usual nodal groups, such as retropharyngeal, mediastinal, and even contralateral nodes, should be carefully assessed.

SUMMARY

Staging OC tumors requires knowledge of OC anatomy, the OC subsites, and tumor spread patterns. Radiologists should always assess for features that would upstage to a T4a disease, including invasion of the extrinsic tongue muscles or mandible, and features that upstage to T4b disease, including involvement of the masticator space, skull base, and encasement of the internal carotid artery. Although it is also important to assess for nodal metastasis, most surgeons perform a prophylactic neck dissection for T2-T4 disease and T1 disease with a depth of invasion greater than 4 mm. Radiologists should be familiar with important pitfalls and the complementary roles of CT, MR imaging, and PET-CT in the staging and surveillance of OC SCC.

REFERENCES

1. Cooper JS, Porter K, Mallin K, et al. National Cancer Database report on cancer of the head and neck: 10-year update. Head Neck 2009;31(6):748–58.
2. Landis SH, Murray T, Bolden S, et al. Cancer statistics, 1999. CA Cancer J Clin 1999;49(1):8–31, 1.
3. Llewellyn CD, Johnson NW, Warnakulasuriya KA. Risk factors for squamous cell carcinoma of the oral cavity in young people: a comprehensive literature review. Oral Oncol 2001;37(5):401–18.
4. Hennessey PT, Westra WH, Califano JA. Human papillomavirus and head and neck squamous cell carcinoma: recent evidence and clinical implications. J Dent Res 2009;88(4):300–6.
5. Jemal A, Thun MJ, Ries LA, et al. Annual report to the nation on the status of cancer, 1975–2005, featuring trends in lung cancer, tobacco use, and tobacco control. J Natl Cancer Inst 2008;100(23):1672–94.
6. Steele TO, Meyers A. Early detection of premalignant lesions and oral cancer. Otolaryngol Clin North Am 2011;44(1):221–9, vii.
7. Laine FJ, Smoker WR. Oral cavity: anatomy and pathology. Semin Ultrasound CT MR 1995;16(6):527–45.
8. Chong V. Oral cavity cancer. Cancer Imaging 2005;5(Spec No A):S49–52.
9. Leslie A, Fyfe E, Guest P, et al. Staging of squamous cell carcinoma of the oral cavity and oropharynx: a comparison of MRI and CT in T- and N-staging. J Comput Assist Tomogr 1999;23(1):43–9.
10. Stambuk HE, Karimi S, Lee N, et al. Oral cavity and oropharynx tumors. Radiol Clin North Am 2007;45(1):1–20.
11. Curtin HD, Ishwaran H, Mancuso AA, et al. Comparison of CT and MR imaging in staging of neck metastases. Radiology 1998;207(1):123–30.
12. Genden EM, Ferlito A, Silver CE, et al. Contemporary management of cancer of the oral cavity. Eur Arch Otorhinolaryngol 2010;267(7):1001–17.
13. Pohar S, Brown R, Newman N, et al. What does PET imaging add to conventional staging of head and neck cancer patients? Int J Radiat Oncol Biol Phys 2007;68(2):383–7.
14. Stuckensen T, Kovacs AF, Adams S, et al. Staging of the neck in patients with oral cavity squamous cell carcinomas: a prospective comparison of PET, ultrasound, CT and MRI. J Craniomaxillofac Surg 2000;28(6):319–24.
15. Mack MG, Vogl TJ. MR imaging of the head and neck. Eur Radiol 1999;9(7):1247–51.
16. Kirsch C. Oral cavity cancer. Top Magn Reson Imaging 2007;18(4):269–80.
17. Escott EJ, Rao VM, Ko WD, et al. Comparison of dynamic contrast-enhanced gradient-echo and spin-echo sequences in MR of head and neck neoplasms. AJNR Am J Neuroradiol 1997;18(8):1411–9.
18. Curtin HD. Detection of perineural spread: fat suppression versus no fat suppression. AJNR Am J Neuroradiol 2004;25(1):1–3.
19. Yuen AP, Lam KY, Wei WI, et al. A comparison of the prognostic significance of tumor diameter, length, width, thickness, area, volume, and clinicopathological features of oral tongue carcinoma. Am J Surg 2000;180(2):139–43.
20. Asakage T, Yokose T, Mukai K, et al. Tumor thickness predicts cervical metastasis in patients with stage I/II carcinoma of the tongue. Cancer 1998;82(8):1443–8.
21. Coughlin A, Resto VA. Oral cavity squamous cell carcinoma and the clinically N0 neck: the past, present, and future of sentinel lymph node biopsy. Curr Oncol Rep 2010;12(2):129–35.

22. Kligerman J, Lima RA, Soares JR, et al. Supraomohyoid neck dissection in the treatment of T1/T2 squamous cell carcinoma of oral cavity. Am J Surg 1994;168(5):391–4.

23. Goerkem M, Braun J, Stoeckli SJ. Evaluation of clinical and histomorphological parameters as potential predictors of occult metastases in sentinel lymph nodes of early squamous cell carcinoma of the oral cavity. Ann Surg Oncol 2010;17(2):527–35.

24. Takes RP, Rinaldo A, Silver CE, et al. Future of the TNM classification and staging system in head and neck cancer. Head Neck 2010;32(12):1693–711.

25. Cohen EE, Baru J, Huo D, et al. Efficacy and safety of treating T4 oral cavity tumors with primary chemoradiotherapy. Head Neck 2009;31(8):1013–21.

26. Trotta BM, Pease CS, Rasamny JJ, et al. Oral cavity and oropharyngeal squamous cell cancer: key imaging findings for staging and treatment planning. Radiographics 2011;31(2):339–54.

27. Kimura Y, Sumi M, Sumi T, et al. Deep extension from carcinoma arising from the gingiva: CT and MR imaging features. AJNR Am J Neuroradiol 2002;23(3):468–72.

28. Moore KL. Clinical oriented anatomy. 3rd edition. Baltimore (MD): Williams and Wilkins; 1992.

29. Ginsberg LE, DeMonte F. Imaging of perineural tumor spread from palatal carcinoma. AJNR Am J Neuroradiol 1998;19(8):1417–22.

30. Ong CK, Chong VF. Imaging of tongue carcinoma. Cancer Imaging 2006;6:186–93.

31. Tytor M, Olofsson J. Prognostic factors in oral cavity carcinomas. Acta Otolaryngol Suppl 1992;492:75–8.

32. Lane AP, Buckmire RA, Mukherji SK, et al. Use of computed tomography in the assessment of mandibular invasion in carcinoma of the retromolar trigone. Otolaryngol Head Neck Surg 2000;122(5):673–7.

33. Brockenbrough JM, Petruzzelli GJ, Lomasney L. DentaScan as an accurate method of predicting mandibular invasion in patients with squamous cell carcinoma of the oral cavity. Arch Otolaryngol Head Neck Surg 2003;129(1):113–7.

34. Imaizumi A, Yoshino N, Yamada I, et al. A potential pitfall of MR imaging for assessing mandibular invasion of squamous cell carcinoma in the oral cavity. AJNR Am J Neuroradiol 2006;27(1):114–22.

35. van den Brekel MW, Castelijns JA, Snow GB. Detection of lymph node metastases in the neck: radiologic criteria. Radiology 1994;192(3):617–8.

36. van den Brekel MW, Stel HV, Castelijns JA, et al. Cervical lymph node metastasis: assessment of radiologic criteria. Radiology 1990;177(2):379–84.

37. Don DM, Anzai Y, Lufkin RB, et al. Evaluation of cervical lymph node metastases in squamous cell carcinoma of the head and neck. Laryngoscope 1995;105(7 Pt 1):669–74.

38. Wein R, Webber R. Malignant neoplasms of the oral cavity. In: Cummings C, Flint P, Harker L, editors. Cummings otolaryngology: head and neck surgery. Philadelphia: Elsevier Mosby; 2005. p. 1591–607.

39. Som P, Brandwein M. Lymph nodes. In: Som P, Curtin H, editors. Head and neck imaging. 4th edition. St Louis (MO): Mosby; 2003. p. 1912.

40. Ryan WR, Fee WE Jr, Le QT, et al. Positron-emission tomography for surveillance of head and neck cancer. Laryngoscope 2005;115(4):645–50.

41. Hudgins PA. Flap reconstruction in the head and neck: expected appearance, complications, and recurrent disease. Eur J Radiol 2002;44(2):130–8.

Pitfalls in the Staging of Cancer of the Oropharyngeal Squamous Cell Carcinoma

Amanda Corey, MD

KEYWORDS

- Oropharyngeal squamous cell carcinoma • Oropharynx • Human papilloma virus
- Transoral robotic surgery

KEY POINTS

- Oropharyngeal squamous cell carcinoma (OPSCC) has a dichotomous nature with 1 subset of the disease associated with tobacco and alcohol use and the other having proven association with human papilloma virus infection.
- Imaging plays an important role in the staging and surveillance of OPSCC.
- A detailed knowledge of the anatomy and pitfalls is critical.
- This article reviews the detailed anatomy of the oropharynx and epidemiology of OPSCC, along with its staging, patterns of spread, and treatment.

Anatomic extent of disease is central to determining stage and prognosis, and optimizing treatment planning for head and neck squamous cell carcinoma (HNSCC). The anatomic boundaries of the oropharynx (OP) are the soft palate superiorly, hyoid bone, and vallecula inferiorly, and circumvellate papilla anteriorly. The OP communicates with the nasopharynx superiorly and the hypopharynx and supraglottic larynx inferiorly, and is continuous with the oral cavity anteriorly. The palatoglossus muscle forms the anterior tonsillar pillar, and the palatopharyngeus muscle forms the posterior tonsillar pillar. The OP has 4 subsites:

- Base of tongue including pharyngoepiglottic and glossoepiglottic folds
- Palatine tonsils including tonsillar fossa and anterior and posterior tonsillar pillars
- Ventral soft palate including the uvula
- Posterior and lateral pharyngeal walls at the oropharyngeal level[1]

Contents of the OP include mucosa, lingual and palatine tonsillar lymphoid tissue, minor salivary tissue, constrictor muscles, and fascia. The overwhelming tumor pathology is squamous cell carcinoma (SCC), arising from the mucosal surface. As the OP contents include lymphoid tissue and minor salivary glands, lymphoma and nonsquamous cell tumors of salivary origin can occur.[2]

In understanding spread of disease from the OP, it is helpful to remember the fascial boundaries subtending the OP, to recall the relationship of the pharyngeal constrictor muscles with the pterygomandibular raphe and the deep cervical fascia, and to be aware of the adjacent spaces and structures. In staging of OP lesions, extension of malignancy to the larynx (but not the lingual surface of the epiglottis), oral cavity, masticator space, nasopharynx, and skull base or tumors with internal carotid artery encasement upstage the disease, regardless of tumor size.[3] Note that mucosal extension to the lingual surface of the epiglottis does not constitute invasion of the larynx.

The OP is bounded deeply by the middle layer of deep cervical fascia (buccopharyngeal fascia), which is deep to the middle and superior

Department of Radiology and Imaging Sciences, Emory University School of Medicine, BG-21, 1364 Clifton Road, Northeast, Atlanta, GA 30322, USA
E-mail address: acorey@emory.edu

Neuroimag Clin N Am 23 (2013) 47–66
http://dx.doi.org/10.1016/j.nic.2012.08.005
1052-5149/13/$ – see front matter © 2013 Elsevier Inc. All rights reserved.

constrictor muscles. The superficial (mucosal) surface of the OP is not bounded by fascia. To attach to the skull base, the superior constrictor muscle attaches to the pharyngobasilar fascia. The buccopharyngeal fascia is deep to the pharyngobasilar fascia. Tumors can potentially spread along the muscle and fascial routes from the OP to the skull base.

The middle pharyngeal constrictor muscle is connected with the buccinator muscle via the pterygomandibular raphe, which extends from the posterior mylohyoid line of the mandible to the hamulus of the medial pterygoid plate. This connection provides a potential route of tumor spread between the OP and the OC, between the OP and the central skull base (sphenoid bone), and between the OP and the pterygoid muscles in the masticator space (**Figs. 1–3**).

EPIDEMIOLOGY

SCC accounts for 95% of neoplasms arising in the OP, and OP cancers represent over 50% of all head and neck cancers in the United States. Annually, 5000 OP cancers are newly diagnosed.[4–7] The proportion of HNSCC arising in the OP increased from 18% in 1973 to 32% in 2005.[8] Minor salivary tumors (adenomas/adenocarcinomas), lymphoid lesions (including lymphoma), undifferentiated malignancy, and sarcomas make up the balance of the tumors arising in the OP.[9] While overall incidence of other HNSCCs has been declining since the 1980s, the incidence of OP SCC has been stable or increasing. Decline in smoking is the reason for the decline in overall numbers of HNSCC, while human papilloma virus (HPV)-associated malignancy explains the increase in otopharyngeal squamous cell carcinoma (OPSCC), particularly in younger patients.[7]

OPSCCs occur most frequently in men over the age of 40. Tumors are often insidious, growing in an infiltrative pattern, clinically silent until reaching a large size. The base of the tongue lacks pain fibers, and tumors in this location are often asymptomatic until quite large.[10] Symptoms vary from site to site, but most commonly patients complain of throat discomfort. Small lesions can present as painless ulcerations. When the lesions are larger, the local extent is greater, and/or metastatic adenopathy is present, patients may complain of difficulty swallowing, ear pain, trismus, or neck mass from metastatic adenopathy.[6,11]

Alcohol abuse and tobacco use, in a dose-dependent fashion, together and independently, are associated with increased incidence of OPSCC. Alcohol abuse has been found to potentiate the cancerous effects of tobacco exposure in the OP.[12,13] In fact, it has been reported that synergistic action between alcohol and tobacco could increase relative risk of HNSCC by as much as 30-fold.[14] Other factors implicated in the development of OPSCC include: history of SCC of the head and neck in a first-degree relative, history of cancer in a sibling, history of oral papillomas, poor oral hygiene, regular marijuana use, heavy tobacco use (20 pack–years or more), or history of heavy alcohol use (15 drinks or more per week for 15 years or more).[13] Other risk factors identified for development of OPSCC are: a diet poor in fruits and vegetables,[15] drinking mate, a brewed herb,[16] and chewing betel quid.[17]

In developed countries, OPSCC makes up 15% to 30% of head and neck cancers. In the past 25 years, the incidence of OPSCC has increased in the United States, Scandinavia, Canada, Netherlands, and Scotland in spite of stability or decline in overall HNSCC incidence.[5,18] Three percent to 9% of OPSCC in these countries occurs in patients denying a history of tobacco/alcohol exposure, especially in young patients (10% to 30% non-smokers and nondrinkers).[5] HPV exposure and infection are responsible for the rise in OPSCC in western countries. Of the HPV-associated HNSCC, over 90% of cases arise in the OP and most commonly in the palatine tonsil, followed distantly by the lingual tonsil/base of tongue. HPV-negative tumors, on the other hand, are found in all subsites of the OP.[18] HPV-associated tumors represent a separate subset of OPSCC with unique epidemiology, etiology and biologic characteristics, and prognosis.

HPV is an epithelliotropic DNA virus that primarily infects transitional epithelium that is found in the upper aerodigestive tract and anogenital regions. Over 120 different HPV types have been identified, but the subtypes implicated in OPSCC include HPV-16, 18, 31, 33, and 35, with HPV-16 identified in approximately 90% of HPV-positive tumors. The malignant potential of the HPV infection lies in the expression of viral oncoproteins E6 and E7; which, in turn, are able to inactivate 2 human tumor-suppressor proteins, p53 and pRb.[18]

HPV is predominately a sexually transmitted disease, and infection is an independent risk factor for development of OPSCC. Its association with the development of cervical cancer and other anogenital malignancies is well known. People with HPV-16 oral infection are at a 15-fold higher risk for OPSCC and a 50-fold increased risk for HPV-positive HNSCC.[8] As reported in the *New England Journal of Medicine* in 2007, lifetime number of vaginal sex partners of 26 or more was associated with development of OPSCC; so too was a lifetime number of oral-sex partners of 6 or more (with

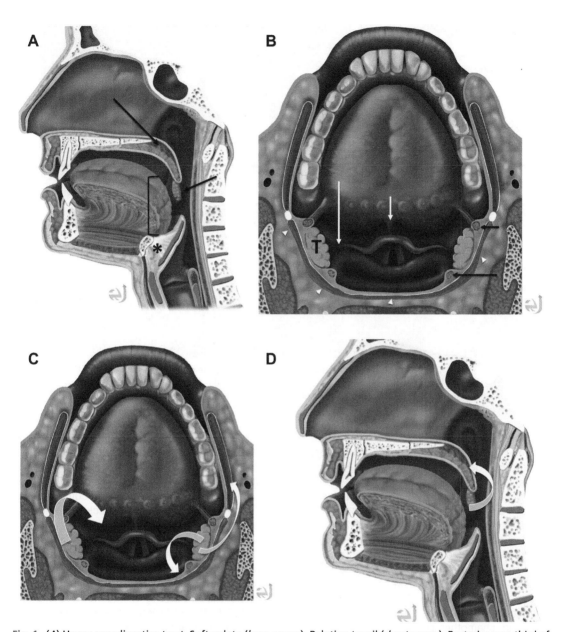

Fig. 1. (*A*) Upper aerodigestive tract. Soft palate (*long arrow*). Palatine tonsil (*short arrow*). Posterior one-third of the tongue (*brackets*). Pre-epiglottic fat (*asterisk*). (*B*) Superior view of oropharynx. Pharyngeal constrictor muscles (superior and upper fibers of middle) (*arrowheads*). Pharyngoepiglottic folds (*long white arrow*) and glossoepiglottic (*midline*) fold (*short white arrow*). Palatoglossus (*anterior*) (*short black arrow*) and palatophar-yngeal (*posterior*) (*long black arrow*) muscles forming the anterior and posterior tonsillar pillars. Palatine tonsil (T). (*C*) Superior view of oropharynx. Pattern of tumor spread from the tonsillar fossa (*arrow*). (*D*) Midline sagittal. Pattern of tumor spread from the tonsillar fossa (*arrow*). (*Courtesy of* Eric Jablonowski.)

a 9-fold increase in relative risk). Synergy between tobacco and alcohol abuse/use and HPV infection with increased odds of OPSCC was not found.[13,19]

HPV-positive OPSCC patients have been found to have significantly better outcomes as compared to HPV-negative patients, with a 28% lower risk of death than the HPV-negative patients.[8,20,21] Also, nonsmoking patients with HPV- positive tumors

have better disease-specific survival rates as compared with smokers with HPV-positive tumors.[22] Black patients with head and neck cancer live significantly shorter periods after treat-ment than white patients, at least in part due to the fact that the black population in the United States has dramatically lower rates of HPV infection than Caucasian population. HPV status directly

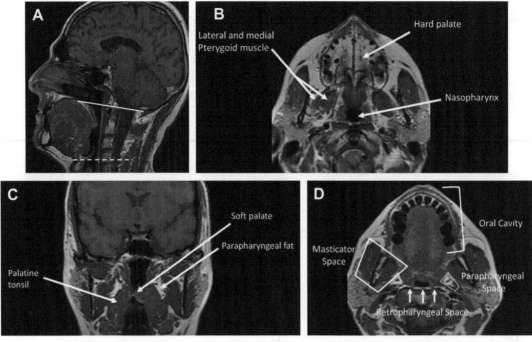

Fig. 2. Normal anatomy. (*A*) Boundaries of the oropharynx. Superiorly, the solid line at the level of the palate and inferiorly, the dashed line at the level of the hyoid bone and vallecula. (*B*) Axial T1-weighted image at level of hard palate and nasopharynx. (*C*) Coronal T1-weighted image. Nasopharynx and oropharynx. (*D*) Spaces adjacent to the oropharynx.

correlates with the significant survival disparities between the 2 patient groups.[23,24] When survival is compared between black and white HPV-negative patients, survival is similar.[23]

HPV-positive tonsillar cancers have been shown to have a lower number of chromosomal alterations as compared to HPV-negative OPSCC.[25,26] HPV-associated OPSCCs are more likely to be undifferentiated and have basaloid histology and more frequent nodal metastasis.[27] HPV-negative tumors, in contrast, have keratinized rather than nonkeratinized histology. Improved overall and disease-free survival after surgery, radiation therapy, and chemotherapy have been reported in HPV-positive OPSCC.[28–32]

AMERICAN JOINT COMMITTEE ON CANCER STAGING

Appropriate staging of cancer at the time of presentation is important, as stage predicts survival rate and guides management. Prognosis and treatment are directly linked to cancer stage (based largely on anatomic factors) as well as other nonanatomically based patient or tumor-specific factors such as overall health, age, sex, race, and the tumor type or biology of malignancy. Evidence-based treatment paradigms are defined by reported outcomes relative to stage and

treatment received. Interdisciplinary and inter-institutional reporting of results needs to be reproducible, clear, consistent, and comparable. With accurate staging, careful follow-up, and multidisciplinary input, treatment outcomes can be compared and related back to stage at presentation.

With the American Joint Committee on Cancer (AJCC) 7 staging of OP cancer, as with all head and neck cancers, staging is primarily based upon anatomic information (Tables 1 and 2). For OP, the AJCC 7 has only one change as compared to AJCC 6. The T4 lesions have been divided into T4a and T4b categories. T4a lesions are moderately advanced local disease, and T4b lesions are very advanced local disease. In association with the new stratification of T4 lesions, stage IV has been subdivided into stage IVA (moderately advanced local/regional disease), stage IVB (very advanced local/regional disease), and stage IVC (distant metastatic disease). For head and neck cancers, in general, the terms resectable and unresectable are replaced with moderately advanced and very advanced in the current staging manual. Extracapsular spread (ECS) of nodal disease is specifically denoted as ECS + (present) or ECS – (absent).[3]

The importance of a thorough physical examination and clinical assessment of the primary lesion

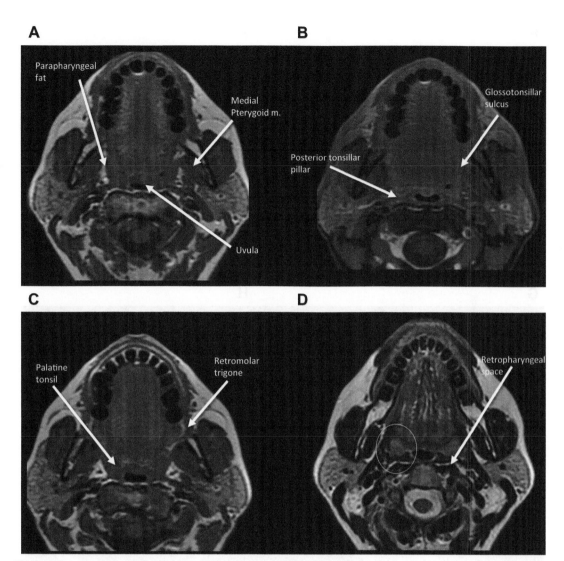

Fig. 3. Normal anatomy. (*A*) Axial T1-weighted image. (*B*) Axial fat-saturated T1-weighted image. Note enhancement of the tonsil. (*C*) Axial T1-weighted image. (*D*) Axial T2-weighted image. Note the hyperintensity of the palatine tonsil (*circle*).

cannot be overemphasized. Cross-sectional and metabolic imaging is complementary, and can further define the T, N, and M status of the patient. In AJCC 7, general rules for tumor node metastases (TNM) staging after include

Microscopic confirmation of malignancy is needed.

When uncertainty exists with assignation of T, N, or M status, the lower category should be assigned.

Separate staging and independent reporting of synchronous primary tumors is necessary.

The guidelines also state that the clinical (pretreatment) stage assigned prior to institution

of therapy (surgery, radiation, chemotherapy, or a combination thereof) is not changed on the basis of new information obtained at the time of pathologic examination.[3]

The T portion of the TNM staging classification defines the malignancy by size or contiguous extension. T designation in the OP is mainly size-based for tumors confined to the OP and includes T1: a tumor 2 cm or less in size, T2: a tumor 2 to 4 cm in size (**Fig. 4**), and T3: a tumor larger than 4 cm in size or with extension to the lingual surface of the epiglottis. T4 tumors have extension into adjacent structures. Moderately advanced local disease, T4a, is defined as tumor invasion of larynx (**Fig. 5**), extrinsic tongue muscles (**Fig. 6**), medial pterygoid muscle, hard palate, or mandible. T4b

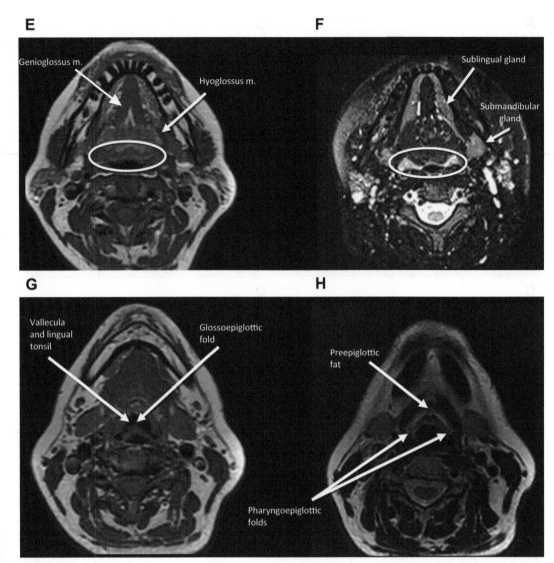

Fig. 3. (*E*) Axial T1-weighted image with 2 of the extrinsic tongue muscles identified. Circled structures are the lingual tonsils. (*F*) Axial fat-saturated T2-weighted image shows lingual tissue (*circled*) is normally T2 hyperintense. (*G*) Axial T1-weighted image. Inferior oropharynx landmarks. (*H*) Axial T2-weighted image. Inferior oropharynx landmarks.

classification is used with very advanced local disease when tumor encases the internal carotid artery (ICA), invades the lateral pterygoid muscle or pterygoid plates, or extends into the lateral nasopharynx or skull base (Fig. 7).

The N component addresses the status of the regional lymph nodes. The OP and hypopharynx have identical nodal classification. Nx refers to situations where the lymph nodes cannot be assessed. N0 is the absence of regional lymph node metastasis. N1, N2, N3 describes increasing number or extent of regional lymph node involvement. Further description of nodal staging can be found in the article by Amit Saindane, entitled Imaging and Staging of Lymph Node Metastases

in this issue. Lymph node status is of great prognostic significance. The more distant the spread in the lymphatic system, the worse the prognosis. Similarly, the presence of ECS worsens the prognosis. ECS is characterized by marginal irregularity and matting of nodes on imaging studies and by the adherence of nodes to adjacent structures on physical examination and imaging (Fig. 8). With OPSCC, the key nodal stations are levels II and III. Levels IA and IB are less commonly involved.[3]

At the time this manuscript was written, the American College of Radiology (ACR) did not have appropriateness criteria for generally accepted standards for diagnostic (imaging) evaluation to aid in staging of the OP cancers. Appropriateness

Table 1			
AJCC 7th edition oropharynx staging			
	Primary Tumor (T)		
TX	Primary tumor cannot be assessed		
T0	No evidence of primary tumor		
Tis	Carcinoma in situ		
T1	Tumor 3 cm or less in greatest dimension		
T2	Tumor more than 2 cm but not more than 4 cm in greatest dimension		
T3	Tumor more than 4 cm in greatest dimension or extension to the lingual surface of the epiglottis		
T4a	Moderately advanced local disease Tumor invades the larynx, extrinsic muscle of tongue, medial pterygoid, hard palate, or mandible[a]		
T4b	Very advanced local disease Tumor invades lateral pterygoid muscle, pterygoid plates, lateral nasopharynx, or skull base or encases carotid artery		
	Regional Lymph Nodes (N)		
NX	Regional lymph nodes cannot be assessed		
N0	No regional lymph node metastasis		
N1	Metastasis in a single ipsilateral lymph node, 3 cm or less in greatest dimension		
N2	Metastasis in a single ipsilateral lymph node, more than 3 cm but not more than 6 cm in greatest dimension; or in multiple ipsilateral lymph nodes, none more than 6 cm in greatest dimension; or in bilateral or contralateral lymph nodes, none more than 6 cm in greatest dimension		
N2a	Metastasis in single ipsilateral lymph node more than 3 cm but not more than 6 cm in greatest dimension		
N2b	Metastasis in multiple ipsilateral lymph nodes, none more than 6 cm in greatest dimension		
N2c	Metastasis in bilateral or contralateral lymph nodes, none more than 6 cm in greatest dimension		
N3	Metastasis in a lymph node more than 6 cm in greatest dimension		
	Distant Metastasis (M)		
M0	No distant metastasis		
M1	Distant metastasis		

[a] Mucosal extension to lingual surface of epiglottis from primary tumors of the base of tongue and vallecula does not constitute invasion of larynx.

From Edge S, Byrd D, Compton C, et al. AJCC Cancer staging manual, 7th edition. Chicago: Springer; 2010. p. 41–56; with permission.

Table 2			
Final tumor stage using the AJCC staging system for oropharyngeal carcinoma, 7th edition			
Group	**T**	**N**	**M**
0	Tis	N0	M0
I	T1	N0	M0
II	T2	N0	M0
III	T3	N0	M0
	T1	N1	M0
	T2	N1	M0
	T3	N1	M0
IVA	T4a	N0	M0
	T4a	N1	M0
	T1	N2	M0
	T2	N2	M0
	T3	N2	M0
	T4a	N2	M0
IVB	T4b	Any N	M0
	Any T	N3	M0
IVC	Any T	Any N	M1

From Edge S, Byrd D, Compton C, et al. AJCC Cancer Staging Manual, 7th edition. Chicago: Springer; 2010. p. 41–56; with permission.

criteria do exist for the work-up of neck mass/adenopathy.[33] Variant scenarios include the adult presenting with a nonpulsatile solitary neck mass, the adult presenting with multiple neck masses, and the adult with a history of treatment for cancer presenting with a neck mass. In the first 2 cases,

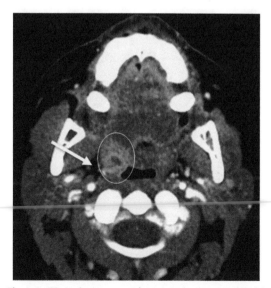

Fig. 4. T2 primary oropharyngeal cancer (*circle*) affecting right lateral soft palate, right anterior tonsillar pillar and right posterior tonsillar pillar. The parapharyngeal fat is normal (*arrow*).

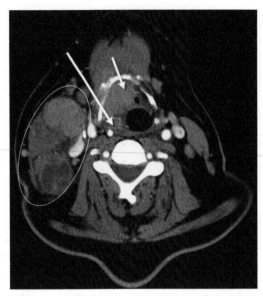

Fig. 5. T4a primary tumor with invasion of the larynx. Tumor (*short arrow*) fills the pre-epiglottic fat and abuts the lingual surface of the epiglottis at the level of the hyoid bone and extends into the pyriform sinus on the right (*long arrow*). N3 necrotic nodal conglomerate measured over 6 cm (*circle*).

contrast-enhanced computed tomography (CECT) or magnetic resonance imaging (MRI) without and with contrast is recommended. In the post-treatment case, CECT of the neck with positron emission tomography (PET) are considered complementary. MRI without and with contrast is an alternative to computed tomography (CT).[33]

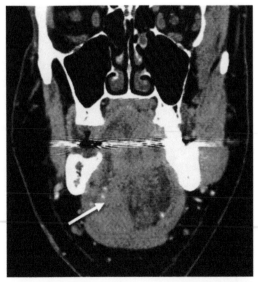

Fig. 6. T4a disease with invasion of the extrinsic tongue muscles. Tumor (*arrow*) surrounds the lingual artery and invades the genioglossus–geniohyoid complex on the right.

Guidelines are available at the National Comprehensive Cancer Network (NCCN) Clinical Practice Guidelines in Oncology site with recommendations for work-up of OP cancer. Work-up should begin with complete history and physical examination to include mirror and fiberoptic examination (as clinically indicated). The tumor should be biopsied, and immunohistochemical staining for p16 is recommended. Chest imaging and CT with contrast and/or MRI with contrast of the primary and of the neck are the next step. PET-CT for stage III to IV disease is recommended, but PET-CT should not replace anatomic imaging. PET-CT is not designed to assess the primary tumor, but rather to assess node status and identify distant metastasis. The patient should complete consultations for oral surgery, nutrition, speech, and swallowing for evaluation/therapy and audiogram as indicated. Examination under anesthesia with endoscopy may be performed prior to treatment to confirm extent of disease.[34] Both the NCCN and ACR have guidelines for therapeutic intervention in OP cancer. The ACR criteria apply to resectable OPSCC.[34,35]

TRENDS IN TREATMENT AFFECTING STAGING

The OP has intricate anatomy, rich lymphatic drainage, and provides critical function central to optimal quality of life. Approximately 60% of patients present with stage III to IV disease.[7] At least 70% of patients have ipsilateral cervical nodal metastases, and 30% or less have bilateral cervical nodal metastases.[1]

The treatment approach for OPSCC is typically multidisciplinary, with the goal to maximize cure potential while minimizing toxicity and preserving functionality. The NCCN and ACR Guidelines separate treatment paradigms on basis of TNM clinical stage. The ACR guidelines further categorize patients by HPV status, smoking history, and age.[34,35] Key to correctly placing the patient in a treatment regimen is accurate staging, pathologic findings (including HPV status), and patient condition.

Treatment options for OPSCC include surgical and nonsurgical regimens. With the more aggressive, but successful, nonsurgical treatments, the risk of swallowing difficulty, salivary gland dysfunction, and other quality-of-life issues exists. Surgical approaches have cosmetic and functional implications. In light of the distinctly different biologic behavior of HPV-positive OPSCC, treatment de-intensification in select patients is considered.[35]

Chemotherapy, radiation therapy, brachytherapy, transoral laser microsurgery, transoral robotic surgery (TORS), open surgery, and bioradiotherapy are current treatment options.[36] TORS and transoral

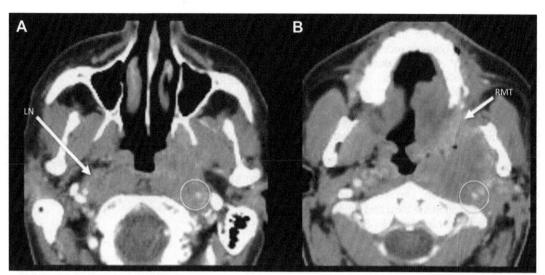

Fig. 7. (*A*, *B*), T4b tumor extends to encircle and narrow the left internal carotid artery (*circle*) and into left naso-pharynx and adjacent prevertebral muscles. Tumor invades the left medial pterygoid muscle and extends into the left retromolar trigone (RMT) (*short arrow*) and soft palate. A right (contralateral) retropharyngeal node is partly necrotic (LN) (*long arrow*).

laser microsurgery offer the benefits of surgical exci-sion of primary tumor without the morbidity of tradi-tional open surgery. Also, patients treated to cure (with de-escalation of adjuvant therapy) avoid some of the toxicities of traditional radiation and chemotherapy. This minimally invasive approach to local control, used in T1 and T2 tumors, is associ-ated with improved quality of life (avoiding

permanent feeding tube or tracheostomy tube and preserving swallowing and speech function) (**Fig. 9**). However, bulky or locally invasive cancers, and cancers located in the inferior OP are not typi-cally suited to TORS.[37]

Early stage (I-II) OPSCC can be handled with definitive radiotherapy; surgical excision of the primary and neck dissection as needed; or for T2, N1 patients, chemotherapy and radiation. Pathologic features such as positive margins, ECS, perineural invasion, or vascular embolism discovered at surgery could necessitate further

Fig. 8. Extracapsular spread of disease and right level 2A/B nodal conglomerate (*arrows*). Nodal disease is inseparable from the sternocleidomastoid muscle, effaces the right jugular vein (J), and displaces the internal and external carotid artery (*circle*) medially. In the floor of mouth, oropharynx primary surrounds the lingual artery (L) and invades the extrinsic tongue muscles. Primary tumor fills the right vallecula and crosses midline posteriorly at base of tongue.

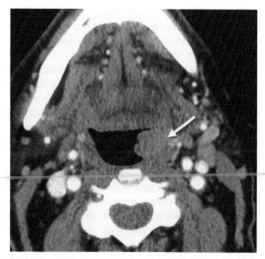

Fig. 9. 2.0 cm mass (*arrow*) centered in the left tonsil. The lesion is localized and somewhat exophytic. Patient underwent TORS procedure with negative margins.

treatment with radiation, chemotherapy, and radiation or re-excision (in the setting of positive margins). For the patients receiving radiation and chemotherapy or definitive radiation who show evidence of persistent disease, salvage surgery is recommended.

More advanced cancers (T3–4a, N0–1; or any T, N2-3) can be managed with concurrent systemic therapy/radiation therapy with cisplatin as the preferred method according to 2011 NCCN guidelines. Surgery of the primary and neck dissection is another provided option. Induction chemotherapy followed by radiation and concurrent chemotherapy and radiation are third and fourth possibilities. In the surgical patients, if ECS and/or positive margins are found at pathologic assessment, additional therapy with chemotherapy and radiation therapy is recommended. NCCN states that the best management of any cancer patient is in a clinical trial and encourages participation in clinical trials.

In cases of newly diagnosed (M0), T4B, any N, or unresectable nodal disease, the NCCN guidelines suggest enrollment in an appropriate clinical trial or treatment arm, and those paradigms include chemotherapy and radiation therapy, alone or in combination.[34]

Ideally, imaging together with clinical findings will define tumor margins, determine lymph node status, and assess for distant disease. Local disease extent that would preclude curative therapy at surgery such as invasion of the lateral pterygoid muscle, pterygoid plates, lateral nasopharynx, skull base, or ICA encasement needs to be established. Imaging findings of ECS, level IV or V disease, or contralateral nodal disease impact treatment.

The evidence-based treatment models reported in the NCCN and ACR guidelines depend upon accurate and consistent definition of primary tumor size and extent, presence and character of nodal disease, and more recently, the HPV status of the patient. The ACR guidelines describe 3 recognized prognostic groups of OPSCC and their fundamentally different treatment objectives. HPV-positive tumors in patients without a smoking history are found to have the most favorable prognosis with mature disease-free survival rates of 80% or higher. The group with intermediate risk is HPV-positive tumors in patients with a smoking history. Disease-free survival in this group is between 55% and 65%. The third group, with worst prognosis, is made up of patients with HPV-negative OPSCC; survival is 50% or less. Clearly establishing HPV status of the tumor is of great clinical and outcome importance.[35] OPSCC is considered a curable cancer, and the

therapeutic options expand with greater understanding of disease biology and as new treatment techniques emerge.[7]

PATTERN OF SPREAD

Local tumor extension occurs in a predictable fashion. Tumors with multiple subsite involvement have a worse response to therapy and higher rates of recurrence as compared with similar T lesions without extension outside the tonsillar fossa.[12] Lymphatic drainage shows slight variation between the different sites, but is predictable.

Tonsillar Pillars

The anterior tonsillar pillar and tonsil are the most common locations for primary tumors of the OP.[1,6] Cancers arising at the anterior tonsillar pillar can spread along the palatoglossus muscle superiorly to the lateral soft palate. The tumor may spread to the masticator space (pterygoid muscles), nasopharynx, and the skull base (pterygoid plates and sphenoid bone or along palatine muscles). Once a tumor is in the pterygoid musculature, pain and trismus are present. Inferior extension along the palatoglossus muscle course results in tumor at the base of tongue. If the tumor spreads laterally and anteriorly, it can travel along the pharyngeal constrictor muscles and pterygomandibular raphe to the oral cavity at the retromolar trigone and into the buccinator muscle.[1,6,12,38–40] Lymphatic drainage from the anterior tonsillar pillar is to levels I, II, and III. Forty-five percent of patients have positive nodes at presentation. Higher T lesions are more likely to have positive nodes. Contralateral nodal involvement is found in 5% of lesions.[6,38]

The posterior tonsillar pillar is the mucosa over the palatopharyngeus muscle. Tumor can spread to the soft palate, posterior thyroid cartilage, middle constrictor muscle (and from there, along the pterygomandibular raphe to the oral cavity), posterior pharyngeal wall and pharyngoepiglottic fold to the top of the pyriform sinus.[6,12,38–40] Lymphatic drainage from the posterior tonsillar pillar is to level II. Once a tumor reaches the posterior oropharyngeal wall, level V and retropharyngeal nodal stations are in the drainage pathway.[6,38]

Tonsillar Fossa

Cancers of the tonsillar fossa are often clinically silent and may present as a neck mass from malignant adenopathy. From the tonsillar fossa, a tumor can spread directly into the parapharyngeal space and from there to the carotid space, into the masticator space, and into the mandible. Additionally a tumor can spread along the anterior and posterior tonsillar pillars with routes of extension as discussed previously.[6,12,38–40]

Lymphatic drainage from the tonsillar fossa is to levels I–IV. Parotid lymph nodes and level V nodes can rarely be affected. Tonsillar primaries have between a 71% and 89% chance of having nodal metastasis with increasing likelihood of nodal disease with increasing T designation. Contralateral nodal disease is found in up to 22% of patients. Tumors with tongue base or soft palate extension have an increased chance of contralateral nodal disease.[6,38]

Soft Palate

Soft palate tumors are typically found on the ventral surface and are generally small at time of diagnosis. Patients complain of odynophagia. These tumors are often well differentiated and have the best prognosis of the oropharyngeal cancers. Local extension can occur anteriorly onto the hard palate; laterally into palatine muscles and the parapharyngeal space, and from there to skull base and nasopharynx; and inferiorly onto the tonsillar pillars. Additionally, perineural extension of disease can occur along the palatine nerves and retrograde to pterygopalatine fossa and cavernous sinus along V2.[6,12,38–40] Lymphatic drainage from the soft palate is to levels II and III as well as the retropharyngeal nodes. Twenty percent to 45% of patients with soft palate primary SCC will present with positive lymph nodes.[6,38]

Base of Tongue

Base of tongue cancers are difficult to diagnosis with imaging when small, and mucosal lesions are best assessed with direct inspection. Of the subsites in the OP, the base of tongue is associated with the highest rate of regional (nodal) disease.[41] These tumors are more aggressive and as such, the advanced stage cancers have a poor overall survival of approximately 20%.[6] Tumors arising in this location spread anteriorly into root of tongue and extrinsic tongue muscles, and into the sublingual space and neurovascular bundle of the oral cavity. Caudal extension is into the vallecula and potentially the pre-epiglottic fat. If the pre-epiglottic fat is invaded, surgical management includes a supraglottic laryngectomy. Lateral extension is potentially into the lateral wall, pterygomandibular raphe, and mandible. More posteriorly, a tumor can invade the parapharyngeal fat and from there, the carotid space. Tumors can extend superiorly along the tonsillar pillars.[6,12,38–40]

Lymphatic drainage of the base of tongue is complicated by cross-drainage. At presentation,

20% to 30% of patients have bilateral nodal disease.[41] Nodal drainage is to levels II to IV. Occasionally level V disease is also found. If the cancer invades the floor of mouth, level I malignant nodes can be seen. As at the other sites, presence of cervical nodal disease decreases survival by more than 50%. At presentation, 70% of T1 lesions have nodal disease, while 84% of T4 lesions do.[6,38]

Posterior Pharyngeal Wall

The last subsite of the OP is the posterior pharyngeal wall. The patient may complain of dysphagia and odynophagia. Tumors here are often large at the time of diagnosis and can spread superiorly to the nasopharynx, laterally into the parapharyngeal space, inferiorly into the hypopharynx, and anteriorly into the tonsil. If the tumor has deep extension, it invades the prevertebral musculature (longus colli and capitus). Recognition of prevertebral muscle invasion is important, as this finding renders the patient unresectable. However, unresectability should be determined at surgery, as imaging is limited in detecting prevertebral muscle invasion. Many of these tumors extend past midline.[6,12,38–40] Lymphatic drainage of the posterior pharyngeal wall includes bilateral jugular chain lymph nodes and the retropharyngeal lymph nodes (**Fig. 10**).[6,38]

PITFALLS IN STAGING

Difficulties encountered in staging of OPSCC are not unique to this location. CECT with adequate mucosal enhancement is a widely used staging tool. Unfortunately, streak artifact from dental amalgam and metal surgical hardware can limit evaluation of the adjacent structures. (**Fig. 11**). Postcontrast fat-saturation MRI is particularly useful in the assessment of the primary lesions and in the search for perineural tumor extension (**Fig. 12**).[12] Motion artifacts are more likely with MRI than with CT given the time it takes to acquire the images. PET-CT can be useful in identifying the primary lesion and malignant adenopathy, but has limitations when evaluation of the skull base, cranial nerves, or small lesions (<1 cm) is necessary.

Mucosal and smaller lesions are best assessed clinically. Lesions arising in areas of lymphoid tissue can be obscured by the normal enhancement/fluorodeoxyglucose (FDG) uptake of the lingual and palatine tonsils. Normal asymmetry in lymphoid tissue further makes staging smaller tumors difficult. The importance of knowing the clinical examination findings while reviewing

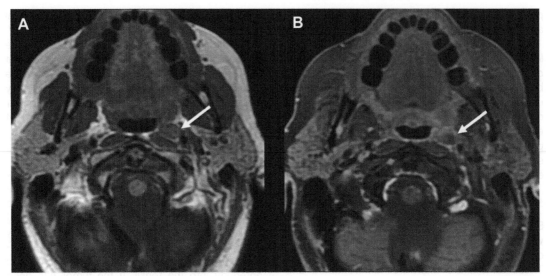

Fig. 10. Metastatic retropharyngeal lymph node (*arrows*) on axial T1-weighted (*A*) and axial fat-saturated post-contrast T1-weighted images (*B*).

imaging studies cannot be overemphasized. (Fig. 13).

The overall size/volume of the tumor needs to be measured. When tumors are discrete and exo-phytic in nature, this is more easily accomplished. However, tumors of the OP are more commonly infiltrative, invasive, and extend along muscle and fascial planes, thus making accurate size determination difficult. Base of tongue cancers can be particularly problematic, as dense interdigitation of muscle without intervening fat to define the tissue planes can obscure lesion margins.[41]

Extension of tumor into the larynx (pre-epiglottic fat), root of tongue, masticator space, skull base, nasopharynx, and carotid space can change the staging to T4 regardless of lesion size. Clues of deep invasion can be found in the clinical note. Trismus suggests pterygomaxillary space extension, and trismus often complicates the clinical

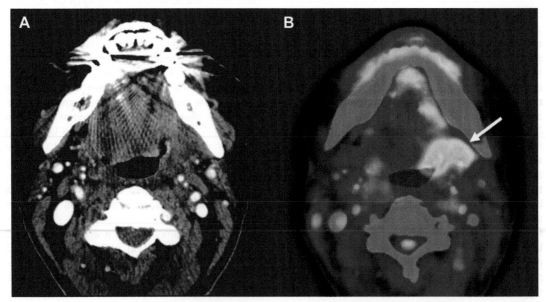

Fig. 11. (*A*) CT with significant dental amalgam artifact. The oropharyngeal primary is partly obscured. (*B*) PET-CT image performed concurrently demonstrating abnormal FDG uptake at the site of recurrent oropharyngeal tumor (*arrow*).

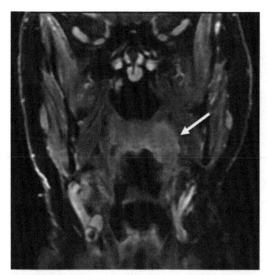

Fig. 12. Coronal fat-saturated postcontrast T1-weighted image of a soft palate and anterior tonsillar pillar primary tumor with extension into pharyngeal constrictor muscles and parapharyngeal fat (*arrow*).

assessment of the primary lesion. The physical examination should also test for intact cranial nerves, especially 5, 7, 9, 10, and 12. Decreased mobility of the tongue suggests deep tongue muscle invasion.[6] Tumor extension into the masticator space and retromolar trigone region can be overlooked and on CT be obscured by streak artifact from dental amalgam, particularly when re-angled views (15° off parallel line to hard palate) are not obtained. MRI is less susceptible to dental amalgam artifacts and often provides superior soft tissue assessment.

Attempts should be made to determine whether the tumor crosses midline, as midline extension increases the likelihood of bilateral/contralateral nodal involvement. At the base of tongue, cross-midline extension changes the surgical plan, as the contralateral neurovascular bundle is at risk.

Because osseous invasion upstages the patients to T4, the mandible, maxilla and pterygoid plates must be carefully evaluated. On CT, cortical and medullary extension can often be appreciated by erosive changes, periosteal reactions, lucency centrally, and/or pathologic fractures (**Fig. 14**). MRI can be used to assess medullary cavity and cartilage. Caution should be exercised, however, as not all marrow signal changes result from infiltrating tumor. Marrow signal changes consisting of low signal on T1 and relative hyperintensity on fat saturation T2 images can be seen with fibrosis from radiation, osteoradionecrosis, and non-neoplastic reactive changes related to dental disease.[41] Regardless, bony invasion can change the surgical plan and needs to be prospectively determined.

With cross-sectional imaging, structures parallel to the plane of the image acquisition are more difficult to appreciate. For example, in the assessment of the soft palate, coronal and sagittal images are often superior to axial images. Reconstruction of thin-slice axial CT image data into the coronal and sagittal planes can accomplish this multiplanar approach. The inherent multiplanar nature of MRI with its superior soft tissue contrast lends itself well to soft palate staging and evaluation of the structures abutting the skull base.

MRI is superior to CT in the assessment for perineural spread (PNS). Clues on CT to perineural extension of tumor include loss of fat in the neural foramen (eg, mandibular foramen, foramen ovale, pterygopalatine fossa), widening of the osseous canals through which the nerves travel, and denervation changes in muscle. Affected nerves are enlarged and enhanced on MRI. Findings of tumor extension along cranial nerves almost always change treatment and prognosis.[41]

Identification of tumor extension into adjacent structures that would render the patient nonoperative should be made. Posterior pharyngeal wall tumor extending into the prevertebral space is one such finding. With imaging, invasion of the prevertebral muscles can sometimes be difficult to determine. Muscular enhancement can occur with direct extent as well as with inflammation. Broad interface of tumor with the prevertebral structures does not necessarily mean invasion of the prevertebral structures, as the deep and middle layers of deep cervical fascia may still be intact. Loss of the normal fat density/signal in the retropharyngeal space is particularly concerning.[38,42,43] If normal fat signal of the retropharyngeal space is preserved, there is probably no invasion of prevertebral muscles. Contiguous aggressive changes in the vertebral body confirm perivertebral space invasion. Tumor encasing the carotid artery (270° or greater) is another example of tumor extension into adjacent spaces, rendering the patient nonsurgical.

Overall, approximately 65% of OPSCC patients present with metastatic lymphadenopathy. Lesions of the base of tongue are the most likely to present with malignant lymph nodes (**Fig. 15**).[41] Accepted imaging criteria for metastatic adenopathy is reviewed in the article on nodal disease by Amit Saindane in this issue. Any node with irregular borders as seen in extracapsular disease extension or with necrosis is considered pathologic. ECS is associated with a 3.5-fold increase in the local recurrence rate.[44]

Lack of recognition of skip and contralateral nodal metastases and/or pathologic retropharyngeal lymph nodes provides other potential staging

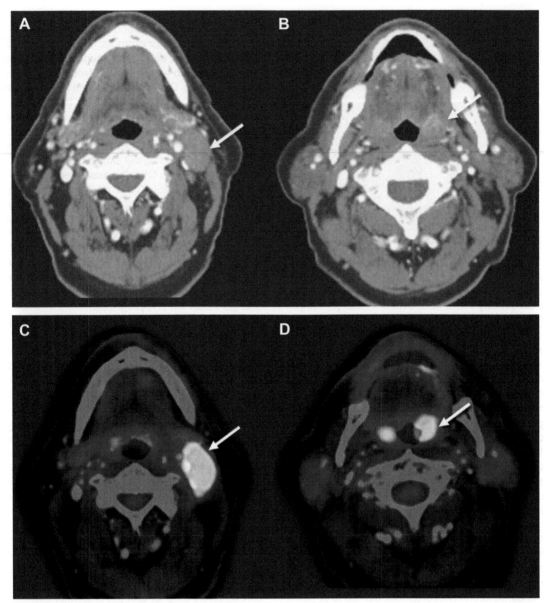

Fig. 13. (A) CE-CT neck performed for palpable left neck mass (arrow) of level IIA adenopathy. (B) Palatine tonsillar tissue is mildly asymmetric on the left (arrow). This finding corresponded to physical examination abnormality and metabolic activity on PET-CT. (C) PET-CT image showing metastatic lymphadenopathy (arrow). (D) PET-CT image showing the left palatine tonsil primary (arrow) with asymmetric FDG uptake.

pitfalls. Fifteen percent to 30% of patients initially staged as N0 will be proven to have regional nodal metastases. In light of that fact, treatment of the neck with either nodal dissection or radiation therapy is part of the therapeutic paradigm.[12] PET alone may miss cystic nodal metastasis and necrotic lymph nodes, reinforcing the need for anatomic imaging as well as PET (Fig. 16). At the author's institution, diagnostic quality CECT is performed in conjunction with the PET, and nuclear medicine physicians and the head and neck radiologists perform consensus interpretation.

As with all HNSCCs, synchronous and second primary tumors can occur (Fig. 17). The risk of developing a second primary tumor in patients with tumors of the upper aerodigestive tract has been estimated to be 3% to 7% per year.[45,46] The radiologist must be vigilant in the imaging assessment and critically examine the images to prevent missing the second lesion.

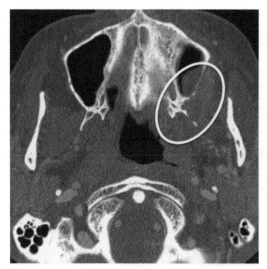

Fig. 14. Axial CT bone windows showing oropharyngeal T4b primary lesion has eroded the pterygoid plates and posterior wall of the maxillary sinus on the left (*circle*).

PITFALLS IN SURVEILLANCE

For a patient with OPSCC, surveillance is lifelong but is especially important in the first 2 years following treatment, when locoregional failure is most likely.[47,48] Patients may have local or regional (neck) failure with persistent or recurrent disease following definitive treatment or even present with distant metastases during follow-up. The development of a second primary is a risk in patients with either HPV-positive tumors or HPV-negative tumors.[45]

In HPV-negative tumors, the second primary lesions are more likely in the upper and lower aerodigestive tract and bladder with a rate of 15% to 30%. This risk can be cut in half by abstaining from alcohol and tobacco products.[49,50] HPV-positive tumors have a lower risk of second primary at 5% to 10%. In addition to sites of second primary in the upper aerodigestive tract and bladder, these patients are at risk for SCC of the anogenital regions.[50]

Surveillance imaging of the neck following definitive treatment for OPSCC can be done with CECT, MRI without and with contrast, PET-CECT, ultrasound, or a combination thereof. The NCCN guidelines stress the importance of regular history and physical examinations with attention to signs or symptoms of recurrent, progressive or metastatic disease and for the development of a second primary lesion. Assessment for locoregional failure on physical examination as well as with imaging is complicated by post-treatment changes in the neck and loss of the normal tissue planes following surgery and radiation treatment, scar and fibrotic tissue, sterile/treated disease residua, and loss of symmetry (**Fig. 18**).

The assessment of any muscle flap and tissues adjacent to the flap can be complex, with fluctuation in flap appearance over time. In the acute postoperative setting, confounding tissue and muscle edema can cause false-positive imaging findings with MRI and PET-CECT. Following chemotherapy and radiation therapy, false-negative findings can be found on PET-CECT when imaged early (1 month vs 4 months following therapy).[51] Therefore, it is recommended that post-treatment MRI and/or PET-CECT be performed at least 3 months following radiation therapy.

False-positive PET-CECT can occur from fasciculation in myocutaneous flaps, fibrosis at the surgical site, aspiration or fungal pneumonia, and normal activity in Waldeyer ring, muscle, mucosa, and salivary tissue. False-negative PET-CECT may occur when there are necrotic or cystic lymph nodes or when the lesion is small, beneath the resolution of the PET. Radiation damage

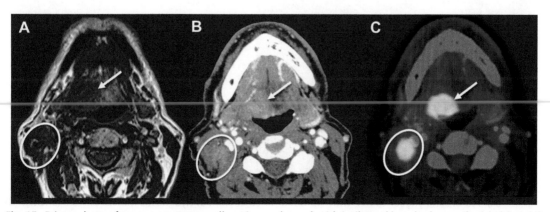

Fig. 15. Primary base of tongue squamous cell carcinoma (*arrow*) with ipsilateral lymphadenopathy (*circle*) on (*A*) Axial T1-weighted MRI. (*B*) CE-CT. (*C*) PET-CT.

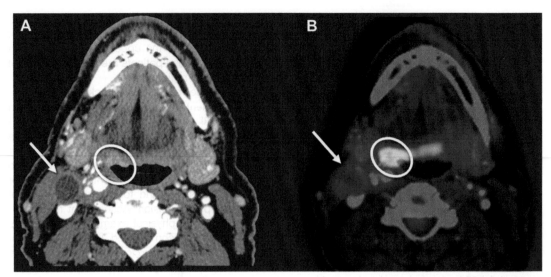

Fig. 16. Cystic lymph nodes (*arrow*) can be a source of false negative PET-CT findings. Contrast enhanced neck CT (*A*) Performed with the PET-CT (*B*) For staging of a base of tongue primary cancer (*circle*).

decreases background physiologic uptake to the affected side, creating asymmetric uptake. Infection and inflammation can cause otherwise normal lymph nodes to show increased FDG avidity, potentially the result of upregulation of glycolysis.[51]

Recurrences can be as subtle as progressive thickening and enhancement in the tumor bed or as obvious as a new mass. After neck surgery, lymphatic drainage will shift to the contralateral side and therefore the lymph node stations in both the ipsilateral and contralateral sides of the neck relative to the site of primary tumor warrant equally close scrutiny. Tumor recurrence/implant

can be recognized by nodular enhancement in the flap, skin, or musculature.

PET-CECT has shown promise in assessment of the post-treatment population. Sensitivity of FDG PET-CECT for detection of residual or recurrent cancer is between 84% and 100% when the scan is obtained more than 12 weeks following the end of therapy. The specificity of this test is 61% to 93%. PET-CT has been shown to be superior in detection of regional or distant disease as compared to local recurrence. PET-CT has a high negative predictive value after treatment for head and neck cancer, especially in assessment of the

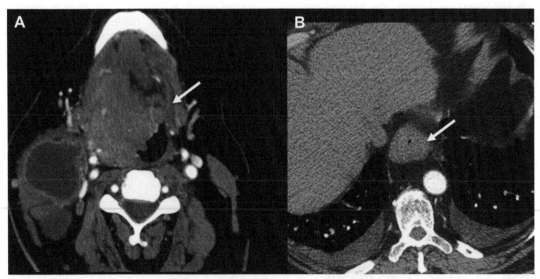

Fig. 17. (*A*) T4a oropharyngeal cancer with N3 nodal disease. Normal hyoglossus muscle on left (*arrow*). (*B*) Staging chest CT noted abnormal distal esophagus (*arrow*). This mass is a biopsy-proven adenocarcinoma, the patient's second primary cancer.

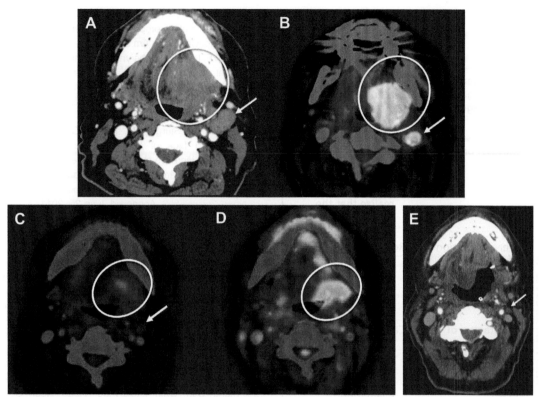

Fig. 18. (*A, B*). Presentation CE-CT (*A*) and PET-CT (*B*) of a T4 oropharynx cancer. Tumor invades sublingual space and adjacent musculature (*circle*). Left level IIA malignant adenopathy (*arrow*). (*C*) PET-CT obtained 3 months following combined modality therapy with significant interval decrease in activity in the tumor bed (*circle*). The previously hot IIA lymph node no longer shows FDG avidity (*arrow*). (*D*) Subsequent surveillance scan with new activity of recurrent disease 1 year following diagnosis (*circle*). (*E*) Postoperative baseline scan following TORS to the site of recurrent tumor. Note the IIA lymph node is now normal in size and appearance (*arrow*).

lymph nodes. It is still debated whether a negative PET-CECT can be used to defer a planned neck dissection. If findings are indeterminate on PET-CECT, ultrasound-guided fine needle aspiration (UG-FNA) could be performed. For evaluation of distant disease, PET-CT is preferred.[51]

While standardized imaging follow-up regimens are not yet supported by evidence-based data, recommendations are available in the NCCN literature. In summary, these guidelines suggest post-treatment baseline imaging of the primary tumor bed (and neck if treated) within 6 months for patients with T3 to T4 or N2 to N3 disease and by re-imaging as indicated based on signs or symptoms concerning for recurrence. Imaging is not routinely recommended in asymptomatic patients.[34]

In patients who have undergone multimodality treatment regimen of surgery, radiation and chemotherapy, the NCCN Guidelines suggest clinical assessment at 4 to 8 weeks. If there are signs or symptoms of persistent or progressive disease, CECT or MRI is recommended. PET is listed as optional. In patients with no clinical signs of disease, PET-CT with anatomic assessment is recommended at a minimum of 12 weeks after treatment. If PET-CT is not available, the guidelines recommend CE-CT or MRI. Close clinical follow-up is encouraged with scheduled history and physical examimnations every 1 to 3 months in the first year, every 2 to 4 months in the second year, every 4 to 6 months in the third to fifth years, and every 6 to 12 months thereafter.[34]

It is not yet proven whether surveillance imaging leads to earlier detection of treatment failure and whether earlier detection actually improves outcome and survival. Salvage treatment success does appear to be better in local and regional recurrences as compared to distant recurrences.[48]

SUMMARY

The face of OPSCC is changing. It has a dichotomous nature, with 1 subset of the disease associated with tobacco and alcohol use and the other having proven association with HPV infection. Imaging plays an important role in the staging and

Table 3	
Pitfalls in staging of oropharyngeal carcinoma	
Pitfall	**Advice**
Streak artifact on CE-CT degrades axial images	Obtain additional reangled images (15° off parallel line to hard palate)
Inability to see small mucosal primary lesion	Recognize limitations of all imaging techniques for evaluation of mucosal lesions, and realize that the clinical examination is complementary
Under-recognition of extension of a tonsillar primary to the soft palate on axial CE-CT	Reconstruct the thin CT image data into the coronal and sagittal planes to better evaluate the soft palate
Understaging of the primary site by failure to recognize skull base involvement on CE-CT	Carefully evaluate the ptergyoid plates for erosion on bone windows; consider MRI for further evaluation
Understaging of lymphadenopathy by not recognizing retropharyngeal metastatic lymph nodes	Evaluate the retropharyngeal nodes ipsilateral and contralateral to the primary, particularly if the primary crosses midline

surveillance of OPSCC, and a detailed knowledge of the anatomy and pitfalls is critical (Table 3).

REFERENCES

1. Hu KS, Harrison LB, Culliney B, et al. Cancer of the Oropharynx. In: Harrison LB, Sessions RB, Hong WK, editors. Head and neck cancer: a multidisciplinary approach. 2nd edition. Philadelphia: Lippincott Williams & Wilkins; 2004. p. 285–315.
2. Harnsberger HR. Handbook of head and neck imaging. 2nd edition. St Louis (MO): Mosby –Year Book; 1995.
3. Edge S, Byrd D, Compton C, et al. AJCC Cancer Staging Manual, 7th edition. Chicago: Springer; 2010.
4. Siegel R, Ward E, Brawley O, et al. Cancer statistics, 2011. CA Cancer J Clin 2011;61(4):212–36.
5. Van Monsjou HS, Balm AJ, van den Brekel MM, et al. Oropharyngeal squamous cell carcinoma: a unique disease on the rise? Oral Oncol 2010; 46(11):780–5.
6. Lin DT, Cohen SM, Coppit GL, et al. Squamous cell carcinoma of the oropharynx and hypopharynx. Otolaryngol Clin North Am 2004;38:59–74.
7. Filion E, Le QT. Oropharynx: epidemiology and treatment outcome. In: Harari PM, Connor NP, Grau C, editors. Functional preservation and quality of life in head and neck radiotherapy. Berlin: Springer-Verlag; 2009. p. 16–29.
8. Gillison M, Sturgis EM, Ramos CA. HPV is the changing face of head and neck cancers. A dramatic increase in the prevalence of HPV-related oropharynx cancers will change current practice. Available at: http://www.hemonctoday.com/article.aspx?rid=65853. Accessed June 25, 2011.
9. Osborne RG, Brown JJ. Carcinoma of the oral pharynx: an analysis of subsite treatment heterogeneity. Surg Oncol Clin N Am 2004;13:71–80.
10. Oropharyngeal cancer treatment (PDQ) from the National Cancer Institute at the National Institutes of Health. Available at: http://www.cancer.gov/concertopics/pdq/treatment/oropharyngeal. Accessed June 23, 2011.
11. Beil CM, Keberle M. Oral and oropharyngeal tumors. Eur J Radiol 2008;66:448–59.
12. Cohan DM, Popat S, Kaplan SE, et al. Oropharyngeal cacner: current understanding and management. Curr Opin Otolaryngol Head Neck Surg 2009;17:88–94.
13. D'Souza G, Kreimer AR, Viscidi R, et al. Case–control study of human papillomavirus and oropharyngeal cancer. N Engl J Med 2007;356:1944–56.
14. Castellsague X, Quintana MJ, Martinez MC, et al. The role of type of tobacco and type of alcoholic beverage in oral carcinogenesis. Int J Cancer 2004;108:741–9.
15. Sánchez MJ, Martínez C, Nieto A, et al. Oral and oropharyngeal cancer in Spain: influence of dietary patterns. Eur J Cancer Prev 2003;12(1):49–56.
16. Goldenberg D, Golz A, Joachims HZ. The beverage maté: a risk factor for cancer of the head and neck. Head Neck 2003;25(7):595–601.
17. Ho PS, Ko YC, Yang YH, et al. The incidence of oropharyngeal cancer in Taiwan: an endemic betel quid chewing area. J Oral Pathol Med 2002;31(4):213–9.
18. Gillison ML. Human papillomavirus-associated head and neck cancer is a distinct epidemiologic, clinical and molecular entity. Semin Oncol 2004; 31(6):744–54.
19. Sturgis EM, Cinciripini PM. Trends in head and neck cancer incidence in relation to smoking prevalence: an emerging epidemic of human papillomavirus-associated cancers? Cancer 2007;110(7):1429–35.
20. Fakhry C, Westra WH, Li S, et al. Improved survival of patients with human papillomavirus-positive head and neck squamous cell carcinoma in a prospective clinical trial. J Natl Cancer Inst 2008; 100:261–9.

21. Ragin CC, Taioli E. Survival of squamous cell carcinoma of the head and neck in relation to HPV infection: review and meta-analysis. Int J Cancer 2007; 121:1813–20.

22. Hafkamp HC, Manni JJ, Haesevoets A, et al. Marked differences in survival rate between smokers and nonsmokers with HPV 16-associated tonsillar carcinomas. Int J Cancer 2008;122(12):2656–64.

23. Settle K, Posner M, Schumaker LM, et al. Racial survival disparity in head and neck cancer results from low prevalence of human papillomavirus infection in black oropharyngeal cancer patients. Cancer Prev Res (Phila) 2009;2(9):776–81.

24. Chernock RD, Zhang Q, El-Mofty SK, et al. Human papillomavirus-related squamous cell carcinoma of the oropharynx: a comparative study in whites and African Americans. Arch Otolaryngol Head Neck Surg 2011;137(2):161–9.

25. Dahlgren L, Mellin H, Wangsa D, et al. Comparative genomic hybridization analysis of tonsillar cancer reveals a different pattern of genomic imbalances in human papillomavirus-positive and -negative tumors. Int J Cancer 2003;107(2):244–9.

26. Dahlstrand HM, Dalianis T. Presence and influence of human papillomaviruses (HPV) in tonsillar caner. Adv Cancer Res 2005;93:59–89.

27. Fakhry C, Gillison M. Clinical implications of HPV in head and neck cancers. J Clin Oncol 2006;24:2606–11.

28. Maru S, D'Souza G, Westra WH, et al. HPV-associated head and neck cancer: a virus-related cancer epidemic. Lancet Oncol 2010;67(10):781–9.

29. Licitra L, Perrone F, Bossi P, et al. High-risk human papillomavirus affects prognosis in patients with surgically treated oropharyngeal squamous cell carcinoma. J Clin Oncol 2006;24(36):5630–6.

30. Lindquist D, Romanitan M, Hammarstedt L, et al. Human papillomavirus is a favourable prognostic factor in tonsillar cancer and its oncogenic role is supported by the expression of E6 and E7. Mol Oncol 2007;1(3):350–5.

31. Lassen P, Eriksen JG, Hamilton-Dutoit S, et al. Effect of HPV-associated p16INK4A expression on response to radiotherapy and survival in squamous cell carcinoma of the head and neck. J Clin Oncol 2009;27(12):1992–8.

32. Kumar B, Cordell K, Lee JS, et al. Response to therapy and outcomes in oropharyngeal cancer are associated with biomarkers including human papillomavirus, epidermal growth factor receptor, gender, and smoking. Int J Radiat Oncol Biol Phys 2007;69(2 Suppl 1):S109–11.

33. American College of Radiology. ACR appropriateness criteria: neck mass/adenopathy. Available at: http://www.acr.org/SecondaryMainMenuCategories/quality_safety/app_criteria/pdf/ExpertPanelonNeurologicImaging/NeckMassAdenopathy.aspx. Accessed June 10, 2011.

34. National Comprehensive Cancer Network. Clinical practice guidelines in oncology: head and neck cancers. Version 2.2011. Available at: http://www.nccn.org/professionals/physician_gls/f_guidelines.asp. Accessed June 11, 2011.

35. American College of Radiology. ACR Appropriateness Criteria: Local-regional therapy for resectable oropharyngeal squamous cell carcinomas. Available at: http://www.acr.org/SecondaryMainMenuCategories/quality_safety/app_criteria/pdf/ExpertPanelonRadiationOncologyHeadNeckWorkGroup/ResectableOropharyngealSquamousCellCarcinomas.aspx. Accessed June 26, 2011.

36. Haignetz M, Silver CE, Corry J, et al. Current trends in initial management of oropharyngeal cancer: the declining use of open surgery. Eur Arch Otorhinolaryngol 2009;266:1845–55.

37. Moore EJ, Olsen KD, Kasperbauer JL. Transoral robotic surgery for oropharyngeal squamous cell carcinoma: a prospective study of feasibility and functional outcomes. Laryngoscope 2009;119:2156–64.

38. Wesolowski JR, Mukherji S. Pathology of the pharynx. In: Som PM, Curtin HD, editors, editors. Head and neck imaging. 5th edition. St. Louis: Elsevier; 2011. p. 1749–810.

39. Stambuk HE, Karimi S, Lee N, et al. Oral cavity and oropharynx tumors. Radiol Clin North Am 2007;45:1–20.

40. Evan RM, Hodder SC. Oral cavity and oropharynx. In: Ahuja A, Evans R, King A, et al, editors. Imaging in head and neck cancer: a practical approach. London: Greenwich Medical Media Limited; 2003. p. 69–88.

41. Trotta BM, Pease CS, Rasamny JJ, et al. Oral cavity and oropharyngeal squamous cell cancer: key imaging findings for staging and treatment planning. Radiographics 2011;31:339–54.

42. Hsu WC, Loevner LA, Karpati R, et al. Accuracy of magnetic resonance imaging in predicting absence of fixation of head and neck cancer to the prevertebral space. Head Neck 2005;27:95–100.

43. Loevner LA, Ott IL, Yousem DM, et al. Neoplastic fixation to the prevertebral compartment by squamous cell carcinoma of the head and neck. AJR Am J Roentgenol 1998;170:1389–94.

44. Brasilino de Carvalho M. Quantitative analysis of the extent of extracapsular invasion and its prognostic significance: a prospective study of 170 cases of carcinoma of the larynx and hypopharynx. Head Neck 1998;20(1):16–21.

45. Khuri FR, Lippman SM, Spitz MR, et al. Molecular epidemiology and retinoid chemoprevention of head and neck cancer. J Natl Cancer Inst 1997;89(3):199–211.

46. León X, Quer M, Diez S, et al. Second neoplasm in patients with head and neck cancer. Head Neck 1999;21(3):204–10.

47. Hu K, Harrison LB. Cancer of the oral cavity and oropharynx. In: Halperin EC, Perez CA, Brady LW, editors. Principles and practice of radiation oncology. Philadelphia: Lippincott Williams and Wilkins; 2008. p. 38–59.

48. Wang SJ, Eisele DW. Role of surveillance radiologic imaging after treatment of oropharyngeal cancer. Internet J Otorhinolaryngol 2010;11(2). Available at: http://www.ispub.com/journal/the_internet_journal_of_otorhinolaryngology/volume_11_number_2_9/article/role-of-surveillance-radiologic-imaging-after-treatment-of-oropharyngeal-cancer.html. Accessed February 2, 2011.

49. Spector JG, Sessions DG, Haughey BH, et al. Delayed regional metastases, distant metastases and second primary malignancy in squamous cell carcinomas of the larynx and hypopharynx. Laryngoscope 2001;111:1079–87.

50. Sikora AG, Morris LG, Sturgis EM. Bidirectional association of anogenital and oral cavity/pharyngeal carcinomas in men. Arch Otolaryngol Head Neck Surg 2009;135(4):402–5.

51. King KG, Kositwattanarerk A, Genden E, et al. Cancers of the oral cavity and oropharynx: FDG PET with contrast enhanced CT in the post-treatment setting. Radiographics 2011;31:355–73.

Pitfalls in the Staging Squamous Cell Carcinoma of the Hypopharynx

Amy Y. Chen, MD[a], Patricia A. Hudgins, MD[b],*

KEYWORDS

- Squamous cell carcinoma • Hypopharynx • Aryepiglottic fold • Larynx

KEY POINTS

- To accurately interpret pretreatment and posttreatment imaging in patients with hypopharyngeal squamous cell carcinoma (SCC), one must understand the complex anatomy of this part of the aerodigestive system.
- Common patterns of spread must be recognized.
- Pitfalls in imaging must be understood.
- This article reviews the epidemiology, anatomy, staging, treatment and pitfalls in imaging of hypopharyngeal SCC.

INTRODUCTION AND EPIDEMIOLOGY

Compared with laryngeal neoplasms, primary hypopharyngeal (HP) tumors, especially those exclusively in the HP subsites, are relatively uncommon, accounting for about 4% of all head and neck tumors. Tumors of the hypopharynx are generally advanced stage when detected, and have often already extended to the larynx or cervical esophagus. Imaging is critical in staging these advanced primary tumors for guiding treatment planning, and because locoregional control may be difficult to attain, accurate staging is especially critical.

Epidemiology is difficult to report, as laryngeal and oral-cavity squamous cell carcinoma (SCC) statistics are often lumped together with HP numbers.[1] Patients are generally older than 50 years, and men are more commonly affected than women at a rate of 3:1. Tobacco and alcohol abuse are the risk factors responsible for SCC, statistically the most common malignancy of the hypopharynx. Alcohol potentiates the mutagenic effects of tobacco. The biology of HP SCC is interesting, and an area of ongoing study. Mutations in the *p53* tumor suppressor gene are more common in HP SCC than in other head and neck sites.[2,3] Field carcinogenesis, the concept that carcinogens affect surrounding tissue that has yet to be transformed to tumor, also is common in HP SCC. Thus tumors may be multicentric, spread submucosally, and be very difficult to stage with imaging or endoscopy alone. At presentation tumors are often at an advanced stage, and the rich lymphatic drainage of the hypopharynx and cervical esophagus result in frequent nodal metastases. The role of human papillomavirus (HPV) in HP SCC is still being determined, but early evidence suggests HPV infection is less commonly involved in SCC of HP than are oropharyngeal subsites.[4,5]

[a] Department of Otolaryngology-Head & Neck Surgery, Emory University School of Medicine, 1364 Clifton Road, Northeast Atlanta, GA 30322, USA; [b] Department of Radiology and Imaging Sciences, Division of Neuroradiology, Head & Neck Section, Emory University School of Medicine, BG-27, 1364 Clifton Road, Northeast, Atlanta, GA 30322, USA
* Corresponding author. Department of Head and Neck Radiology, Emory University School of Medicine, Atlanta, GA 30322.
E-mail address: phudgin@emory.edu

Neuroimag Clin N Am 23 (2013) 67–79
http://dx.doi.org/10.1016/j.nic.2012.08.007

A rare but well-described syndrome of upper esophageal webs, iron-deficiency anemia, and postcricoid HP SCC is Plummer-Vinson syndrome. Patients are usually Caucasian women between 40 and 70 years of age. Better nutrition including iron supplementation has led to a marked decrease in this syndrome.[6]

NORMAL ANATOMY AND BOUNDARIES

To conceptualize HP anatomy, one must understand that the larynx and the hypopharynx are so interrelated that it is impossible to know the anatomy of one without understanding the other. A simplified concept is that the larynx is immediately anterior with respect to the hypopharynx, forms the anterior wall of the hypopharynx, and the larynx "bulges into" the anterior aspect of the hypopharynx. Boundaries of the hypopharynx are often described as they relate to laryngeal subsites. The craniocaudal boundaries are quite specific: the superior boundary is at a plane at the hyoid bone level, and the inferior boundary is the lower border of the cricoid cartilage (Fig. 1). As such, the hypopharynx is that portion of the aerodigestive tract between the oropharynx (superior) and the proximal cervical esophagus (inferior). The hyoid bone and cricoid are parts of the laryngeal skeleton. Immediately posterior and deep to the hypopharynx is the retropharyngeal space.

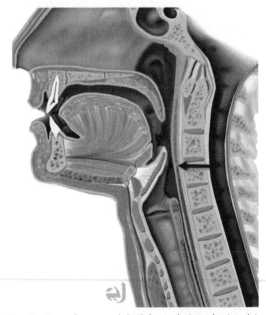

Fig. 1. Hypopharyngeal (HP) boundaries, depicted in orange. The hypopharynx extends from the posterior pharyngeal wall (*arrow*) at the level of the hyoid bone, to the proximal cervical esophagus. The hypopharynx is posterior to the larynx and anterior to the retropharyngeal space. (*Courtesy* of Eric Jablonowski.)

Another helpful way to understand HP anatomy is to know the individual subsite anatomy. The 3 HP subsites are the pyriform sinuses, lateral and posterior HP walls, and the postcricoid region. The pyriform sinuses are paired, right and left, and they extend from the pharyngoepiglottic folds of the suprahyoid epiglottis to the inferior cricoid cartilage. For each pyriform sinus, the lateral border is the lateral pharyngeal wall and the medial border is the aryepiglottic fold, specifically the HP surface of the aryepiglottic fold. The pyriform sinuses are shaped like upside down pyramids, with the apex located at the true vocal cord level. So even if they are collapsed and not filled with air, if the axial image is at the true vocal cord or arytenoid cartilage level, each pyriform sinus apex is posterior and lateral. The pyriform sinus is the most common location for HP SCC, accounting for about 60% of all cases.

The second subsite, the posterior HP wall, is the inferior extension of the posterior wall of the oropharynx. This portion extends to the postcricoid subsite of the hypopharynx.

The postcricoid portion of the hypopharynx, also the caudalmost region, is accurately named as located posterior to the cricoid cartilage, extending from the posterior wall of the hypopharynx at the cricoarytenoid joint level to the inferior cricoid cartilage and proximal cervical esophagus. On axial images, therefore, the mucosal overlying the posterior cricoid cartilage is the anterior aspect of the postcricoid HP. The posterior portion of the postcricoid HP is the cricopharyngeus muscle, which merges with the cervical esophagus. Postcricoid tumors are the least common of HP SCC.

AMERICAN JOINT COMMITTEE ON CANCER STAGING

The American Joint Committee on Cancer (AJCC) staging manual should be used as a guide, as it clearly lays out the anatomic details necessary to accurately stage tumors of the hypopharynx (Table 1). Like other subsites, the difference between AJCC sixth and seventh editions is primarily the division of T4 lesions into T4a or moderately advanced disease and T4b, or very advanced local disease.[7]

Staging HP tumors requires both clinical and radiologic information.[8] Knowledge of the specific subsites and the maximum diameter of the tumor are essential (see Table 1). A T1 tumor involves one subsite (posterior pharyngeal wall, pyriform sinus, or postcricoid hypopharynx) or is 2 cm or smaller in greatest dimension (Figs. 2–4). A T2 tumor invades another HP subsite or an adjacent site (for example, a laryngeal subsite), or is greater than

Table 1
AJCC 7: hypopharynx

	Primary Tumor (T)
	Primary Tumor (T)
TX	Primary tumor cannot be assessed
T0	No evidence of primary tumor
Tis	Carcinoma in situ
T1	Tumor limited to one subsite of hypopharynx and/or 2 cm or less in greatest dimension
T2	Tumor invades more than one subsite of hypopharynx or an adjacent site, or measures more than 2 cm but not more than 4 cm in greatest dimension without fixation of hemilarynx
T3	Tumor more than 4 cm in greatest dimension or with fixation of hemilarynx or extension to esophagus
T4a	Moderately advanced local disease Tumor invades thyroid/cricoid cartilage, hyoid bone, thyroid gland or central compartment soft tissue (includes prelaryngeal strap muscles and subcutaneous fat)
T4b	Very advanced local disease Tumor invades prevertebral fascia, encases carotid artery, or involves mediastinal structures
	Regional Lymph Nodes (N)
NX	Regional lymph nodes cannot be assessed
N0	No regional lymph node metastasis
N1	Metastasis in a single ipsilateral lymph node, 3 cm or less in greatest dimension
N2	Metastasis in a single ipsilateral lymph node, more than 3 cm but not more than 6 cm in greatest dimension; or in multiple ipsilateral lymph nodes, none more than 6 cm in greatest dimension; or in bilateral or contralateral lymph nodes, none more than 6 cm in greatest dimension
N2a	Metastasis in single ipsilateral lymph node more than 3 cm but not more than 6 cm in greatest dimension
N2b	Metastasis in multiple ipsilateral lymph nodes, none more than 6 cm in greatest dimension
N2c	Metastasis in bilateral or contralateral lymph nodes, none more than 6 cm in greatest dimension
N3	Metastasis in a lymph node more than 6 cm in greatest dimension
	Note: Metastases at level VII are considered regional lymph node metastases
	Distant Metastasis (M)
M0	No distant metastasis
M1	Distant metastasis

From Edge SB, Byrd DR, Compton CC, et al. Editorial Board. AJCC Cancer staging manual. 7th edition. Chicago: Springer; 2010. p. 41–56; with permission.

2 cm but less than 4 cm (**Fig. 5**). By definition, there is no fixation of the hemilarynx for a T1 or T2 tumor.

Fixation of the hemilarynx is defined as impaired motion of the true vocal cord. For HP SCC, this can be a result of tumor invading the larynx at the cricoarytenoid joint or the intrinsic laryngeal muscles. Thus, the vocal cord paralysis is from tumor extending from the hypopharynx into the larynx. Other mechanisms for vocal cord dysfunction from HP SCC are invasion of the recurrent laryngeal nerve or direct invasion of the posterior cricoarytenoid muscle.[9] Tumor on the medial pyriform sinus wall often involves the hemilarynx, usually at the insertion of the aryepiglottic fold to the arytenoid cartilage (**Fig. 6**). Therefore, vocal cord motion is often impaired when the tumor is in the medial pyriform sinus. Bulky pyriform sinus carcinomas may cause hemilarynx fixation owing to a weight effect. The tumor may cause arytenoid cartilage immobility at the top of the cartilage, but the base is still mobile. The arytenoid appears immobile to the endoscopist, but there is really no histologic tumor invasion of the arytenoid cartilage. Vocal cord, and not just arytenoid cartilage mobility, should be reported by the endoscopist.[9]

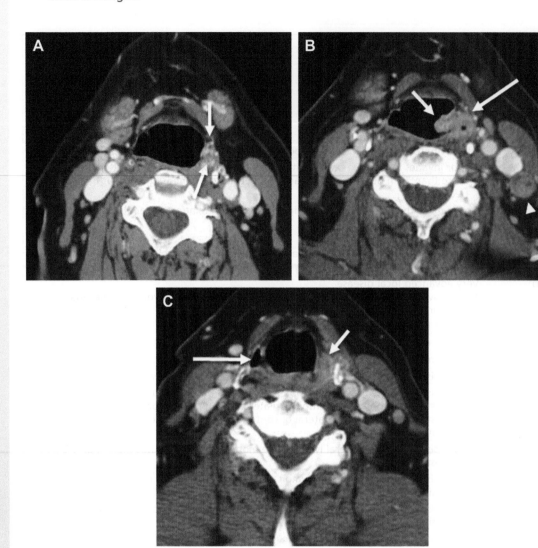

Fig. 2. T1 pyriform sinus SCC on left, missed on initial image interpretation. (*A*) Axial contrast-enhanced computed tomography (CECT) shows left SCC (<2 cm) at the superior pyriform sinus (*arrows*). This study was interpreted as "Normal neck CT. No tumor." (*B*) Axial CECT obtained 16 months after *A* shows increase in size of the mass filling the pyriform sinus, and involvement of the laryngeal surface of the left aryepiglottic fold (AEF) (*arrow*). Note extension to the posterior paraglottic fat (*long arrow*). Posterior left level III node is now larger with unequivocal necrosis (*arrowhead*). (*C*) Axial CECT at low pyriform sinus level shows normal right air-filled sinus (*long arrow*). Note tumor in left pyriform sinus (*short arrow*). On subsequent images tumor was present in the apex of the sinus, a finding that was not present on the initial study. Pyriform apex involvement carries a poor prognosis when compared with tumor only at the superior aspect of the pyriform sinus.

Staging a tumor as T3 or T4 requires knowing whether the true vocal cord is mobile. Because this is best determined clinically by direct visualization of the larynx, it is not possible to accurately stage an HP tumor with imaging alone. In their practice, the authors usually describe the extent and size of an HP tumor, but do not always report a T stage because knowledge of the cord mobility may not be available at the time of image interpretation.

Three criteria define a T3 HP tumor: greater than 4 cm, fixation of the hemilarynx, or extension to the

cervical esophagus (Fig. 7). By definition, if the hemilarynx is "fixed," the tumor has extended from the boundaries of the hypopharynx and involves part of the larynx or the recurrent laryngeal nerve.

T4 tumor is subdivided, as with all other subsites, into T4a or moderately advanced local disease and T4b, very advanced local disease. Criteria for T4a tumor involves invasion of the thyroid or cricoid cartilage, the hyoid bone, thyroid gland, or central compartment including the infrahyoid prelaryngeal strap muscles and subcutaneous fat. T4b tumor

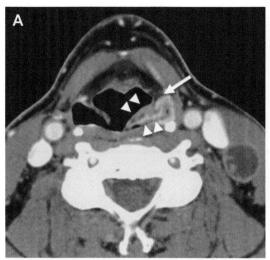
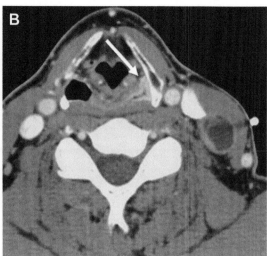

Fig. 3. T1 left pyriform sinus SCC. (*A*) Axial CECT image at superior AEF shows tumor encircling pyriform sinus (*arrowheads*), with extension into posterior paraglottic fat (*arrow*). (*B*) Image is slightly lower, but tumor is still present in sinus and posterior paraglottic fat (*long arrow*). The laryngeal surface of the AEF is normal and symmetric with right side.

invades the prevertebral fascia, extending through the retropharyngeal space, encases the common carotid artery, or extends inferiorly to the mediastinum.

The hypopharynx has a rich lymphatic drainage system, and nodal metastases are common. Neck disease is staged as all other head and neck subsites: N1 through N3. The primary nodal stations are high, mid, and low jugular chains, or levels II, III, and IV. Tumors on the posterior wall of the hypopharynx may metastasize to the retropharyngeal nodes. Bilateral nodal disease, or

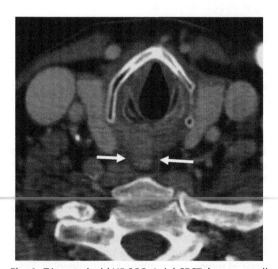

Fig. 4. T1 postcricoid HP SCC. Axial CECT shows a small mass (*arrows*) of the postcricoid hypopharynx. There is a crescent of normal fat around the posterior portion of the tumor, suggesting no invasion of retropharyngeal space or prevertebral muscles.

N2c, increases with increasing tumor stage. Distant metastasis is either M0 (no distant disease) or M1 (definite distant disease). Lungs are the most common site for distant disease, and mediastinal nodal metastases are considered distant disease.[7]

Because staging HP SCC requires imaging and endoscopic information, a multispecialty tumor board is ideally the best way to stage and recommend treatment for the patient with HP SCC.

IMAGING PROTOCOLS

No randomized prospective trial has been done to compare contrast-enhanced computed tomography (CECT), magnetic resonance imaging (MRI), positron emission tomography/CT (PET-CT), or PET-CECT for HP SCC. Early evidence suggests that PET-CT was more sensitive than 3.0-T whole-body MRI for detecting distant metastases and second primary cancers.[10] However, there is no current consensus as to which modality is best for staging HP SCC, but the argument for PET-CECT is strong. In the authors' practice, all patients with HP SCC undergo a staging combined PET-CECT (see Fig. 7). The advantages of this combined anatomic and metabolic study are accurate staging of the primary tumor via CECT, while PET is superior for detecting nodal disease, distant metastases, and second primary tumors, which are common in HP SCC. The authors use at least 100 mL nonionic iodinated contrast, with variable injection protocols but at least a 75-second delay before the CT is performed. This delay makes both mucosal and vascular enhancement optimal, and

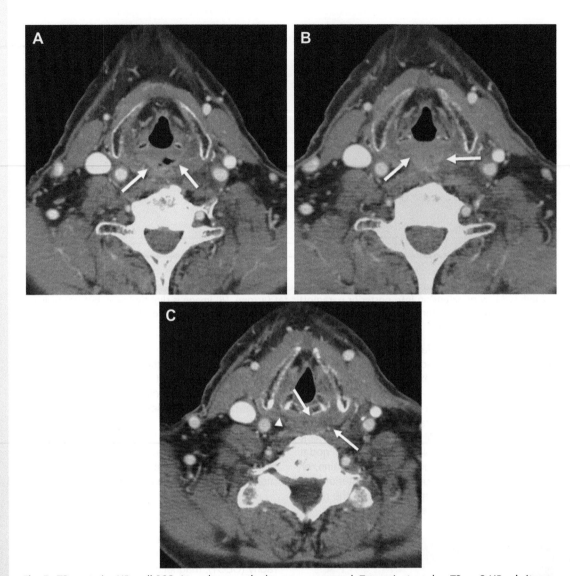

Fig. 5. T2 posterior HP wall SCC. At endoscopy the larynx was normal. Tumor is staged as T2, as 2 HP subsites are involved. (*A*) CECT shows a peripherally enhancing mass (*arrows*) on the posterior wall, with air in a central ulceration. (*B*) CECT obtained 3 mm inferior to *A* shows anterior displacement of the larynx by the HP mass (*arrows*). (*C*) CECT image at postcricoid hypopharynx shows subtle but definite asymmetric fullness on left (*arrows*). Note normal intramural fat planes (*arrowhead*) on right.

also is long enough to detect necrosis. Detailed technical parameters for the PET portion are beyond the scope of this article, but 15 to 18 mCi of ^{18}F-fluorodexoyglucose is administered intravenously and then whole-body imaging is performed 60 minutes later. Standardized uptake values (SUV) of the tumor and nodes are measured and reported. The staging PET-CECT provides a baseline for comparison to a posttreatment PET-CECT at 8 to 10 weeks after therapy.

The CECT is interpreted by the Head and Neck Imaging section, the PET by the Nuclear Medicine section, and 2 separate dictations are generated. If the interpretations are discordant, a consensus discussion comes up with a recommendation on how to resolve the issue in question.

MRI is rarely requested, and is reserved for problem solving. The most common indications for MRI are questionable cartilage penetration, confirming extrapharyngeal or extralaryngeal tumor extension, and to determine if the prevertebral fascia is clear of tumor. The authors' MRI protocol includes imaging through the area of question only, as the neck has already been staged with PET-CECT. Standard neck phased-array surface coils are used. T1-weighted images in all 3 planes are always

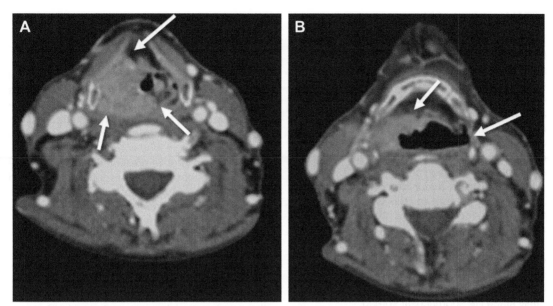

Fig. 6. T3 laryngohypopharyngeal SCC based on tumor (>4 cm) and fixation of right hemilarynx. (*A*) Large bulky right laryngohypopharyngeal SCC involves right AEF, pyriform sinus, and posterior laryngeal and HP walls (*short arrows*). Note tumor extending into right paraglottic fat (*long arrow*). (*B*) At hyoid bone level, there is invasion of right pre-epiglottic fat (*short arrow*). Note normal left lateral HP wall (*long arrow*), and compare with right lateral wall, which is filled with tumor.

performed, followed by T2-weighted images with fat saturation, in the axial and sagittal planes. After gadolinium is injected, the 3 T1-weighted sequences are repeated, and at least 2 have fat saturation.

On staging workup, indeterminate lymph nodes are described and are generally treated with neck dissection, or the chain is included in the neck radiation field. Ultrasound-guided fine-needle aspiration (UG-FNA) is used frequently to resolve discordant CECT and PET findings. Most aspirations, however, are for indeterminate nodal disease after treatment, and rarely is pretreatment nodal sampling performed.

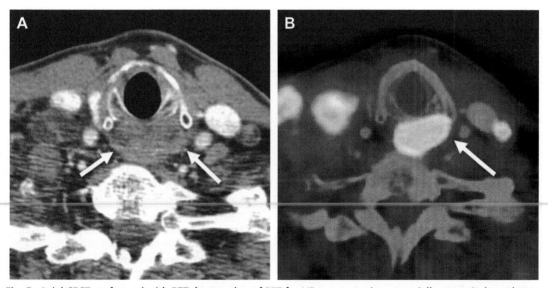

Fig. 7. Axial CECT performed with PET shows value of PET for HP tumor staging, especially at cervical esophagus. (*A*) Postcricoid hypopharynx (*arrows*) is greater than 10 mm anteroposterior, and there is anterior displacement of larynx by the mass. Bilateral metastatic adenopathy is consistent with N2c disease. (*B*) Fused positron emission tomography (PET)-CECT portion of the study at same level confirms increased metabolic activity in mass (*arrow*).

PITFALLS

Most pitfalls in staging HP SCC can be overcome by knowing the anatomy of the hypopharynx and surrounding structures, high-quality imaging with either CECT, PET-CECT, or MRI, and close communication with other members of the Head and Neck Tumor Board (Table 2). Patient care is improved when imaging interpretation is not done in a vacuum without clinical information, but rather when closely coordinated with the head and neck surgeon or endoscopist.

Hypopharyngeal tumor commonly extends in a submucosal pattern, and this behavior accounts for one of the most important staging pitfalls.[11–13] One histopathologic study showed 60% incidence of submucosal extension.[13] Imaging, therefore, is extremely important as the endoscopist may only see the proverbial tip of the iceberg. However, even metabolic imaging, like PET, may inaccurately stage HP submucosal spread.

Each HP subsite has its own difficulties or pitfalls with imaging and staging, and by knowing the subsites the radiologist can anticipate patterns of disease.

Extension and complications of pyriform sinus SCC, the most common location for HP SCC, depends on location of the tumor: medial wall versus lateral wall, and apex versus high pyriform sinus tumor. Tumors on the medial wall, or the HP surface of the aryepiglottic fold, may extend caudally to the arytenoid cartilage and cricoarytenoid joint. Tumors arising on the lateral pyriform sinus wall often spread anteriorly and laterally to involve the laryngeal paraglottic fat and the posterior thyroid cartilage (see Fig. 6). Tumor in the pyriform sinus apex may spread anteriorly between the thyroid and arytenoid cartilages. It is essential to describe extension across the midline, as this has significant surgical implications. More pharyngeal mucosa will need to be resected, and thus free-flap reconstruction will be necessary.

Tumors of the second subsite, the posterior HP wall, are often large at presentation, as symptoms are similar to those of gastroesophageal reflux and there is a delay in diagnosis. Posterior HP wall tumors extend superiorly to involve the posterior oropharyngeal wall and base of the tongue (Fig. 8). When this occurs, the tumor has by definition involved a second site: the oropharynx. Inferior extension from the postcricoid hypopharynx to the cervical esophagus is another pattern of spread that by definition involves another subsite: the esophagus. Likewise, postcricoid HP extension from a cervical esophageal SCC is, in the authors' experience, often overlooked on staging imaging (Fig. 9). It is critical to identify posterior extension into the retropharyngeal and prevertebral spaces, as in the AJCC seventh edition invasion of prevertebral fascia is T4b stage. Patients may present with the neck in a fixed position, and a barium esophagogram shows lack of normal motion during the swallowing phase. MRI has been shown to have excellent negative predictive value (Fig. 10). If the retropharyngeal fat between the tumor and the prevertebral compartment is

Table 2
Pitfalls in staging of HP SCC

Pitfall	Advice
HP SCC frequently spread via submucosal route	Careful contrast technique on CECT MRI may be more accurate PET combined with CECT or MRI probably best technique
Medial pyriform sinus wall tumor	Assess for laryngeal extension to arytenoid cartilage and cricoarytenoid joint
Lateral pyriform sinus wall tumor	Assess for supraglottic laryngeal extension to paraglottic fat or thyroid cartilage
Pyriform sinus apex tumor	Assess for extension through thyroarytenoid space
Posterior wall tumor	Assess posterior wall at oropharyngeal level, about level of epiglottis
Missing esophageal extension	Assess verge and proximal cervical esophagus PET-CECT may be best technique
Upstaging to T4b	Prevertebral fascia invasion can only be determined directly during surgery
PET-CT too early after surgery or biopsy	Wait at least 8 wks

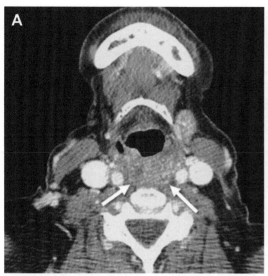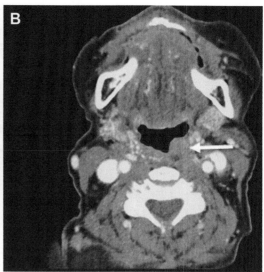

Fig. 8. Posterior HP wall tumor with superior extension to posterior oropharyngeal wall. (*A*) Axial CECT shows symmetric fullness of posterior HP wall (*arrows*). Image is noisy, as patient was scanned with arms over head. (*B*) Axial CECT at oropharyngeal level, above the epiglottis. Note asymmetric mass on left lateral posterior wall (*arrow*). Although this did not change the final stage, it affected treatment, as the patient was deemed unresectable and was treated with chemoradiation.

preserved on T1-weighted sagittal and axial images, there is no invasion of the prevertebral space (**Fig. 11**).[14] However, if the fat signal is interrupted the converse is not true.[15] The only reliable

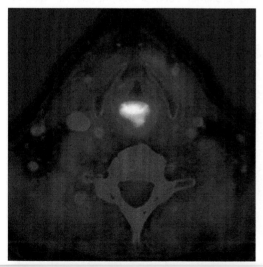

Fig. 9. Fused PET-CECT image in a patient who "recurred" after radiation for cervical esophageal SCC. Within 1 month following treatment for cervical esophageal SCC, the patient underwent PET-CECT because of persistent dysphagia and pain. A pretreatment PET had not been performed. The initial tumor was probably understaged and likely already involved the postcricoid hypopharynx. In the authors' experience, understaging HP SCC at the proximal cervical esophagus is a common pitfall.

way to determine prevertebral compartment tumor extension, based on personal experience and the literature, is direct surgical inspection (**Fig. 12**).

Tumors in the third subsite, the postcricoid HP, are relatively uncommon, and almost always locally invasive at the time of diagnosis. With high-resolution cross-sectional imaging the anatomy at the postcricoid HP can clearly be delineated. Intramural fat planes are commonly

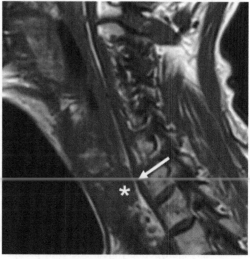

Fig. 10. Sagittal T1-weighted image in a patient with a small postcricoid SCC of hypopharynx (*asterisk*). Preservation of high signal intensity retropharyngeal fat (*arrow*) is strong evidence that there is no invasion.

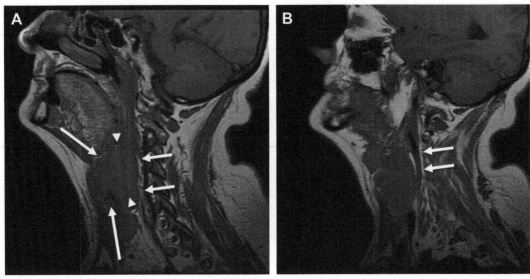

Fig. 11. Parasagittal (*A*) and further lateral parasagittal (*B*) T1-weighted MR images of bulky laryngohypophar-yngeal tumor. Note bulky tumor involving both larynx (*long arrows*) and hypopharynx (*arrowheads*). Fat stripe is preserved (*short arrows*), implying no involvement of the retropharynx or prevertebral fascia.

present in the HP walls, and loss of the planes is seen with tumor (see **Fig. 5**C). The anteroposterior (AP) diameter of the postcricoid region is normally less than 10 mm, and if greater than 10 mm, in a patient with HP SCC, should be considered abnormal.[16] In a patient with cervical esophageal tumor, a postcricoid AP diameter greater than 10 mm implies extension of the tumor to the hypopharynx. Variability in the width or transverse dimension on the postcricoid HP is broad, so that this measurement is not reliable for staging. The proximal cervical esophagus AP diameter

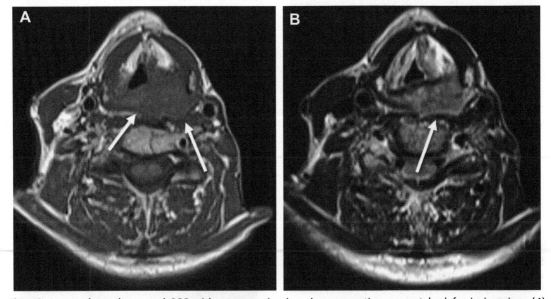

Fig. 12. Laryngohypopharyngeal SCC with preoperative imaging suggesting prevertebral fascia invasion. (*A*) T1-weighted axial image shows apparent obliteration of fat in the retropharyngeal space (*arrows*). (*B*) T2-weighted axial image at the same level shows loss of fat in retropharyngeal space but smooth interface between posterior aspect of tumor and prevertebral muscles (*arrow*). At surgery the fascia over prevertebral muscles was intact and the tumor was completely resected.

should be no greater than 16 mm. Of course, these measurements should not be used in a patient who has undergone radiation or in the setting of gastroesophageal reflux disease, as mucosal edema will affect these measurements.

Postcricoid tumors can cause vocal cord dysfunction by recurrent laryngeal nerve spread or direct anterior extension to the posterior larynx. Inferior extension through the cricopharyngeus muscle into the proximal cervical esophagus has enormous treatment implications.

The extra-HP surrounding structures most commonly invaded by HP SCC are the posterior oropharyngeal wall (superior), the larynx (anterior), and the proximal cervical esophagus (inferior). Posterior extension through the retropharyngeal space occurs less commonly and is only accurately detected at surgery, but is important because the patient is then truly nonoperable.

TREATMENT

No randomized trial comparing surgical with nonsurgical management of SCC of the hypopharynx has been reported, and treatment data have been extrapolated from studies of laryngeal SCC. Treatment of HP SCC has evolved significantly in the past decade. The goal of any treatment plan, whether surgical or chemoradiation

(CRT), is the same: local control of disease while preserving, maintaining, or improving voice quality and swallowing, and avoiding aspiration and airway compromise. Treatment considerations must include subsite, stage, presence of distant metastases, laryngohypopharyngeal function at presentation, status of laryngeal cartilage, and patient preference (Fig. 13). Patient preference is, of course, always a consideration, but especially in laryngeal and HP SCC. A review of treatment in the 1980s and 1990s showed that surgery was the primary treatment 42% of the time, and radiotherapy or CRT without surgery was used 41% of the time, with relatively similar survival outcomes.[17] Radiation therapy and surgery have similar outcomes for early-stage disease.[18]

Two arguments are used to advocate for CRT or radiation alone. First, there is high propensity for HP SCC to spread submucosally, with the likelihood of positive surgical margins. Second, even with a clinical and radiologic N0 neck, the chance of micrometastases has been reported to be as high as 40%.[19] In general, T1 or T2 disease is treated much like supraglottic laryngeal carcinoma, and treatment depends on function. The 20% of patients who present with T1 or T2 disease can be treated with surgery, radiation, chemotherapy, or CRT. The role of transoral endoscopic

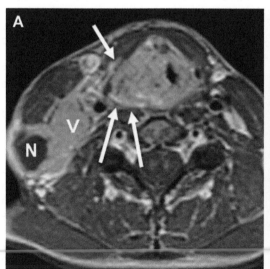
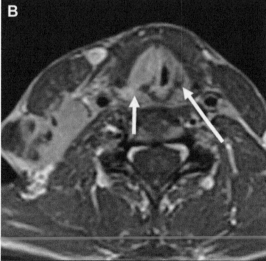

Fig. 13. Large laryngohypopharyngeal SCC with extralaryngeal spread. The patient ultimately underwent laryngohypopharyngectomy and radical neck dissection. (A) Postcontrast T1-weighted axial image shows enhancing tumor, with direct extension through the right thyroid cartilage (*short arrow*) into infrahyoid strap muscle. Note smooth interface (*long arrows*) with prevertebral fascia, which was uninvolved at surgery. Nodal disease fills the right jugular vein (V). Necrotic nodal mass (N) is present immediately beneath the skin. (B) Postcontrast T1-weighted axial image at glottic level shows extralaryngeal extension through right thyroarytenoid space (*short arrow*). Note normal left space (*long arrow*) between posterior thyroid ala and arytenoid cartilage. The tumor enhances robustly, but there is no enhancement in the cartilage, suggesting it is not invaded at this location.

resection (TORS) is still unknown, but may be a significant addition to the surgical armamentarium.[20] If there is significant laryngeal or HP dysfunction, radical resection or laryngohypopharyngectomy with reconstruction is chosen. In general, partial hypopharyngectomy is reconstructed with a myocutaneous flap, whereas a free jejunal flap is used to reconstruct a total or circumferential hypopharyngectomy. Posterior pharyngeal wall tumors are almost always treated nonsurgically with CRT, as the oropharyngeal wall is often involved as well (see Fig. 8).

SURVEILLANCE

Well-designed prospective studies determining sensitivity and specificity of different imaging modalities for assessing treatment response in HP SCC are lacking. Most available studies are retrospective and are not sufficiently careful with uniform adherence to imaging technique or protocol. However, relapse rate in advanced SCC of the head and neck, including the hypopharynx, is more than 50%.[21] In the authors' practice, the initial study posttreatment is PET-CECT. Because of the chance for false-positive findings, this is generally obtained 8 to 10 weeks following surgery or at the end of CRT. Mucosal edema after CRT can be particularly difficult to differentiate from residual disease. Thickened aryepiglottic folds with collapse of the entire pyriform sinus from the superior inlet to the apex are an expected and universal finding following CRT. The posterior pharyngeal wall and postcricoid hypopharynx also have a boggy edematous appearance, making submucosal residual disease especially difficult to identify with cross-sectional imaging. Enhancement on CECT helps differentiate edema from tumor, as tumor tends to enhance in a homogeneous pattern, and only the mucosal surface should enhance with edema. However, current accepted chemotherapeutic regimens may include a monoclonal antibody such as cetuximab, an epidermal growth factor receptor inhibitor, or bevacizumab, a vascular endothelial growth factor A inhibitor, and both agents directly or indirectly affect tumor angiogenesis, potentially changing contrast enhancement appearances on CECT. PET is very helpful in this regard. Posttreatment mucosal edema generally has a lower SUV than residual tumor.

As with pretreatment PET-CECT, the 2 components of the examination are interpreted separately, then in a consensus fashion. When there are discordant findings in the primary tumor bed or neck, for example, CECT shows a large necrotic node but PET shows no increased metabolic activity in the node, UG-FNA or neck dissection is performed. No findings should be interpreted in isolation, however. Symptoms such as ear pain or dysphagia strongly suggest persistent or residual disease. Posttreatment image interpretation should not be performed by the radiologist without sufficient history, especially as it relates to treatment.

FUTURE DIRECTIONS AND ADVANCED IMAGING

There are many unanswered questions regarding the staging of HP SCC, surveillance imaging, and the role of the various imaging techniques. Prospective comparison of both staging and surveillance modalities must be performed to determine the most accurate modalities. Because treatment is often nonsurgical, and it is therefore impossible to know the accurate extent of disease, both surgical and clinical outcome measures need to be used as end points. For example, without pathologic confirmation, imaging could overstage or understage tumor size and local invasion, or nodal disease could be inaccurately determined. If tumor is treated with radiation therapy or systemic therapy, we may not know how accurate the imaging staging is unless clinical outcomes are used to compare modalities. The prospective imaging trials, therefore, must include surgeons, radiation therapists, and oncologists in addition to radiologists.

To understand postoperative changes in the larynx and hypopharynx, the radiologist will need to be familiar with new reconstructive flap techniques, innovative methods to reconstruct the HP mucosal surface, and the expected appearance after TORS for small T1 and T2 HP resections.

Radiologists also need to stay current and abreast in developments in molecular-targeted therapy, which will have a significant effect on tumor metabolic activity and thus imaging appearance of HP SCC on conventional modalities. Neuroradiologists are already experienced with incorporating new knowledge about treatment in imaging interpretations. In neurooncology, changes in size and enhancement of glioblastoma multiforme on brain MRI can no longer be used to imply tumor progression or regression, but may be due to "pseudoprogression" or "pseudoregression."[22] Interpreting brain tumor imaging can no longer be performed without knowing details of treatment: whether the patient is on steroids, which chemotherapeutic agents were used and at what doses, and how the patient is doing clinically. As new CRT regimens are developed for SCC of the hypopharynx, we will also need to know the treatment details to recognize toxicities and tumor recurrence.

In summary, to accurately interpret pretreatment and posttreatment imaging in patients with HP SCC, one must understand the complex anatomy of this part of the aerodigestive system, recognize common patterns of spread, and know the pitfalls in imaging. With this infrastructure and foundation, even the most complex new developments will make sense.

REFERENCES

1. Surveillance Epidemiology and End Results (SEER) cancer statistics review. 1975-2008. Available at: http://seer.cancer.gov. Accessed March, 2012.

2. Karsai S, Abel U, Roesch-Ely M, et al. Comparison of p16INK4a expression with p53 alterations in head and neck cancer by tissue microarray analysis. J Pathol 2007;211:314–22.

3. Somers KD, Merrick MA, Lopez MF, et al. Frequent p53 mutations in head and neck cancer. Cancer Res 1992;52(21):5997–6000.

4. Boscolo-Rizzo P, Da Mosto MC, Fuson R, et al. HPV-16 E6 L83V variant in squamous cell carcinomas of the upper aerodigestive tract. J Cancer Res Clin Oncol 2009;135(4):559–66.

5. Rodrigo JP, Gonzalez MV, Lazo PS, et al. Genetic alterations in squamous cell carcinomas of the hypopharynx with correlations to clinicopathological features. Oral Oncol 2002;38:357–63.

6. Song L-M. Plummer-Vinson syndrome. Medscape reference. Available at: http://emedicine.medscape.com/article/187341-overview#a0199. Accessed March, 2012.

7. Edge SB, Byrd DR, Compton CC, et al. Editorial Board. AJCC cancer staging manual. 7th edition. Chicago: Springer; 2010. p. 41–56.

8. Thabet HM, Sessions DG, Gado MY, et al. Comparison of clinical evaluation and computed tomographic diagnostic accuracy for tumor of the larynx and hypopharynx. Laryngoscope 1996;106:589–94.

9. Katilmis H, Ozturkcan S, Ozdemir I, et al. A clinicopathological study of laryngeal and hypopharyngeal carcinoma: correlation of cord-arytenoid mobility with histopathologic involvement. Otolaryngol Head Neck Surg 2007;136:291–5.

10. Chan SC, Wang HM, Yen TC, et al. ^{18}F-FDG PET/CT and 3.0 T whole-body MRI for the detection of distant metastases and second primary tumours in patients with untreated oropharyngeal/hypopharyngeal carcinoma: a comparative study. Eur J Nucl Med Mol Imaging 2011;38:1607–19.

11. Gourin CG, Terris DJ. Carcinoma of the hypopharynx. Surg Oncol Clin N Am 2004;13:81–98.

12. Ho CM, Lam KH, Wei WI, et al. Squamous cell carcinoma of the hypopharynx—analysis of treatment results. Head Neck 1993;15:405–12.

13. Ho CM, Ng WF, Lam KH, et al. Submucosal tumor extension in hypopharyngeal cancer. Arch Otolaryngol Head Neck Surg 1997;123:959–65.

14. Hsu WC, Loevner LA, Karpati R, et al. Accuracy of magnetic resonance imaging in predicting absence of fixation of head and neck cancer to the prevertebral space. Head Neck 2005;27:95–100.

15. Loevner LA, Ott IL, Yousem DM, et al. Neoplastic fixation to the prevertebral compartment by squamous cell carcinoma of the head and neck. AJR Am J Roentgenol 1998;170:1389–94.

16. Schmalfuss IM, Mancuso AA, Tart RP. Postcricoid region and cervical esophagus: normal appearance at CT and MR Imaging. Radiology 2000;213:237–46.

17. Hoffman HT, Karnell LH, Shah JP, et al. Hypopharyngeal cancer patient care evaluation. Laryngoscope 1997;107:1005–17.

18. Wei WI. The dilemma of treating hypopharyngeal carcinoma: more or less. Arch Otolaryngol Head Neck Surg 2002;128:229–32.

19. Pfister DG, Hu KS, Lefebvre JL. Chapter 17. Cancer of the hypopharynx and cervical esophagus. In: Harrison LB, Sessions RB, Hong WK, editors. Head and neck cancer. 3rd edition. Philadelphia: Lippincott Williams & Wilkins; 2009. p. 397–435.

20. Genden EM, Desai S, Sung CK. Transoral robotic surgery for the management of head and neck cancer: a preliminary experience. Head Neck 2009;31:283–9.

21. Machiels JP, Schmitz S. Molecular-targeted therapy of head and neck squamous cell carcinoma: beyond cetuximab-based therapy. Curr Opin Oncol 2011; 23:241–8.

22. Fatterpekar GM, Galheigo D, Narayana A, et al. Treatment-related change versus tumor recurrence in high-grade gliomas: a diagnostic conundrum—use of dynamic susceptibility contrast-enhanced (DSC) perfusion MRI. AJR Am J Roentgenol 2012; 198:19–26.

Pitfalls in the Staging of Cancer of the Laryngeal Squamous Cell Carcinoma

Kristen L. Baugnon, MD[a],*, Jonathan J. Beitler, MD, MBA[b]

KEYWORDS

- Squamous cell carcinoma • Larynx • Intensity-modulated radiation therapy

KEY POINTS

- Laryngeal carcinoma is a devastating malignancy that severely affects patients' quality of life, with compromise of ability to talk, breathe, and swallow.
- Accurate tumor staging is imperative, because treatment plans focus on laryngeal conservation therapy whenever possible.
- Although the mucosal extent of tumor and vocal cord mobility is best assessed with endoscopic evaluation, cross-sectional imaging is essential for accurate T-staging, because only cross-sectional imaging can assess the submucosal extent of the tumor, cartilage invasion, and extralaryngeal spread.
- This article reviews topics crucial for interpreting imaging studies of patients with laryngeal squamous cell carcinoma.

Laryngeal carcinoma is a devastating malignancy that severely affects patients' quality of life, with compromise of ability to talk, breathe, and swallow. Accurate tumor staging is imperative, because treatment plans focus on laryngeal conservation therapy, whenever possible. Although the mucosal extent of tumor and vocal cord mobility is best assessed with endoscopic evaluation, cross-sectional imaging is essential for accurate T-staging, because only cross-sectional imaging can assess the submucosal extent of the tumor, cartilage invasion, and extralaryngeal spread. This article reviews topics crucial for interpreting imaging studies of patients with laryngeal squamous cell carcinoma (SCC).

EPIDEMIOLOGY OF LARYNGEAL SCC

The incidence of laryngeal SCC ranges from 0.3 to 9.8 per 100,000 people annually and represents approximately 1% to 2% of all adult malignancies. Men are affected 3 times more frequently than women, and incidence increases with advancing age, with the median age at diagnosis of 65 years, from 2004 to 2008.[1]

The patient population is similar to that affected by lung cancer, with a strong association with smoking and alcohol use in up to 95% of patients, and reported increased incidence in patients of low socioeconomic status.[2] Other potential risk factors for laryngeal carcinoma include passive tobacco smoke exposure, occupational exposure to chemical irritants, chronic irritation caused by reflux, and possibly viral exposure (see later). Nonsmokers with laryngeal SCC are uncommon but tend to be older and the primary subsite is more often glottis, compared with smokers with SCC.[3]

Laryngeal neoplasms are associated with human papillovirus (HPV) infection, particularly

[a] Department of Radiology and Imaging Sciences, Emory University School of Medicine, BG-32, 1364 Clifton Road Northeast, Atlanta, GA 30322, USA; [b] Department of Radiation Oncology, Winship Cancer Institute, Emory University School of Medicine, 1701 Uppergate Drive, Atlanta, GA 30322, USA
* Corresponding author.
E-mail address: kmlloyd@emory.edu

Neuroimag Clin N Am 23 (2013) 81–105
http://dx.doi.org/10.1016/j.nic.2012.08.008

with benign laryngeal papillomatosis, most often associated with the low-risk HPV subtypes, HPV 6 and 11. Patients with laryngeal papillomatosis have an approximately 2% risk of developing laryngeal malignancy, particularly if the patient is diagnosed as an adult.[4] The association of HPV infection with the development of SCC has not been well established, and this contrasts with oropharyngeal cancers, in which the clinical significance of and association with the development of SCC and HPV infection have been well documented. There is a broad range of prevalence of HPV infection in laryngeal carcinoma in the literature, present in up to 25% of patients on meta-analysis, with malignancy most commonly associated with the high-risk subtypes 16 and 18. However, the clinical significance and implication of these infections are unclear at this time and require further investigation.[5]

ANATOMY AND BOUNDARIES OF THE LARYNX

The larynx is a mucosa-lined tube that is responsible for phonation and airway protection. The laryngeal structural framework is composed of the thyroid, cricoid, and arytenoid cartilages; ligaments connecting the cartilaginous framework; and a series of 7 separate paired intrinsic laryngeal muscles, surrounded by fat-containing spaces and lined internally by squamous epithelial mucosa.

The superior border of the larynx is the free edge of the epiglottis, dividing it from the oropharynx, and the inferior extent is to the lower border of the cricoid cartilage. Posteriorly, the larynx is separated from the hypopharynx by the aryepiglottic (AE) folds. The larynx is divided into supraglottic, glottic, and infraglottic (or subglottic) components (Fig. 1A).

The supraglottic larynx extends from the tip of the epiglottis (lingual and laryngeal surfaces) and AE folds superiorly to the apex of the laryngeal ventricle (see Fig. 1B, C). The supraglottic larynx can be subdivided into suprahyoid and infrahyoid regions, divided by the hyoid bone, and the suprahyoid epiglottis contains the free edge of the epiglottis. The petiole of the epiglottis is another term for the base of the infrahyoid epiglottis, at its attachment with the thyroid cartilage (overlying the thyroepiglottic ligament) (Fig. 2A). The subsites of the supraglottic larynx, therefore, include the epiglottis (suprahyoid and infrahyoid components), the AE folds, the arytenoids, and the false vocal cords.[6] The AE folds sweep down laterally from the epiglottis and extend to the arytenoid cartilages, and contain 2 small prominences,

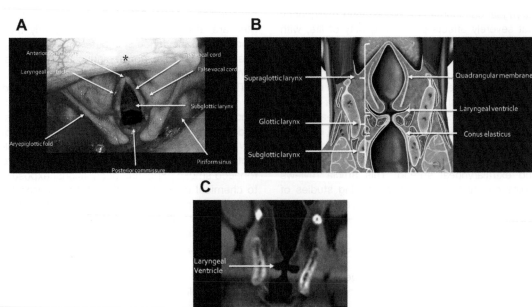

Fig. 1. Normal larynx anatomy. (A) Endoscopic view of normal larynx. Asterisk denotes the epiglottis. Note the relationship of the larynx to the hypopharynx (piriform sinus). (B) Coronal illustration of the larynx, showing the division into supraglottic, glottic, and subglottic larynx. (C) Coronal CE-CT scan dividing the larynx into supraglottic, glottic, and subglottic larynx. Division between supraglottic and glottic larynx is at the apex of the lateral ventricle. Glottic larynx is the extent of the true vocal cords (1 cm anteriorly, and 5 mm posteriorly). (*Courtesy of* Eric Jablonowski.)

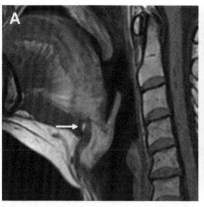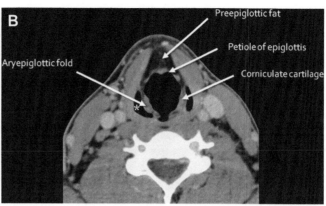

Fig. 2. Supraglottic larynx. (*A*) Mid-sagittal T1-weighted image of a normal supraglottic larynx. The hyoid bone (*arrow*) divides the epiglottis into a suprahyoid and infrahyoid portion. (*B*) Axial CE-CT through the levels of the AE folds, as they extend toward the arytenoid cartilage (not shown). The AE folds separate the larynx from the hypopharynx (piriform sinuses). The small protruberances along the medial AE folds overlie the corniculate cartilage.

which denote the location of the cuneiform and corniculate cartilages. The corniculate cartilage may be seen on imaging perched on top of the arytenoid cartilage; however, the cuneiform cartilage is often too small to resolve (see **Fig. 2**B).[7] The lateral aspect of the AE folds forms the medial wall of the piriform sinus, actually part of the hypopharynx. On axial cross-sectional imaging, the false vocal cords are at the level of the adjacent paraglottic fat (**Fig. 3**A). The interarytenoid space forms the posterior border of the larynx, dividing it from the hypopharynx.

The glottic larynx is composed of the true vocal folds, extending from the apex of the lateral ventricle (the inferior boundary of the supraglottic larynx and the superior margin of the true vocal fold) to the inferior margin of the true vocal folds (the beginning of the subglottic larynx). The glottis should be an area 1 cm in height, extending caudal to the plane of the mid ventricle (see **Fig. 1**B, C). The subsites of the glottic larynx include the anterior and posterior commissures and the right and left true vocal cords.

Histologically, the vocal fold has a surface of stratified squamous epithelium, and beneath the epithelium is the lamina propria, formed of 3 layers. The most superficial layer, Reinke space, can be crucial for transoral laser resections. Beneath Reinke space are the intermediate and deep layers of the lamina propria, which make up the vocal ligament. The true vocal cord is made up of the epithelial layer, Reinke space, the vocal ligament (a thin fibrous band medially within the free margin of the vocal fold, extending the full length of the cord from the vocal process of the arytenoid cartilage to the anterior commissure), and the thyroarytenoid muscle, which also forms the vocalis muscle medially. The anterior commissure is the site of attachment of the vocal ligaments to the thyroid cartilage, via Broyles ligament. The area of anterior attachment is devoid of perichondrium and relatively vulnerable to early cartilaginous invasion.[7] The posterior commissure is the posterior space between the vocal cords, at the vocal process of each arytenoid cartilage.

On axial cross-sectional imaging, the true vocal cord level is identified by the lack of adjacent submucosal fat and the presence of all 3 cartilages (thyroid, cricoid, and vocal process of the arytenoid cartilages) in 1 cross-sectional image (see **Fig. 3**B).

The subglottic larynx extends from the inferior margin of the true vocal cord (approximately 1 cm below the laryngeal ventricle anteriorly), through the inferior border of the cricoid cartilage (see **Fig. 1**B, C). On axial cross-sectional imaging, the immediate subglottic mucosa is usually smooth, thin, and symmetric, without any significant soft tissue between the cricoid cartilage and the air column (see **Fig. 2**C). Any abnormal soft tissue in the subglottic lumen should raise the possibility of tumor extension. Subglottic tumor is difficult to assess endoscopically and is important for the radiologist to detect, because it will impact treatment planning and prognosis.

The preepiglottic space is a pyramid-shaped (in the sagittal plane) or C-shaped (in the axial plane), fat-containing, potential space anterior to the epiglottis, extending superiorly to the hyoid bone. It is bordered posteriorly by the infrahyoid epiglottis and anteriorly by the thyrohyoid membrane and anterior and superior lamina of the thyroid cartilage. Cranially, the preepiglottic space is bounded by the hyoepiglottic ligament and

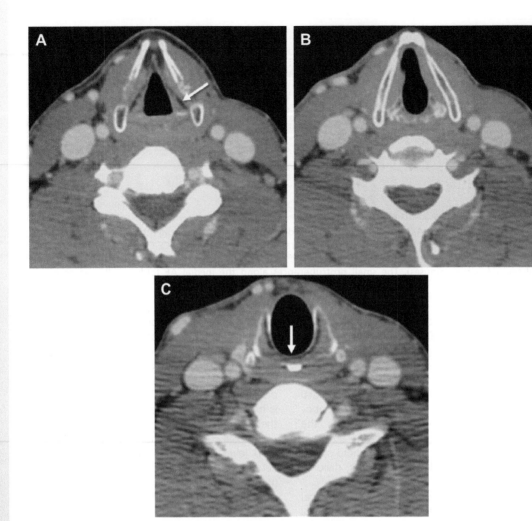

Fig. 3. Axial larynx anatomy. (*A*) Normal axial CE-CT of the larynx at the level of the false vocal cords. Note the paraglottic fat (*arrow*). (*B*) Normal axial CE-CT of the larynx at the level of the true vocal cords. Despite slight volume averaging through the laryngeal ventricle on the right, one can appreciate the linearity of the TVCs, the absence of paraglottic fat, and can see all 3 cartilages on one axial image. (*C*) Normal axial CE-CT of the larynx at the level of the subglottic larynx. Note the normal absence of endoluminal soft tissue at the level of the cricoid cartilage (*arrow*).

caudally by the petiole of the epiglottis. Inferiorly and laterally, the preepiglottic space is contiguous with the paraglottic space. Both spaces are important potential paths of submucosal tumor spread from both laryngeal and oropharyngeal tumors and cannot be identified on clinical examination, and involvement by tumor will upstage the lesion. Although this space can easily be seen in the axial plane, the preepiglottic space is best evaluated in the sagittal plane, on both reformatted contrast-enhanced computed tomography (CE-CT) and sagittal T1-weighted magnetic resonance (MR) imaging (**Fig. 4**).

The paraglottic space is a paired, fat-filled potential space, between the mucosa and laryngeal cartilage framework, and is contiguous superiorly

with the preepiglottic space. The paraglottic space is mostly fat containing at the level of the supraglottis, surrounding the laryngeal ventricle, and contains the thyroarytenoid (or vocalis) muscle at the level of the glottis, with a thin sliver of fat laterally deep to the thyroid cartilage. The paraglottic space can be seen in the axial plane but is seen better in the coronal plane on both CT reformations and MR imaging (**Fig. 5**).

Two thin fibrous structures, the quadrangular membrane and the conus elasticus, are not resolved on imaging but dictate the pattern of tumor spread (see **Fig. 1**B). The medial border of the paraglottic space is formed by the quadrangular membrane, a thin fibrous structure just beneath the mucosa of the supraglottic larynx, which gives

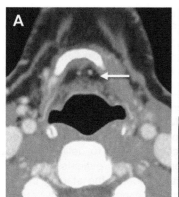
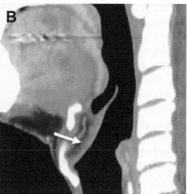
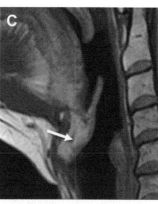

Fig. 4. Preepiglottic space. Axial CE-CT (A), sagittal CE-CT (B), and sagittal T1-weighted MR imaging (C) demonstrating the fatty preepiglottic space (*arrow*) that normally contains vascular structures and lymphatics.

support to the AE fold, and the conus elasticus inferiorly at the glottis and sublottic level, a thicker fibrous layer that extends inferiorly from the vocal ligament of the true cord and attaches along the upper inner margin of the cricoid cartilage, which becomes the cricothyroid membrane anteriorly.[7]

The thyroid cartilage is a triangular shield-shaped cartilage made of paired edges called the thyroid ala, which may or may not be fused anteriorly. It is connected to the hyoid bone by the thyrohyoid membrane, through which the paired external laryngeal arteries and nerves pierce laterally to provide sensation to the supraglottic larynx for airway protection. The cricoid cartilage is a round, ring-shaped cartilage inferior to the thyroid cartilage, separated from the thyroid cartilage by the cricothyroid membrane. The cricoid is the only complete cartilaginous ring in the airway, is much thicker posteriorly, and provides the foundation for the larynx. The paired arytenoid cartilages are triangular in shape and articulate with the cricoid cartilage via the cricoarytenoid joint, a synovial joint. The vocal process of the arytenoid attaches to the true vocal cord, and its mobility is necessary for phonation.[7]

The thyroid, cricoid, and arytenoid cartilages are made of varying amounts of ossified and nonossified hyaline cartilage. Ossified cartilage appears similar to bone on CT, with a peripheral hyperdense

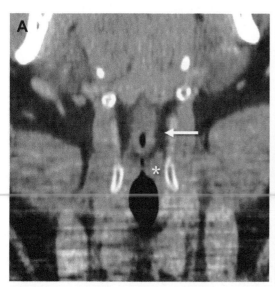
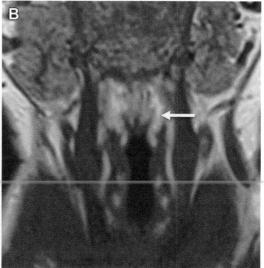

Fig. 5. Paraglottic space. Coronal CE-CT (A) and T1-weighted (B) images demonstrating the fat containing paraglottic space at the level of the supraglottic larynx, wrapping around the lateral aspect of the thyroarytenoid muscle at the true vocal cord (*asterisk*).

cortex and central hypodense medullary cavity, whereas nonossified bone has an appearance of soft tissue. On MR imaging, ossified cartilage is hypointense peripherally on all sequences (similar to cortical bone), with the medullary cavity similar to fat on all sequences. Conversely, nonossified hyaline cartilage appears intermediate to low signal on both T1- and T2-weighted sequences. On MR imaging, there should be no postcontrast enhancement within the medullary cavity of either ossified or nonossifed cartilage. The trend is toward increased cartilage ossification with advancing age; however, these findings are extremely variable and irregular, often making determination of laryngeal cartilage erosion or penetration by adjacent tumor difficult, particularly on CT (Fig. 6). The epiglottis and vocal process of the arytenoid are composed of yellow fibrocartilage and do not ossify.[8]

LYMPHATIC DRAINAGE

There is often significant and bilateral supraglottic lymphatic drainage to the high jugular nodes (levels II and III).[9] Rarely, supraglottic neoplasms can involve submandibular and retropharyngeal nodes. The subglottic larynx initially may also drain in a cephalad direction, and a characteristic lymph node draining the subglottic region is the node anterior to the cricothyroid membrane, the delphian node (Fig. 7). However, the low subglottic lymphatics drain to the paratracheal and pretracheal lymph nodes (level VI). There is almost no lymphatic drainage of the submucosa of the true vocal cord, but once tumor infiltrates the preepiglottic or paraglottic spaces, there is a higher likelihood of nodal disease.[7,10]

American Joint Commission on Cancer Staging and Changes from the 6th Edition to the 7th Edition

Clinically, tumors are staged by the tumor-nodes-metastasis (TNM) staging system, a classification system developed by the American Joint Committee on Cancer and used to define treatment and quantify prognosis for patients. The committee periodically updates the staging system, taking into account changes in clinical practice, and the new 7th edition has been in effect since January 1, 2010. Although staging is done primarily via laryngoscopy, imaging is important in staging the deep extent of tumor and nodal and distant disease. Refer to Table 1 for the most recent TNM staging for laryngeal SCC (Table 1).[6]

The primary change in staging of laryngeal carcinoma is the division of T4 lesions into T4a (resectable lesions, with cartilage penetration and/or extralaryngeal spread of tumor) and T4b (unresectable lesions, invading prevertebral space, encasing carotid artery, or invading the mediastinum), leading to development of stage IVA (any T4a primary or any N2 nodal disease), stage IVB (any T4b), and stage IVC (any M1). Additionally, there has been clarification of cartilage involvement and T4 disease. Prior staging systems were vague with regard to cartilage involvement, because patients with *any* cartilage involvement were potentially overstaged as T4 and underwent laryngectomy. With the current staging system, tumors involving only the inner cortex of thyroid

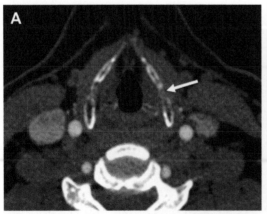
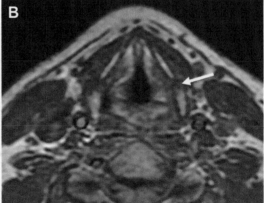

Fig. 6. Thyroid cartilage. Heterogeneous ossification of normal thyroid cartilage on axial CE-CT (*A*) and axial T1-weighted MR imaging (*B*). Note the hypodense fatty marrow (T1 hyperintense), with surrounding hyperdense cortical sclerosis and the intermediate soft tissue density and intensity cartilage. The anterior thyroid ala are often not well ossified.

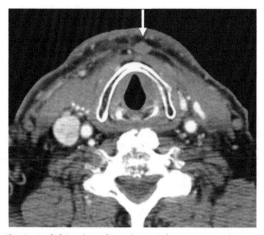

Fig. 7. Delphian lymph node. Axial CE-CT scan demonstrating a small pathologic delphian (prelaryngeal) lymph node, anterior to the cricoid cartilage, which was hypermetabolic on the concordant PET examination (not shown). Note the posttreatment changes from prior radiation therapy in the neck.

cartilage (previously termed "minor cartilage erosion") are classified as T3, but through-and-through cartilage penetration (both inner and outer cortex involvement) and/or extralaryngeal tumor spread are classified as T4a.[1]

TREATMENT TRENDS

The major focus in the management of laryngeal cancer is voice retention. This is precluded when the larynx is functionless or there is aspiration despite working with a speech pathologist. Classic voice preservation operations are the open supraglottic laryngectomy (reserved for those patients with only supraglottic involvement) and the vertical hemilaryngectomy (reserved for patients with lesions predominantly involving one true vocal cord). However, in the past 10 years, there has been a significant decline in the use of open surgery, primarily because of the development of transoral endoscopic laser microsurgery, improvements in radiation therapy, and new combined modality chemotherapy and radiation therapy regimens. Oncologic results, both local control and survival results, are similar to more conventional open surgeries, however, with less morbidity and, overall, improved postoperative function and laryngeal preservation rates. In general, open surgery is now primarily reserved for those patients with persistent or recurrent disease post therapy or for those patients with bulky extralaryngeal extension or cartilage invasion on initial presentation.[11] Specific treatment trends are further discussed with regard to the laryngeal site of involvement.

Site-Specific Evaluation with Imaging

General considerations/pitfalls

The larynx is one of the most difficult organs to image, because the structures are small, it is subject to motion from respiration and swallowing, and early mucosal lesions are difficult to resolve on imaging. Performing thin section images through the larynx (both CT and MR imaging), making every effort to suspend swallowing, and angling the gantry through the plane of the larynx can help with these limitations. Additionally, on CE-CT, delayed imaging after contrast may help improve mucosal enhancement to aid in delineating the extent of tumor.

One of the greatest pitfalls in staging any head and neck cancer is either overstaging or understaging tumors. In the larynx, overstaging may result in unnecessary laryngectomy; however, understaging can result in local treatment failure after radiation (**Table 2**). A study in 2008 demonstrated a false diagnosis rate for detecting the extent of supraglottic laryngeal cancers, and up to 25% of the time, the tumor was overstaged by imaging.[12,13] Becoming familiar with the American Joint Committee on Cancer staging system for the different subsites and the common patterns of spread of laryngeal cancer and pitfalls associated with staging will help the radiologist to avoid these mistakes.

Supraglottic SCC

Because they are initially clinically occult, supraglottic tumors often present later than glottic tumors and are often large. As with other early laryngeal lesions, the T1 and T2 lesions are often best staged with endoscopy. However, imaging is critical for showing the cranial, caudal, and deep extension of supraglottic SCC. Patterns of extension can be anticipated by knowing common pathways of spread.

Small tumors involving the free edge of the epiglottis may be treated with endoscopic surgery, with conservation of a portion of the supraglottic larynx. However, the radiologist must assess the full extent of the tumor and detect submucosal extension. Superior extension with involvement of the vallecula or base of tongue is extremely important to note, because it will upstage to T2 and will likely alter management. Tumor may reach the base of tongue, and even the extrinsic tongue muscles via extension through the preepiglottic space (**Fig. 8**). Spread anteriorly along the glossoepiglottic fold, which overlies the hyoepiglottic ligament, results in extension to the vallecula and base of tongue.

Tumors can extend from the suprahyoid epiglottis laterally along the pharyngoepiglottic fold

Table 1
American Joint Committee on Cancer 7 larynx staging

	Primary Tumor (T)
TX	Primary tumor cannot be assessed
T0	No evidence of primary tumor
Tis	Carcinoma in situ
	Supraglottis
T1	Tumor limited to one subsite of supraglottis with normal vocal cord mobility
T2	Tumor invades mucosa of more than one adjacent subsite of supraglottis or glottis or region outside the supraglottis (eg, mucosa of base of tongue, vallecula, medial wall of pyriformsinus) without fixation of the larynx
T3	Tumor limited to larynx with vocal cord fixation and/or invades any of the following: postcricoid area, pre-epiglottic space, paraglottic space, and/or inner cortex of thyroid cartilage
T4a	Moderately advanced local disease. Tumor invades through the thyroid cartilage and/or invades tissues beyond the larynx (eg, trachea, soft tissues of neck including deep extrinsic muscle of the tongue, strap muscles, thyroid, or esophagus)
T4b	Very advanced local disease. Tumor invades prevertebral space, encases carotid artery, or invades mediastinal structures
	Glottis
T1	Tumor limited to the vocal cord(s) (may involve anterior or posterior commissure) with normal mobility
T1a	Tumor limited to one vocal cord
T1b	Tumor involves both vocal cords
T2	Tumor extends to supraglottis and/or subglottis, and/or with impaired vocal cord mobility
T3	Tumor limited to the larynx with vocal cord fixation and/or invasion of paraglottic space, and/or inner cortex of the thyroid cartilage
T4a	Moderately advanced local disease. Tumor invades through the outer cortex of the thyroid cartilage and/or invades tissues beyond the larynx (eg, trachea, soft tissues of neck including deep extrinsic muscle of the tongue, strap muscles, thyroid, or esophagus)
T4b	Very advanced local disease. Tumor invades prevertebral space, encases carotid artery, or invades mediastinal structures
	Subglottis
T1	Tumor limited to the subglottis
T2	Tumor extends to vocal cord(s) with normal or impaired mobility
T3	Tumor limited to larynx with vocal cord fixation
T4a	Moderately advanced local disease. Tumor invades cricoid or thyroid cartilage and/or invades tissues beyond the larynx (eg, trachea, soft tissues of neck including deep extrinsic muscles of the tongue, strap muscles, thyroid, or esophagus)
T4b	Very advanced local disease. Tumor invades prevertebral space, encases carotid artery, or invades mediastinal structures
	Regional Lymph Nodes (N)
NX	Regional lymph nodes cannot be assessed
N0	No regional lymph node metastasis
N1	Metastasis in a single ipsilateral lymph node, 3 cm or less in greatest dimension
N2	Metastasis in a single ipsilateral lymph node, more than 3 cm but not more than 6 cm in greatest dimension; or in multiple ipsilateral lymph nodes, none more than 6 cm in greatest dimension; or in bilateral or contralateral lymph nodes, none more than 6 cm in greatest dimension
N2a	Metastasis in single ipsilateral lymph node more than 3 cm but not more than 6 cm in greatest dimension
N2b	Metastasis in multiple ipsilateral lymph nodes, none more than 6 cm in greatest dimension
N2c	Metastasis in bilateral or contralateral lymph nodes, none more than 6 cm in greatest dimension
N3	Metastasis in a lymph node more than 6 cm in greatest dimension
	Distant Metastasis (M)
M0	No distant metastasis
M1	Distant metastasis

Table 2
Pitfalls in staging of larynx cancers

Pitfall	Advice
Understaging of a T2 supraglottic tumor as a T1 from failure to recognize BOT extension.	Carefully evaluate the BOT and vallecula on sagittal images.
Understaging from failure to recognize paraglottic space involvement	Look for replacement of the fat just above and lateral to the thyroarytenoid muscle on axial and coronal images
Overstaging of cartilage invasion on CT	Recognize that there is considerable variability and asymmetry in cartilage ossification on CT. Consider MR imaging for further evaluation.
Overstaging of cartilage invasion and extralaryngeal extension on MR imaging	Look for areas isointense in signal to the tumor on T1-, T2-, and fat-suppressed T2-weighted images. Reactive edema will be T2 hyperintense to tumor.
Failure to recognize extralaryngeal tumor extension without laryngeal penetration	Carefully evaluate the thyroid notch, thyrohyoid membrane, and thyroaretenoid gaps. Consider MR imaging for further evaluation.
Understaging of nodal metastasis by PET-CT	Use intravenous CE-CT along with the PET to evaluate for small abnormal lymph nodes that may be below the resolution of PET or have low FDG uptake as a result of necrosis.

to reach the lateral pharyngeal wall. If there is greater than 2 cm of involvement of the base of tongue, the patient may no longer be a candidate for a supraglottic laryngectomy.[7] Additionally, a patient with any advanced laryngeal tumor (T3 or T4) with greater than 1 cm of extension to the base of tongue may not be considered a candidate for laryngeal conservation therapy,[14] and in the event that the patient is undergoing a total laryngectomy, tumor at the base of tongue will require a more extensive resection, possibly a glossectomy, and reconstruction of the neopharynx.

Both suprahyoid and infrahyoid supraglottic tumors are at risk for involvement of the preepiglottic space, because the epiglottis is a poor barrier to tumor spread. Submucosal involvement of the preepiglottic space by tumor cannot be assessed clinically and involvement will upstage a tumor to T3 status. Preepiglottic space spread is associated with a worse prognosis after radiation and an increased risk of nodal metastasis. Although not precluding a supraglottic laryngectomy, involvement of the preepiglottic space may alter the surgical approach, because the surgeon would likely also apply treatment to the neck. Infiltration of the fat within the preepiglottic space is easy to detect on both CT and T1-weighted MR imaging, in both the axial and sagittal plane, with a reported sensitivity of 100% (**Fig. 9**).[15]

Supraglottic laryngeal tumors that involved the AE folds or false cords may extend inferiorly to cross the laryngeal ventricle, becoming "transglottic" tumors. The inferior margin of tumor extension is the most critical for the surgeon considering a voice-conserving partial supraglottic laryngectomy, because tumor cannot involve the ventricle, more than 1 arytenoid, the interarytenoid region, or the anterior commissure. Additionally, glottic tumors can spread cranially, crossing the ventricle, to become a transglottic tumor, which precludes vertical hemilaryngectomy.[7] Therefore, the radiologist staging a primary laryngeal malignancy must closely evaluate the status of the laryngeal ventricle, with coronal images often aiding in determining tumor relationship to the laryngeal ventricle (**Fig. 10**).

If tumor at the ventricle obstructs outflow of the saccule, a small appendage of the anterior aspect of the laryngeal ventricle, it can cause an air-filled laryngocele or saccular cyst, a laryngocele filled with retained secretions. Laryngoceles have been reported to be associated with laryngeal cancer from 5% to 29% of the time.[16] When a laryngocele is present on imaging, the region of the laryngeal ventricle must be carefully evaluated (**Fig. 11**).

Paraglottic space involvement will also upstage tumors to T3, and because of involvement of the thyroarytenoid muscle are often associated with vocal cord paresis or paralysis. Tumor infiltration of the paraglottic space carries a lower response to radiation therapy alone for local control. In fact, a study by Murakami and colleagues[17] in 2005 described deep paraglottic space invasion with the "adjacent sign," a broad interface with the thyroid cartilage, with or without minor inner

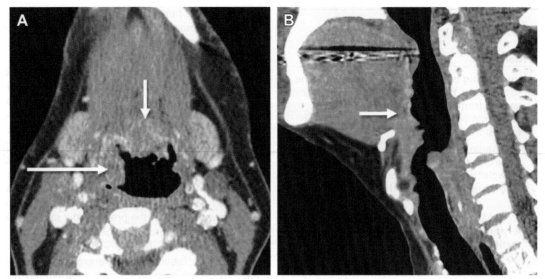

Fig. 8. Supraglottic tumor involving base of tongue. Axial (*A*) and sagittal (*B*) CE-CT scans of a large supraglottic tumor involving the epiglottis and preepiglottic space and extending to involve the right lateral oropharyngeal wall (*long arrow*) and base of tongue (*short arrow*).

cortex erosion, as an independent prognostic factor, heralding lower rates of local control and overall survival rates. Similar to preepiglottic space involvement, tumors in the paraglottic space have a greater risk of transglottic spread and increased risk of cervical nodal metastasis.[10] Axial and coronal imaging demonstrating tumor within the fat just above and lateral to the thyroarytenoid muscle is the characteristic appearance of paraglottic tumor (see **Fig. 10**).

Epiglottic midline tumors may easily extend along the laryngeal surface of the epiglottis to involve the anterior commissure. Involvement of the anterior commissure is frequently associated with early cartilage invasion as a result of extension along Broyle ligament, as well as extralaryngeal spread through the thyrohyoid and cricothyroid membranes. Previously, this was thought to be the overwhelming pattern of extralaryngeal spread, but recent analysis suggests that transthyroid cartilage spread occurs in only 44% of cases with extralaryngeal tumor.[2] Patterns of extralaryngeal spread will be discussed later. Once a tumor extends to the anterior commissure, the

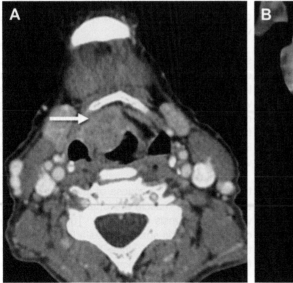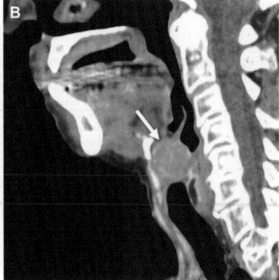

Fig. 9. Axial (*A*) and sagittal (*B*) CE-CT scans of a T3 supraglottic tumor originating in the infrahyoid epiglottis, extending along the right AE fold, with invasion of the right preepiglottic space (*arrow*).

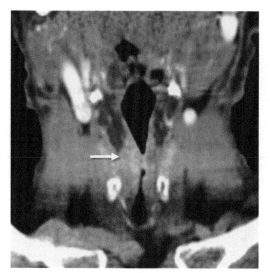

Fig. 10. Coronal CE-CT scan showing a transglottic tumor spanning the right laryngeal ventricle, involving the right false and true vocal cords, and extending into the right paraglottic space (*arrow*).

patient is no longer a candidate for supraglottic laryngectomy, because a 2- to 3-mm separation between tumor and the anterior commissure is necessary to perform that voice-sparing surgery.[7] Axial CT scans through the larynx should be in the plane of the true vocal folds to optimize visualization of these regions (**Fig. 12**).

Subglottic extension is often much better seen on imaging than via laryngoscopy. As described previously, any soft tissue within the airway at the level of the cricoid cartilage should be

concerning for subglottic tumor. The conus elasticus, a thick membrane extending from the free edge of the true vocal cord to the upper margin of the cricoid cartilage, acts as a relative barrier to subglottic extension of tumor, with tumor diverted laterally and anteriorly through the cricothyroid membrane. However, once tumor violates this membrane and extends into the subglottic larynx (at the level of the cricoid ring), there is increased risk for cricoid cartilage erosion.[18] The extent of subglottic disease from the level of the true vocal cords is best assessed in the coronal plane, recalling that the subglottis begins at a level approximately 1 cm below the level of the ventricle, anteriorly (**Fig. 13**).

Cartilage invasion

Detecting cartilage invasion is perhaps the greatest pitfall in laryngeal cancer imaging, and for that reason, much of the conventional radiologic literature discussing laryngeal cancer staging focuses on cartilage invasion. Cartilage invasion by tumor upstages the lesion to at least T3, if not T4a, depending on whether there is full penetration through both the inner and outer cortices. The conventional teaching is that invasion of the cartilage is generally associated with a lower response rate to radiation therapy, with a higher risk of recurrence, and a higher risk of radiation-associated chondronecrosis, which can ultimately lead to a nonfunctional larynx. Thus, historically, patients with only minor cartilage invasion previously underwent laryngectomy. The larynx preservation consensus panel in 2009 recommended that patients with cartilage penetration or

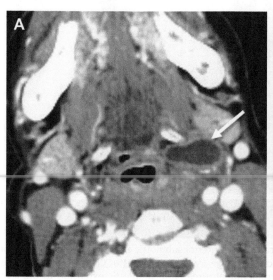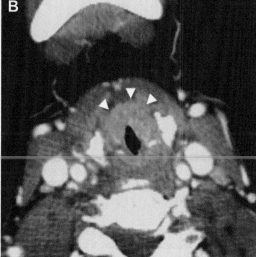

Fig. 11. Axial CE-CT scans showing a left-sided external laryngocele (saccular cyst) (*arrow* in *A*) associated with bilateral true vocal cord and anterior commissure tumor, with transglottic tumor extension (*arrowheads* in *B*).

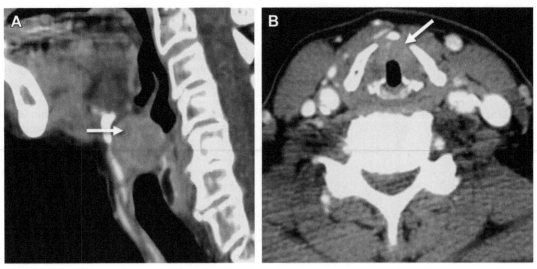

Fig. 12. Sagittal (*A*) and axial (*B*) CE-CT scans showing a supraglottic tumor involving the preepiglottic space (*arrow* in *A*) and extending inferiorly to involve the anterior commissure (*arrow* in *B*).

transcartilaginous extralaryngeal spread of tumor are not candidates for larynx preservation and therefore require initial surgical laryngectomy.[19] In turn, in the absence of frank cartilage penetration or bulky extralaryngeal tumor, laryngeal conservation therapies should be initial treatment. Although still important for staging purposes, and in the assessment of patients who may be a candidate for partial laryngeal resections or laser surgery, the imaging focus should be on determining extralaryngeal extension and frank

cartilage penetration because laryngeal conservation may hinge on those findings.

Another reason that emphasis has been placed on cartilage invasion in the radiology literature is that it is very difficult to assess. There is extensive variability in the degree of cartilage ossification, and focal areas of apparent "erosion" of the cartilage on CT may merely be areas of asymmetric nonossified cartilage. Reactive changes (ie, edema) may occur within adjacent cartilage, without intramedullary tumor invasion, which can cause

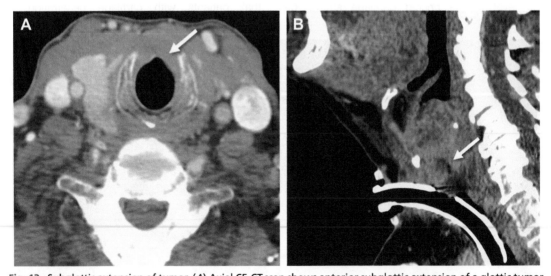

Fig. 13. Subglottic extension of tumor. (*A*) Axial CE-CT scan shows anterior subglottic extension of a glottic tumor. Note the soft tissue anteriorly at the level of the cricoid cartilage (*arrow*). (*B*) Sagittal CE-CT scan of another patient demonstrates a large transglottic SCC with extralaryngeal spread and subglottic extension to the level of a tracheostomy tube (*arrow*). Placement of a tracheostomy tube through tumor increases the risk of parastomal recurrence after laryngectomy.

both sclerosis on CT and T2 hyperintensity on MR imaging. Both CT and MR imaging have limitations in assessment of laryngeal cartilage, with a study from 1995 demonstrating that CT overall seemingly underestimated neoplastic cartilage invasion and MR imaging overestimated cartilage invasion.[20]

CT findings that have been associated with possible cartilage involvement include sclerosis, erosion (focal osteolysis), lysis (more extensive osteolysis), and extralaryngeal tumor extension (cartilage penetration). *Cartilage sclerosis*, initially thought to be a sensitive sign for cartilaginous tumoral involvement, has been found to have a low specificity (40% in the thyroid cartilage, increasing to 76% and 79% in the cricoids and arytenoid cartilages) as a result of the high likelihood of reactive edema and inflammatory change within the adjacent cartilages.[21] Therefore, sclerosis can be caused by tumor adjacent to, but not frankly invading, cartilage.[7] Focal *erosion or lysis* of the adjacent cartilage does increase specificity up to 93%; however, detection of subtle or early erosion is difficult, particularly in the setting of incomplete ossification of cartilage, and focal erosion of the inner cortex still would not upstage from a T3 primary tumor. The most specific finding of cartilage involvement on CT is adjacent *extralaryngeal tumor* extension, with up to 95% specificity (**Fig. 14**).[21] However, CT is only 49% sensitive for the detection of extralaryngeal spread, and in up to 40% of cases, extralaryngeal spread of tumor can be seen in the absence of frank cartilage penetration.[13]

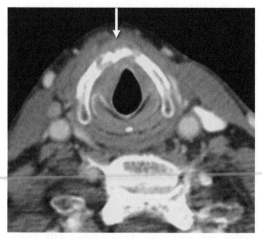

Fig. 14. Axial CE-CT demonstrating sclerosis and lysis of cartilage, with frank cartilage penetration and transcartilaginous extralaryngeal extension. Tumor on the other side of cartilage (*arrow*) is the most specific sign of cartilage involvement.

MR imaging has been reported to be more sensitive for pretreatment determination of laryngeal cartilage involvement. Initial studies demonstrated that peritumoral inflammation and reactive changes causing T2 hyperintensity within the cartilage led to overstaging. However, recent reassessment of imaging criteria for cartilaginous involvement by Becker and colleagues[22] in 2008 demonstrated significantly increased accuracy when describing cartilage involvement based on soft tissue within the cartilage being similar in signal, on both T1- and T2-weighted images, and enhancement to the adjacent tumor (**Fig. 15**). Fat-suppressed T2-weighted images are important to help differentiate tumor from the adjacent fat-containing medullary space. Edema has generally been thought to be higher in signal intensity on the T2-weighted images than the adjacent tumor, whereas frank tumor involvement should be similar in signal to the adjacent tumor on T2-weighted imaging (**Fig. 16**). Additionally, gadolinium-enhanced images through the larynx should be obtained with fat suppression, and any abnormal enhancing soft tissue within the medullary space, similar in signal and enhancement to the tumor, should be considered tumor extension. In summary, current MR criteria for cartilage invasion is that soft tissue in the cartilage should be isointense to the laryngeal component of the tumor on T1, T2, and contrast-enhanced sequences.

Extralaryngeal tumor spread
There are multiple potential pathways for extralaryngeal tumor spread, either through or around laryngeal cartilage (**Fig. 17**).[23] One is direct extension, termed *penetration*, of tumor through the thyroid cartilage into the strap musculature and soft tissues of the anterior and lateral neck (**Fig. 18**). However, tumor can also extend through and widen the thyroid notch between the unfused thyroid ala, without frank cartilage involvement.[23] Tumor can extend into the extralaryngeal anterior soft tissues through the thyrohyoid membrane or through the lateral defects in the thyrohyoid membrane, along the course of the external laryngeal nerve and artery (**Fig. 19**). Superior extension can occur into the base of tongue and oropharynx, along the pharyngoepiglottic or glossoepiglottic fold, or via the preepiglottic space (see **Fig. 8**). Posteriorly, tumor can extend through the arytenoid cartilage or extend from the paraglottic space through the thyroarytenoid gap into the hypopharynx (**Fig. 20**) and then even erode through the pharyngeal constrictors into the soft tissues of the neck. Laterally, tumor can creep over the AE fold into the piriform sinus, and posteriorly, tumor can extend from the interarytenoid space

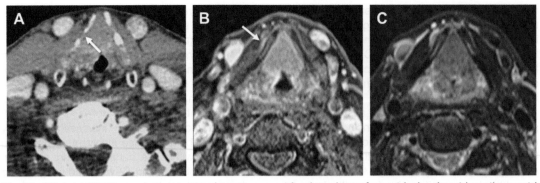

Fig. 15. (*A*) Axial CE-CT scan demonstrating large tumor with a broad interface with the thyroid cartilage, with adjacent heterogeneous ossification of the thryroid cartilage (*arrow*). (*B*) Axial fat-saturated postcontrast T1-weighted image shows enhancing tumor extending through the right thyroid ala into the adjacent strap muscles (*arrow*). (*C*) Axial fat-saturated T2-weighted image shows soft tissue T2 isointense to tumor.

and posterior commissure into the post cricoid hypopharynx and, from there, extend into the proximal cervical esophagus. Finally, as described earlier, tumors can extend inferiorly from the subglottic region through the conus elasticus, through the cricothyroid membrane into the soft tissues of the neck (including the thyroid gland), with or without cricoid or tracheal cartilage erosion, and from there extend inferiorly into the proximal cervical trachea (**Fig. 21**B).[23]

Initially, extralaryngeal tumor was thought to be only transcartilage. In 2011, Chen and colleagues[23] demonstrated that only a minority of pathologically proven extralaryngeal tumor occurred via thyroid cartilage penetration (44% of cases), usually glottic or supraglottic tumors. Additionally, that same study demonstrated that CT may have questionable accuracy when assessing extralaryngeal spread, with only 49% sensitivity and 81% positive predictive value. Tumors may bulge the membranes, without frank invasion of extralaryngeal soft tissues, and there is little discussion in the literature as to whether these are technically T3 versus T4a tumors. In the authors' opinion, they should be staged as T3 (**Fig. 22**). MR imaging may have increased utility but may overestimate extralaryngeal spread.

With the current American Joint Committee on Cancer, 7th edition, all tumors with extralaryngeal spread are staged as T4a. This is a heterogeneous group, and tumors that extend through potential spaces (the thyrohyoid membrane, thyroartyenoid gap, etc) may behave differently than those that penetrate through the cartilage, with the latter being more aggressive and potentially more likely to fail nonsurgical therapy. Chen and colleagues[23] have suggested that this may lead to further subdivision of the T4a category in the future.

With the exception of the patient being a poor surgical candidate or having distant metastatic disease, the only true instances of unresectability are stage T4b tumors that either involve the prevertebral space, encase the carotid artery, or invade the mediastinum.[24] Prevertebral space involvement is most often seen when laryngeal tumors involve the hypopharynx, can be difficult to determine on imaging, and is better assessed surgically. If there is preservation of the retropharyngeal fat plane on T1-weighted MR images between the tumor and prevertebral musculature, there is likely no prevertebral space fixation.[25] However, obliteration of the fat plane does not reliably predict prevertebral tumor extension, and the

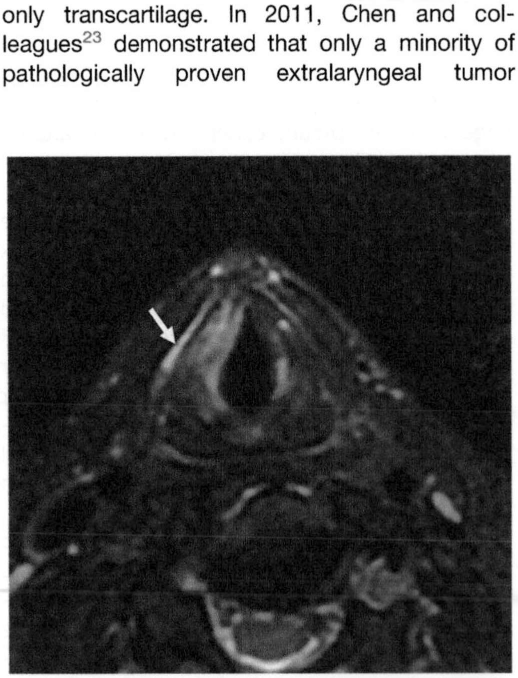

Fig. 16. Axial fat-saturated T2-weighted image showing T2 hyperintense tumor in the right paraglottic space; however the T2 signal in the adjacent thyroid cartilage is hyperintense to the tumor, suggesting reactive edema instead of cartilage invasion.

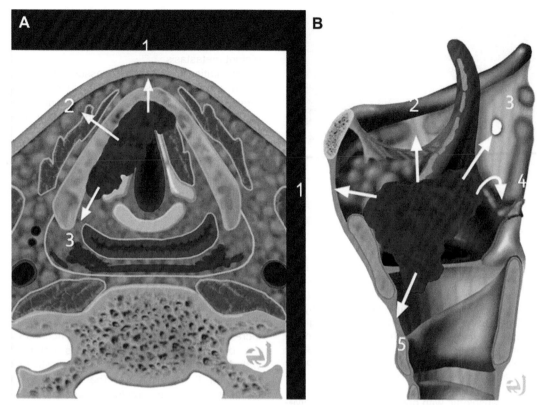

Fig. 17. Extralaryngeal spread of tumor. (*A*) Axial illustration of some of the potential paths of extralaryngeal spread of a glottic tumor. (1) Anteriorly through thyroid notch. (2) Transcartilaginous through the thyroid cartilage. (3) Posteriorly through the thyroartenoid space. (*B*) Sagittal illustration of a large transglottic tumor with some of the potential paths of extralaryngeal spread. (1) Anteriorly through the preepiglottic fat and through the thyrohyoid membrane. (2) Superiorly into the vallecula and base of tongue. (3) Laterally through potential defects in the thyrohyoid membrane. (4) Posteriorly into the hypopharynx. (5) Inferiorly through the cricothyroid membrane. (*Courtesy of* Eric Jablonowski.)

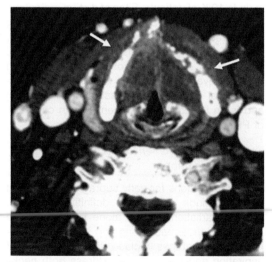

Fig. 18. Bulky laryngeal mass at the level of the true vocal cords with bilateral thyroid cartilage penetration and transcartilaginous extralaryngeal spread of tumor. Not the sclerosis and the frank lysis and obvious tumor outside the margin of the cartilage into the strap musculature bilaterally (*arrows*).

most accurate method of determining prevertebral involvement remains intraoperative assessment.[26] Preoperative determination of carotid arterial encasement is based on imaging findings. Greater than 270° of carotid artery encasement is a reliable predictor for tumor invasion of the adventitia, predicting unresectability reportedly 100% of the time. Contact less than 180° has a low likelihood of tumor invasion, and tumors with contact between 180 and 270° have an intermediate likelihood of fixation (**Fig. 23**).[27] Mediastinal invasion includes laryngeal or hypopharyngeal tumors with extension into the cervical trachea and esophagus below the sternal notch and infiltration of mediastinal fat or involvement of the supra-aortic vessels.[24]

Nodal metastasis

Supraglottic primary laryngeal tumors, or those with preepiglottic or paraglottic space involvement, have a higher propensity for nodal metastasis, particularly to levels II through IV (**Fig. 24**). Purely glottic tumors rarely have nodal metastasis,

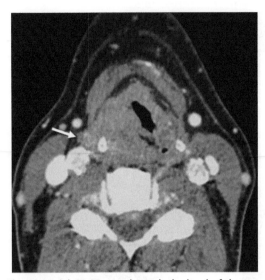

Fig. 19. Axial CE-CT scan through the level of the pre-epiglottic space and thyrohyoid membrane (note hyoid bone anteriorly and superior aspect of thyroid cartilage posteriorly). Circumferential supraglottic tumor, more bulky on the right, with extralaryngeal spread from the preepiglottic and paraglottic space laterally through the right thyrohyoid membrane into the soft tissues of the neck (*arrow*).

unless transglottic with paraglottic space involvement. Subglottic tumors may involve the delphian nodes but most frequently involve level VI (paratracheal) lymph nodes, cephalad to the innominate

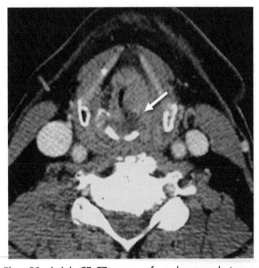

Fig. 20. Axial CE-CT scan of a laryngeal tumor involving the left true vocal cord, extending across the anterior commissure to the right, and extending posteriorly to widen the left thyroarytenoid space, into the left piriform sinus and hypopharynx. Note the lysis of the left arytenoid cartilage, suspicious for involvement (*arrow*), and sclerosis of the left thyroid ala and cricoid cartilage (nonspecific).

artery within the anterior superior mediastinum. Paratracheal lymph node involvement places the patient at a higher risk for mediastinal nodal and distant metastasis.[28,29]

Metastatic adenopathy is associated with a much worse prognosis and with lower survival rates, which is reflected in the staging of any tumor with nodal disease as automatically stage III or higher. N2 disease is automatically stage IVA.[6] A single positive lymph node in laryngeal cancer reportedly decreases survival by 50% and bilateral adenopathy decreases the survival by an additional 25%. Imaging is important in detection of cervical metastasis, particularly with small or deep cervical lymph nodes. CT findings suggestive of nodal metastasis are similar to those used in other head and neck primary site SCCs. Extracapsular extension (including conglomerate lymphadenopathy) and contralateral nodal disease are negative prognostic indicators and may alter treatment regimens. Positron-emission tomography (PET)-CT has been shown to have an increased sensitivity, specificity, and accuracy in the detection of nodal metastasis compared with CT alone, particularly in patients with more advanced T stage tumors. The exceptions are completely necrotic nodes or subcentimeter nodes.[30]

Distant metastasis

Laryngeal SCC is associated with a 10% to 20% risk of distant metastases.[14] Unfortunately, the risk of second primary malignancy in the first 5 years[31] is also high. Lung cancer may develop in up to 10% of patients. Sites of distant metastatic disease include mediastinal lymph nodes, lung (most frequent site of metastasis), bones, liver, skin (ie, dermal metastasis), or brain. Extranodal extension or contralateral or paratracheal lymph node involvement increases the risk for mediastinal nodal and distant metastasis (M1 disease) and is an indication for screening with chest CT or PET-CT.[28]

Trends in Management Affecting Staging of Supraglottic Cancer

Treatment options for early supraglottic laryngeal cancer include surgery or definitive radiation. External radiation therapy alone for supraglottic laryngeal cancer has a long and successful track record. Advantages include the lower risk of aspiration and the ability to address both necks without neck dissection. For patients with smaller supraglottic larynx cancers (ie, tumor volumes <6 mL), local control is 83% to 89%.[32,33]

After the Veterans Administration larynx trial proved that nonsurgical therapy produces survival

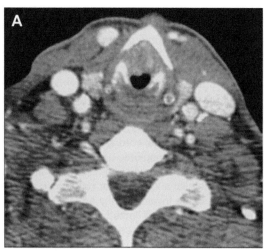
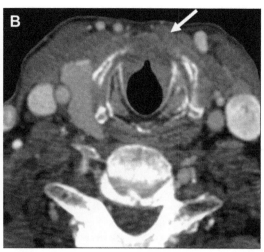

Fig. 21. (A) Axial CE-CT scan showing bulky subglottic primary tumor with nonspecific sclerosis of the adjacent thyroid and cricoid cartilages. (B) Axial CE-CT of another patient demonstrating subglottic tumor with extralaryngeal extension anteriorly (arrow) through the cricothyroid membrane.

rates equivalent to those for surgery plus adjuvant radiation,[34] advanced laryngeal cancer (T3 or higher) not invading more than 1 cm of the base of tongue and without extralaryngeal spread is treated with concurrent chemoradiation.[14] Two-year local control rate with concurrent chemoradiation is 78%.

For patients with adequate pulmonary reserve, the traditional surgery for early supraglottic cancer has been supraglottic laryngectomy. The traditional inferior border of the resection is the apex of the ventricles; however, one arytenoid can also be included in the resection.[35] Bilateral

adenopathy justifies either bilateral neck dissection or bilateral external radiation (while sparing the primary anastomosis in most cases). Additional conservational external surgeries, rarely performed, include the near total laryngectomy (resecting hemilarynx, including ipsilateral cricoid

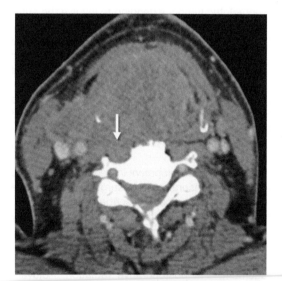

Fig. 23. Axial CE-CT scan of large laryngeal/hypopharyngeal tumor obliterating the airway, with transcartilaginous extralaryngeal spread of tumor into the soft tissues of the neck on the right. There is probable nodal disease within the carotid space on the right, resulting in at least 180° of encasement of the right common carotid artery, and obliteration of the prevertebral fat planes on the right (arrow). Findings are concerning for a T4b unresectable laryngeal tumor. MR imaging may be beneficial in this scenario.

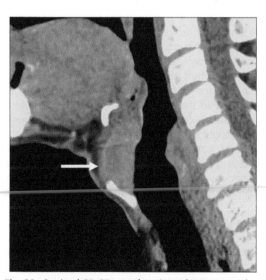

Fig. 22. Sagittal CE-CT scan showing a large supraglottic mass bulging the thyrohyoid membrane (arrow), without definite extralaryngeal tumor.

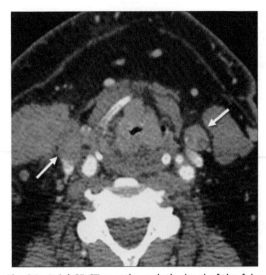

Fig. 24. Axial CE-CT scan through the level of the false cords shows a large circumferential supraglottic tumor with bilateral necrotic level III nodal metastasis (*arrows*), well circumscribed on the left, and with extracapsular extension of disease on the right into the sternocleidomastoid muscle and internal jugular vein.

cartilage) or the supracricoid partial laryngectomy (resecting anterior supraglottic larynx and anterior true vocal cords with or without 1 arytenoid, for supraglottic tumors extending to involve the anterior true vocal cords).

Transoral laser surgery for T1 or T2 supraglottic cancer is very successful in experienced hands if a complete resection can be achieved.[36] One of the limitations of laser surgery is difficult exposure, particularly tumors with anterior commissure involvement. Steiner's series also makes the point that with neck dissection, 5-year survival was 72.9% versus 58.6% without neck dissection (N = 141).[33]

The newest development in treating supraglottic cancer is transoral robotic surgery. Whether the limitations in exposure described with laser surgery are overcome with transoral robotic surgery has yet to be determined.[37]

T4 disease (regardless of nodal status) is usually treated with laryngectomy, appropriate neck management, and postoperative radiation. Adjuvant chemoradiation is administered if there are positive margins or extracapsular nodal extension.[38]

Glottic SCC
Staging/patterns of spread/pitfalls in staging The key points when staging a glottic primary tumor include arytenoid or thyroid cartilage involvement, transglottic (cranial) or subglottic (caudal) extension, paraglottic and preepiglottic extension, and

anterior or posterior commissure tumor. Some of these patterns of spread have been described earlier for supraglottic primary malignancies.

Glottic tumors have a propensity to present at an earlier stage, with very small lesions, because they produce hoarseness or airway compromise. Small but symptomatic tumors may be very difficult to detect on imaging and are much better assessed on laryngoscopy. T1 tumors include those confined to the vocal cord(s) (T1a vs T1b). A tumor is T2 if there is transglottic or subglottic extension, even if there is somewhat impaired mobility. Once there is hemilarynx fixation or paraglottic or preepiglottic space invasion, they are T3 and considered advanced, with limited options for laryngeal conservation. Early T1 or even T2 glottic primary tumors will often not undergo imaging, unless there is clinical concern for deep extension, significant transglottic or subglottic spread, or bulky anterior commissure involvement.

Involvement of the anterior commissure is extremely important for the radiologist to appreciate, because these tumors are frequently associated with early cartilage invasion, subglottic extension, and early extralaryngeal extension. T1 and T2 tumors with anterior commissure involvement are more difficult to treat with either surgery or radiation, are often associated with higher recurrence rates, and are often understaged.[39,40] Additionally, if the anterior commissure is crossed and more than the anterior third or half of the contralateral vocal cord is involved, the patient is no longer a candidate for a vertical hemilaryngectomy or extended vertical hemilaryngectomy. Posterior commissure involvement precludes the possibility of a supracricoid partial laryngectomy and may put the patient at risk for hypopharyngeal extension of tumor.[18]

Thus, although extension to the anterior or posterior commissure may not upstage a patient, it is important to detect, because it may affect survival and choice of treatment. If there is air adjacent to the thyroid lamina anteriorly, there is no anterior commissure involvement. However, one should be careful calling any soft tissue in the anterior commissure tumor, because often the phase of respiration or laryngeal edema can cause the vocal cords to oppose, resulting in soft tissue fullness (**Fig. 25**). Axial CT scans through the larynx should be in the plane of the true vocal folds to optimize visualization of the commissures.

Trends in management affecting staging of glottic cancer Early T1 or T2 glottic cancer can be treated with transoral laser excision as long as the anterior commissure is not involved. Anterior commissure involvement increases the risk of local failure for

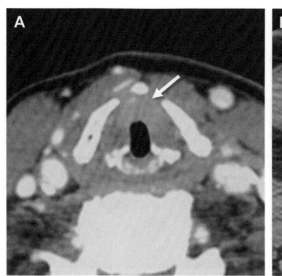
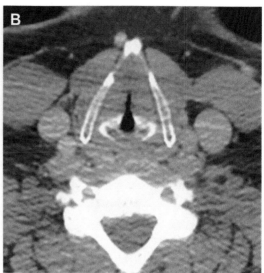

Fig. 25. Pitfall in imaging anterior commissure tumors. (A) Axial CE-CT scan demonstrating enhancing tumor thickening the anterior commissure (arrow). (B) Normal larynx with apparent thickening of the anterior commissure as a result of opposition of the true vocal cords during imaging and limited mucosal enhancement.

transoral laser excision.[41] Generally, the deeper the resection, the worse are the functional results for a surgical approach.[42]

Unilateral disease may be approached with a vertical hemilaryngectomy, but external radiation has a success rate of 90% for T1 glottic disease and of 75% for T2 disease.[43] The disadvantages of radiation include the long course of treatment and the expense. Advantages include superior voice quality for lesions penetrating the lamina propria and the therapeutic effectiveness regardless of anterior commissure location. T1 cancers can be understaged on imaging, especially if subglottic extension is not appreciated, and will result in treatment failure because the radiation fields for T1 and T2 glottic cancer are small.

Advanced glottic cancers (T3 or T4 disease) are treated in a manner similar to advanced supraglottic cancers.

Subglottic SCC
Staging/patterns of spread/pitfalls in staging Primary infraglottic tumors are rare but often present late, because they are relatively asymptomatic until large. Staging depends on the extent of involvement of the true vocal cord, fixation of the hemilarynx, whether there is invasion of the cricoid or thyroid cartilage, or extralaryngeal spread below the cricoid cartilage into the cervical trachea (see Fig. 21).

Trends in management affecting staging of subglottic cancer Most treatment recommendations are total laryngectomy, partial or total thyroidectomy, and an extensive neck dissection that includes the pretracheal, paratracheal, prelaryngeal nodes in level VI and the more conventional level II, III, and IV neck dissection.[44] Postoperative radiation therapy to the primary site is the rule.

PET–CE-CT in staging laryngeal cancer Nonintravenous CE-PET or -PET-CT in the initial T staging of laryngeal cancer is difficult, because resolution is limited. Any vocal cord mobility during the approximately 1-hour uptake phase of fludeoxyglucose F 18 (^{18}F FDG) (ie, talking, coughing, even throat clearing) can cause uptake within the larynx in the vocal cords and adjacent laryngeal musculature. With ipsilateral vocal cord palsy, compensatory hypertrophy and overuse of the contralateral cord can cause increased FDG uptake, with a false-positive PET scan on the contralateral side (Fig. 26).[45] However, initial PET staging can be useful in patients who undergo radiation therapy because it may serve as a baseline study for comparison posttreatment. Additionally, some studies have shown that the standardized uptake value of a primary tumor may have prognostic value, with an standardized uptake value of greater than 9 heralding a potential higher rate of recurrence and lower overall disease-free survival.[46] However, FDG-PET imaging has been found to be very useful in the detection of nodal disease, with a higher sensitivity and specificity than CE-CT alone, particularly for smaller nodal metastasis. The scanner camera resolution for PET is currently only approximately 7 mm.[47] Therefore, in patients with advanced

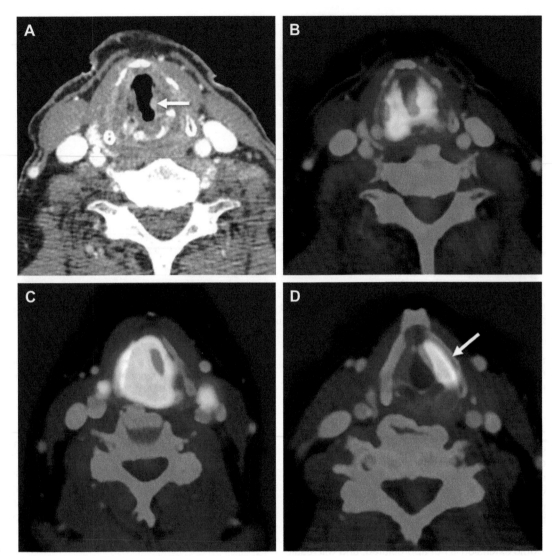

Fig. 26. PET staging pitfall: (*A*) axial CE-CT and (*B*) fused PET–CE-CT scans of a patient with a small polypoid T1 well-differentiated tumor of the posterior third of the left true vocal cord, seen on CT (*arrow*). Note the diffuse laryngeal uptake bilaterally, a false-positive PET result, as a result of phonation during the uptake phase. (*C*) Axial fused PET-CT scans of another patient with a large supraglottic tumor, circumferential, with bilateral nodal metastasis. (*D*) Same patient, more inferiorly. Discontinuous uptake in the contralateral left true vocal cord, without tumor visible on CT or examination as a result of right TVC paralysis, with compensatory hypertrophy and uptake of the contralateral left TVC (*arrow*) as a result of phonation during the uptake phase.

stage primary T3 or T4 tumors, PET should not take the place of a neck dissection if the patient is clinically N0, as the sensitivity for nodal metastasis drops to 50% (from 79%) in patients with a clinically N0 neck.[48] Micrometastases in a T3 or T4 laryngeal tumor are high, and they are beneath the resolution of PET.

PET imaging is critical in detecting both distant disease and synchronous lesions, particularly in patients with more advanced disease on presentation.[30] Overall, PET-CT has been shown to alter

TNM staging approximately 15% to 36% of the time.[49] In our practice, the CT is performed with contrast, using diagnostic CT parameters, and is interpreted by an experienced head and neck radiologist. National Comprehensive Cancer Network guidelines from 2011 state to consider PET-CT for advanced (T3 or T4) stage primary tumors.[50]

The authors have adopted the following strategy for initial staging for a T3 or higher laryngeal lesion on examination: The patient undergoes PET–CE-CT, which is interpreted in conjunction by both a dedicated nuclear medicine physician and a head and neck radiologist, and the images and patient are presented at a multidisciplinary head and neck tumor conference. A consensus regarding the staging is reached, taking into account the findings on endoscopy. If there is concern regarding cartilage invasion or extralaryngeal extension that is not answered on CE-CT and may alter the patient's management, then a dedicated laryngeal protocol MR imaging for problem solving is performed, with thin section T1-weighted, fat-saturated T2-weighted, and postcontrast fat-saturated T1-weighted images through the larynx.

Pitfalls in surveillance and appearance of recurrence Posttreatment follow-up imaging is indicated in patients with clinically suspected residual or recurrent tumor and as routine surveillance in asymptomatic patients with a high risk of recurrence. Local recurrence rates for laryngeal carcinoma range from 15% to 50%, depending on stage of the original tumor.[30] Surveillance imaging is important, particularly in the first 2 to 3 years after therapy, because two-thirds of the local and nodal metastases occur during this period, early detection of recurrence is important as a predictor of survival, and this imaging improves the possibility of performing salvage surgery. However, there is no current evidence-based consensus or guidelines regarding the optimal modality or timing of surveillance imaging. National Comprehensive Cancer Network 2011 guidelines do recommend that some baseline posttreatment imaging be performed at least 6 months posttreatment.[50]

CE-CT has traditionally been the imaging modality of choice to follow patients with head and neck cancer. In general, the literature suggests that CE-CT has good sensitivity and moderate specificity for assessing tumor response to therapy. Recent studies have suggested that FDG–PET–CT may have improved accuracy, particularly within the nodes of the neck.[51–53] One prospective study performed recently on 98 patients showed that PET-CT outperformed CT alone in detecting persistent disease in patients considered high risk for treatment failure but provided little value compared with CE-CT alone for unselected patients with locally advanced disease.[54] Many authors, however, continue to suggest that the combined use of FDG-PET with CE-CT in the posttreatment setting is the most sensitive and specific modality for the detection of recurrent laryngeal carcinoma.[30,47]

CT imaging in the posttreatment setting can be limited because of postradiation edema or postsurgical scarring, fibrosis, flap reconstruction, or streak artifact from surgical clips. Additionally, PET has its own pitfalls in the posttreatment setting. Imaging performed too soon after combined radiation and chemotherapy can elicit false-positive results as a result of postradiation inflammatory changes. Studies and meta-analyses have shown PET-CT to be most accurate at least 2 to 3 months after combined chemotherapy and radiation therapy, and the accuracy increases at 12 weeks or longer.[55] PET-CT has a high (up to 98%) negative predictive value and specificity at this time for excluding residual disease.[53]

Other PET pitfalls in the posttreatment setting include postbiopsy changes and infections, postradiation mucositis, mucosal ulcerations, and pharyngitis, all of which can cause false-positive results. Additionally, radiation-induced chondronecrosis of the laryngeal cartilage can mimic recurrent disease, both on PET imaging and on routine CE-CT. On CT, cartilage necrosis can appear as hypodensity, mixed sclerosis and lysis, with fragmentation of the cartilage, and even air, and these findings can be hypermetabolic on PET imaging. Biopsy, and occasionally laryngectomy, is performed to exclude recurrent disease, particularly if the patient has a nonfunctioning larynx (**Fig. 27**).

After laryngectomy, the most common sites for recurrent tumor are at the margins of the resection, within the neopharynx, or in the parastomal soft tissues (**Fig. 28**). However, postsurgical patients can also have false-positive findings on PET imaging, including uptake around the tracheostomy or laryngectomy site, uptake around a tracheoesophageal speech prosthesis, or uptake around the margins of a neopharyngeal reconstruction.[30]

FUTURE DIRECTIONS/ADVANCED IMAGING

As laryngeal preservation therapies are becoming more prevalent, even in the setting of large-volume T4 disease,[56,57] there is emphasis in the literature on the use of CE-CT, MR, and PET imaging to predict the patient's response to therapy, occasionally in the setting of a cycle of induction chemotherapy.

A technique used frequently by radiation oncologists in treatment planning is measuring gross tumor volume, based on contouring performed around the tumor on a workstation on pretreatment imaging. Based on the subsite, higher gross tumor volume can be one of the strongest independent predictors of outcome and local control. Specific to the larynx, thresholding volumes have been described for supraglottic and T3 glottic carcinomas.[58] Other findings that

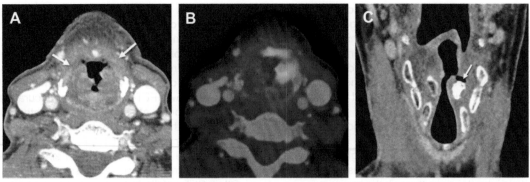

Fig. 27. (*A, B*) Posttreatment PET–CE-CT examination (12 weeks after therapy), demonstrating persistent ulcerated soft tissue within the larynx, extending into the thyroid cartilage bilaterally (*arrows*), with some scattered enhancement and mild FDG uptake. Findings are suspicious for chondronecrosis but may represent persistent tumor. Initial biopsies were negative for tumor; however, patient underwent laryngectomy for nonfunctional larynx, and persistent tumor was noted in the specimen, in addition to areas of chondronecrosis. (*C*) Coronal CE-CT scan of a different patient with persistent pain and ulceration post chemotherapy and radiation demonstrates ulceration extending to a sclerotic and previously infiltrated left arytenoid cartilage (*arrow*). Note sclerosis of the thyroid and cricoid cartilage. Repeat biopsies were negative for persistent tumor. This was thought to be caused by posttreatment chondronecrosis.

predict higher likelihood of local failure include cartilage invasion, hypopharyngeal extension, extralaryngeal tumor, subglottic extension, and preepiglottic and paraglottic space involvement.[58,59]

Tumor or nodal perfusion with CT or MR imaging has been studied, in both a pretreatment and a posttreatment setting (after induction chemotherapy), to help with nodal diagnosis and to help predict response to therapy. For instance, a study by Trojanowska and colleagues[60] in 2011 has

shown a statistically significant difference in the blood volume, blood flow, and permeability surface parameters with CT perfusion imaging between benign and malignant lymph nodes. Perfusion imaging (both CT and MR imaging) has also demonstrated that tumors with elevated blood volume and flow and other pharmacokinetic parameters demonstrate a statistically significant improved response to induction chemotherapy.[61–63]

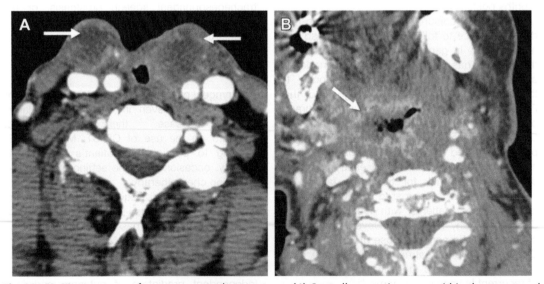

Fig. 28. CE-CT appearance of recurrence post laryngectomy. (*A*) Centrally necrotic masses within the parastomal tissues bilaterally (*arrows*) representing parastomal recurrence. (*B*) Circumferential thick nodular enhancement of the neopharynx at the superior oropharyngeal margin (*arrow*); pathologic examination proved neopharyngeal recurrence.

In addition to improved techniques in FDG-PET scanner resolution and improved PET imaging techniques (such as smaller field of view and high-resolution techniques), new PET radiotracers are in development, including anti–epidermal growth factor receptor antibody imaging.[64]

REFERENCES

1. Howlader N, Noone AM, Krapcho M, et al. SEER cancer statistics review, 1975-2008. Bethesda MD: National Cancer Institute; 2010. Available at: http://seer.cancer.gov/csr/1975_2008/. SEER data submission, posted to the SEER web site, 2011.

2. Hoffman HT, Porter K, Karnell H, et al. Laryngeal cancer in the United States: changes in demographic, patterns of care, and survival. Laryngoscope 2006;116(9 Pt 2 Suppl 111):1–13.

3. Hamzany Y, Hadar T, Feinmesser R, et al. Laryngeal carcinoma in nonsmoking patients. Ann Otol Rhinol Laryngol 2008;117(8):564–8.

4. Jeong WJ, Park SW, Shin M, et al. Presence of HPV type 6 in dysplasia and carcinoma arising from recurrent respiratory papillomatosis. Head Neck 2009;31(8):1095–101.

5. Torrente MC, Rodrigo JP, Haigentz M, et al. Human papillomavirus in infections in laryngeal cancer. Head Neck 2011;33(4):581–6.

6. American Joint Committee on Cancer. AJCC cancer staging manual. 7th edition. New York: Springer-Verlag; 2010.

7. Curtin H. Anatomy, imaging, and pathology of the larynx. Som P, Curtin H. Head and neck imaging. 5th edition. St Louis (MO): Elsevier; 2011. p.1905–2039.

8. Becker M, Burkhardt K, Dulguerov P, et al. Imaging of the larynx and hypopharynx. Eur J Radiol 2008; 66:467–79.

9. Mukherji SK, Armao D, Joshi VM. Cervical nodal metastases in squamous cell carcinoma of the head and neck: what to expect. Head Neck 2001; 23:995–1005.

10. Chijiwa H, Sato K, Umeno H, et al. Histopathological study of correlation between laryngeal space invasion and lymph node metastasis in glottic carcinoma. J Laryngol Otol Suppl 2009;31:48–51.

11. Silver CE, Beitler JJ, Shaha AR, et al. Current trends in initial management of laryngeal cancer: the declining use of open surgery. Eur Arch Otorhinolaryngol 2009;266:1333–52.

12. Kim JW, Yoon SY, Park IS, et al. Correlation between radiological images and pathological results in supraglottic cancer. J Laryngol Otol 2008;122(11): 1224–9.

13. Beitler JJ, Muller S, Grist WJ, et al. Prognostic accuracy of computed tomography findings for patients with laryngeal cancer undergoing laryngectomy. J Clin Oncol 2010;28:2318–22.

14. Forastiere AA, Goepfert H, Maor M, et al. Concurrent chemotherapy and radiotherapy for organ preservation in advanced laryngeal cancer. N Engl J Med 2003;349(22):2091–8.

15. Loevner LA, Yousem DM, Montone KT, et al. Can Radiologists accurately predict preepiglottic space invasion with MR imaging? AJR Am J Roentgenol 1997;169:1681–7.

16. Celin SE, Johnson J, Curtin H, et al. The association of laryngoceles with squamous cell carcinoma of the larynx. Laryngoscope 1991;101:529–36.

17. Murakami R, Nishimura R, Baba Y, et al. Prognostic factors of glottic carcinomas treated with radiation therapy: value of the adjacent sign on radiological examinations in the sixth edition of the UICC TNM staging system. Int J Radiat Oncol Biol Phys 2005; 61(2):471–5.

18. Blitz AM, Aygun N. Radiologic evaluation of larynx cancer. Otolaryngol Clin North Am 2008;41: 697–713.

19. Lefebvre JL, Ang KK. Larynx preservation clinical trial design: key issues and recommendations–a consensus panel summary; Larynx Preservation Consensus Panel. Head Neck 2009;31(4): 429–41.

20. Zbaren P, Becker M, Laeng H. Pretherapeutic staging of laryngeal cancer: clinical findings, computed tomography, and magnetic resonance imaging versus histopathology. Cancer 1996;77: 1263–73.

21. Becker M, Zbaren P, Delavelle J, et al. Neoplastic invasion of the laryngeal cartilage: reassessment of criteria for diagnosis at CT. Radiology 1997;203(2): 521–32.

22. Becker M, Zbaren P, Casselman JW, et al. Neoplastic invasion of laryngeal cartilage: reassessment of criteria for diagnosis at MR imaging. Radiology 2008;249:551–9.

23. Chen SA, Muller S, Chen AY, et al. Patterns of Extralaryngeal spread of laryngeal cancer: thyroid cartilage penetration occurs in a minority of patients with extralaryngeal spread of laryngeal squamous cell cancers. Cancer 2011;117(22): 5047–51.

24. Yousem DM, Gad K, Tufano RP. Resectability issues with head and neck cancer. AJNR Am J Neuroradiol 2006;27(10):2024–36.

25. Hsu WC, Loevner LA, Karpati R, et al. Accuracy of magnetic resonance imaging in predicting absence of fixation of head and neck cancer to the prevertebral space. Head Neck 2005;27:95–100.

26. Loevner LA, Ott IL, Yousem DM, et al. Neoplastic fixation to the prevertebral compartment by squamous cell carcinoma of the head and neck. Am J Roentgenol 1998;170:1389–94.

27. Yousem DM, Hatabu H, Hurst RW, et al. Carotid artery invasion by head and neck masses: prediction with MR imaging. Radiology 1995;195:715–20.

28. Ljumanovic R, Langendijk JA, Hoekstra S, et al. Distant metastasis in head and neck carcinoma: identification of prognostic groups with MR imaging. Eur J Radiol 2006;60:58–66.

29. Som PM. Detection of metastasis in cervical lymph nodes: CT and MR criteria and differential diagnosis. AJR Am J Roentgenol 1992;158:961–9.

30. Chu MM, Kositwattanarerk A, Lee DJ, et al. FDG PET with contrast enhanced CT: a critical imaging tool for laryngeal carcinoma. Radiographics 2010;30(5): 1353–72.

31. Milano MT, Peterson CR, Zhang H, et al. Second primary lung cancer after head and neck squamous cell cancer: population-based study of risk factors. Head Neck 2012. http://dx.doi.org/10.1002/hed. 22006 [online].

32. Freeman DE, Mancuso AA, Parsons JT, et al. Irradiation alone for supraglottic larynx carcinoma: can CT findings predict treatment results? Int J Radiat Oncol Biol Phys 1990;19(2):485–90.

33. Mancuso AA, Mukherji SK, Schmalfuss I, et al. Pre-radiotherapy computed tomography as a predictor of local control in supraglottic carcinoma. J Clin Oncol 1999;17(2):631–7.

34. Induction chemotherapy plus radiation compared with surgery plus radiation in patients with advanced laryngeal cancer. The department of veterans affairs laryngeal cancer study group. N Engl J Med 1991; 324(24):1685–90.

35. Bocca E, Pignataro O, Oldini C. Supraglottic laryngectomy: 30 years of experience. Ann Otol Rhinol Laryngol 1983;92(1 Pt 1):14–8.

36. Iro H, Waldfahrer F, Altendorf-Hoffman A, et al. Transoral laser surgery of supraglottic cancer: follow-up of 141 patients. Arch Otolaryngol Head Neck Surg 1998;124(11):1245–50.

37. Weinstein GS, O'Malley BW, Snyder W, et al. Transoral robotic surgery: supraglottic partial laryngectomy. Ann Otol Rhinol Laryngol 2007;116(1):19–23.

38. Bernier J, Cooper JS, Pajak TF, et al. Defining risk levels in locally advanced head and neck cancers: a comparative analysis of concurrent postoperative radiation plus chemotherapy trials of the EORTC (#22931) and RTOG (#9501). Head Neck 2005; 27(10):843–50.

39. Rodel RM, Steiner W, Muller RM, et al. Endoscopic laser surgery of early glottic cancer: involvement of the anterior commissure. Head Neck 2009;31:583–92.

40. Connor S. Laryngeal cancer: how does the radiologist help? Cancer Imaging 2007;7:93–103.

41. Steiner W, Ambrosch P, Rodel RM, et al. Impact of anterior commissure involvement on local control of early glottic carcinoma treated by laser microresection. Laryngoscope 2004;114(8):1485–91.

42. Beitler JJ, Johnson JT. Transoral laser excision for early glottic cancer. Int J Radiat Oncol Biol Phys 2003;56(4):1063–6.

43. Mendenhall WM, Amdur RJ, Morris CG, et al. T1–T2N0 squamous cell carcinoma of the glottic larynx treated with radiation therapy. J Clin Oncol 2001; 19(20):4029–36.

44. Ferlito A, Rinaldo A. The pathology and management of subglottic cancer. Eur Arch Otorhinolaryngol 2000;257(3):168–73.

45. Lee M, Ramaswamy MR, Lilien DL, et al. Unilateral vocal cord paralysis causes contralateral false positive positron emission tomography scans of the larynx. Ann Otol Rhinol Laryngol 2005;114(3):202–6.

46. Schwartz DL, Rajendran J, Yueh B, et al. FDG-PET prediction of head and neck squamous cell cancer outcomes. Arch Otolaryngol Head Neck Surg 2004;130(12):1361–7.

47. Branstetter BF, Blodgett TM, Zimmer LA, et al. Head and neck malignancy: is PET/CT more accurate than PET or CT alone? Radiology 2005;235:580–6.

48. Kyzas PA, Evangelou E, Denaxa-Kyza D, et al. 18F-Fluorodeoxyglucose positron emission tomography to evaluate cervical node metastases in patients with head and neck squamous cell carcinoma: a meta-analysis. J Natl Cancer Inst 2008;100(10): 712–20.

49. Agarwal V, Branstetter BF. Johnson JT. Indications for PET/CT in the head and neck. Otolaryngol Clin North Am 2008;41:23–49.

50. National Comprehensive Cancer Network. NCCN clinical practice guidelines for oncology: head and neck cancer. [Online] Feb 2011. Available at: http://www.nccn.org/professionals/physician_gls/pdf/head-and-neck.pdf.

51. Chen AY, Vilaseca I, Hudgins PA, et al. PET-CT vs contrast-enhanced CT: what is the role for each after chemoradiation for advanced oropharyngeal cancer? Head Neck 2006;28:487–95.

52. Kao J, Vu HL, Genden EM, et al. The diagnostic and prognostic utility of positron emission tomography/computed tomography-based follow-up after radiotherapy for head and neck cancer. Cancer 2009; 115:4586–94.

53. Ong SC, Schoder H, Lee NY, et al. Clinical utility of F-18-FDG PET/CT in Assessing the neck after concurrent chemoradiotherapy for locoregional advanced head and neck cancer. J Nucl Med 2008;59:532–40.

54. Moeller BJ, Rana V, Cannon BA, et al. Prospective risk-adjusted (F-18) fluorodeoxyglucose positron emission tomography and computed tomography assessment of radiation response in head and neck cancer. J Clin Oncol 2009;27:2509–15.

55. Isles MG, McConkey C, Mehanna HM. A systematic review and meta-analysis of the role of positron emission tomography in the follow up of head and

neck squamous cell carcinoma following radio-therapy or chemoradiotherapy. Clin Otolaryngol 2008;33(3):210–22.

56. Knab BR, Salama JK, Solanki A, et al. Functional organ preservation with definitive chemoradiother-apy for T4 laryngeal squamous cell carcinoma. Ann Oncol 2008;19:1650–4.

57. Worden FP, Moyer J, Lee JS, et al. Chemoselection as a strategy for organ preservation in patients with T4 laryngeal squamous cell carcinoma with cartilage invasion. Laryngoscope 2009;119:1510–7.

58. Mukherji SK, Schmalfuss IM, Castelijns J, et al. Clin-ical applications of tumor volume measurements for predicting outcome in patients with squamous cell carcinoma of the upper aerodigestive tract. AJNR Am J Neuroradiol 2004;25:1425–32.

59. Ljumanovic R, Langendijk JA, Wattingen MV, et al. MR Imaging predictors of local control of glottic squamous cell carcinoma treated with radiation alone. Radiology 2007;244(1):205–12.

60. Trojanowska A, Trojanowski P, Bisdas S, et al. Squa-mous cell cancer of hypopharynx and larynx - eval-uation of metastatic nodal disease based on computed tomography perfusion studies. Eur J Radiol 2012;81(5):1034–9. http://dx.doi.org/10.1016/j.e.jrad.2011.01.084.

61. Zima A, Carlos R, Gandhi D, et al. Can pretreatment CT perfusion predict response of advanced squa-mous cell carcinoma of the upper aerodigestive tract treated with induction chemotherapy? AJNR Am J Neuroradiol 2007;28:328–34.

62. Petralia G, Preda L, Giugliano G, et al. Perfusion computed tomography for monitoring induction chemotherapy in patients with squamous cell carcinoma of the upper aerodigestive tract: corre-lation between changes in tumor perfusion and tumor volume. J Comput Assist Tomogr 2009; 33(4):552–9.

63. Kim S, Loevner LA, Quon H, et al. Prediction of response to chemoradiation therapy in squamous cell carcinomas of the head and neck using dynamic contrast enhanced MRI imaging. AJNR Am J Neuroradiol 2010;31:262–8.

64. Hoeben BA, Molkenboer-Kuenen JD, Oyen WJ, et al. Radiolabeled cetuximab: dose optimization for epidermal growth factor receptor imaging in a head-and-neck squamous cell carcinoma model. Int J Cancer 2011;129(4):870–8.

Pitfalls in the Staging of Cancer of the Major Salivary Gland Neoplasms

Elliott R. Friedman, MD[a],*, Amit M. Saindane, MD[b]

KEYWORDS

- Salivary glands • Adenoid cystic carcinoma • Benign mixed tumor
- Carcinoma ex pleomorphic adenoma

KEY POINTS

- The major salivary glands consist of the parotid, submandibular, and sublingual glands.
- Most neoplasms in other subsites in the head and neck are squamous cell carcinoma, but tumors of the salivary glands may be benign or malignant.
- Surgical treatment differs if the lesion is benign, and therefore preoperative fine-needle aspiration is important in salivary neoplasms.
- The role of imaging is to attempt to determine histology, predict likelihood of a lesion being malignant, and report an imaging stage.
- This article reviews the various histologies, imaging features, and staging of major salivary gland neoplasms.

ANATOMY AND BOUNDARIES

The major salivary glands consist of the parotid, submandibular, and sublingual glands. Submucosal clusters of salivary tissue located in the palate, oral cavity, paranasal sinuses, and upper aerodigestive tract are minor salivary glands, and are variable in distribution. Primary neoplasms arising in the minor salivary glands are staged according to the anatomic site of origin.[1]

The parotid gland is the largest of the salivary glands, the bulk of which lies superficial to the masseter muscle and mandibular ramus and angle (Fig. 1). The investing fascia arises from the superficial layer of the deep cervical fascia. The deep portion of the gland extends through the stylomandibular tunnel into the prestyloid compartment of the parapharyngeal space. The stylomandibular tunnel is formed by the skull base, posterior margin of the mandibular ramus, and styloid process and stylomandibular ligament.[2] Although the parotid

gland is a single contiguous structure, for surgical convenience it has been divided into superficial and deep lobes by the course of the facial nerve, which courses lateral to the retromandibular vein. Most neoplasms arise in the superficial portion of the gland.[3] Considerable variation in intraparotid facial nerve anatomy exists, but most commonly the nerve enters the posteromedial aspect of the gland and divides into 2 main trunks before dividing into 5 main branches: temporal, zygomatic, buccal, mandibular, and cervical. The auriculotemporal nerve, which curves around the mandibular neck, embedded in the gland capsule, connects the mandibular branch of the trigeminal nerve with the facial nerve and serves as a potential route of perineural tumor spread.

Accessory parotid tissue is found in approximately 20% of the population, anterior to the parotid gland, typically overlying the masseter muscle between the zygomatic arch and parotid

[a] Department of Diagnostic & Interventional Imaging, University of Texas Health Science Center at Houston, 6431 Fannin Street, MSB 2.130B, Houston, TX 77030, USA; [b] Department of Radiology and Imaging Sciences, Emory University School of Medicine, BG-22, 1364 Clifton Road Northeast, Atlanta, GA 30322, USA
* Corresponding author.
E-mail address: Elliott.Friedman@uth.tmc.edu

Neuroimag Clin N Am 23 (2013) 107–122
http://dx.doi.org/10.1016/j.nic.2012.08.009
1052-5149/13/$ – see front matter © 2013 Elsevier Inc. All rights reserved.

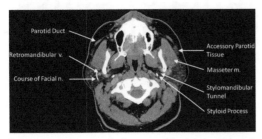

Fig. 1. CT anatomy of the parotid gland. *Abbreviations:* m, muscle; n, nerve; v, vein.

duct.[4] In distinction to other salivary glands, between 3 and 24 lymph nodes are found within the parotid gland, almost all within the superficial portion of the gland.[5] Parotid lymph nodes drain into the level IIA and IIB upper cervical chains.[2] The main parotid duct, Stensen's duct, is approximately 7 cm in length, exiting the anterior aspect of the gland, passing horizontally lateral to the masseter muscle and medial to the zygomaticus major muscle, pierces the buccinator muscle, and opens on a papilla in the buccal mucosa opposite the second maxillary molar tooth.[4]

The submandibular gland occupies most of the submandibular triangle, which is formed by the inferior border of the mandibular body and anterior and posterior bellies of the digastric muscle (**Fig. 2**). The stylohyoid muscle also forms part of the posterior boundary. The submandibular gland is enveloped by a thin fibrous capsule. The stylomandibular ligament, a reflection of the deep cervical fascia, separates the parotid and submandibular glands. The submandibular gland is arbitrarily divided into superficial and deep lobes based on its extension around the posterior margin of the mylohyoid muscle, which divides the submandibular space from the floor of the mouth. No lymph nodes or large nerves are present within the submandibular gland. Lymphatic drainage is into IB or submandibular nodes

and deep cervical lymph nodes, particularly IIA nodes. Wharton's duct, the primary excretory duct, courses anteriorly and superiorly between the genioglossus muscle and sublingual gland to open in the floor of mouth on the sublingual papilla on the side of the tongue.[4]

The anterior facial vein, which runs along the lateral margin of the submandibular gland, can be used to distinguish exophytic submandibular masses from extrinsic lesions, such as lymphadenopathy or soft tissue tumors, that arise adjacent to the gland. A mass separated by the facial vein from the gland must be an extrinsic lesion.[6]

The sublingual gland is the smallest of the major salivary glands and is situated above the mylohyoid muscle, covered by mucosa of the floor of the mouth.[4] No well-defined capsule exists. Numerous small excretory ducts, the Rivinus ducts, open directly into the floor of the mouth. A large duct, Bartholin duct, may empty into the submandibular duct near its orifice.[7] Primary lymphatic drainage is into level I lymph nodes.

IMAGING WORKUP

MR imaging is the preferred cross-sectional imaging modality to assess a noninflammatory salivary gland mass. Rarely, imaging will be definitive of a diagnosis (**Fig. 3**); however, histologic differentiation of neoplasm is generally not possible on CT or T1-weighted images with or without contrast, although noncontrast T1-weighted images are helpful to assess tumor size, margins, depth, and extent.[8] Certain imaging features may suggest malignancy. Bone invasion, perineural

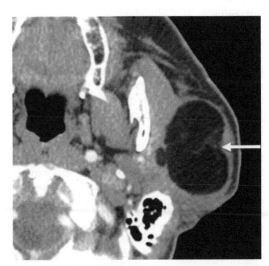

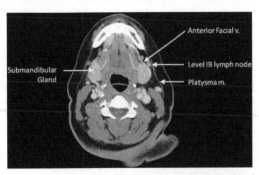

Fig. 2. CT anatomy of the submandibular gland. Whether a mass is glandular or nodal may sometimes be difficult to determine. If the facial vein comes between the gland and the mass, the lesion is nodal.

Fig. 3. Imaging diagnosis of parotid mass. Axial contrast-enhanced CT shows a well-defined fat-density mass within the superficial left parotid gland diagnostic of a lipoma (*arrow*).

spread, and deep extension into the parapharyng-eal space or muscles are highly indicative of malignancy. Although infiltrative margins suggest malignancy, hemorrhage or inflammatory changes on CT can create false-positive results for malignancy (Fig. 4).

Benign and low-grade malignant lesions are likely to exhibit more hyperintense T2 signal, whereas high-grade malignancies tend to have intermediate or lower T2 signal. T2 signal is influenced by intracellular water content and cellularity. Differentiated benign or low-grade malignant lesions are more likely to produce serous or mucous secretions, which have a high water content. Unfortunately, although elevated T2 signal suggests that a lesion is not high-grade, it does not reliably distinguish between benign and low-grade malignant lesions (Fig. 5). Low-grade malignancies, particularly mucoepidermoid and adenoid cystic carcinomas, may exhibit high T2 signal.[9] Some benign lesions can have low T2 signal, including Warthin tumor, which is the second most common benign tumor of the parotid gland, granulomas, and fibrosis. However, for practical purposes, low T2 signal should serve as a warning that a high-grade lesion may be present.[10,11] T1-weighted gadolinium-enhanced fat-saturated sequences should be included to

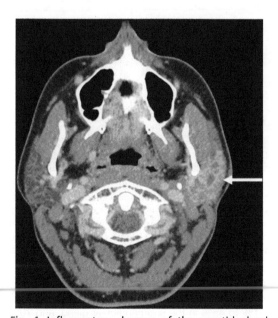

Fig. 4. Inflammatory changes of the parotid gland simulating a malignancy. Axial contrast-enhanced CT demonstrates ill-defined enhancement of the left parotid gland (arrow) with areas of low attenuation that represent segments of a dilated intraparotid duct. This focal parotid inflammation could be mistaken for an infiltrative neoplasm. Findings resolved after antibiotics.

assess for perineural spread, bone invasion, or meningeal involvement if intracranial extension is present. Effacement of fat in the neural foramen on noncontrast T1-weighted images allows for assessment of perineural spread while avoiding artifactual degradation that can be present at the skull base on fat-saturated sequences (Fig. 6). Because almost all salivary gland neoplasms enhance, an important role of contrast in assessing the tumor is distinguishing a T2 hyperintense mass from a cyst.

MR imaging can delineate the intraparotid course of the facial nerve and parotid ducts. One technique acquires T1-weighted images through a 3-dimensional (3D) Fourier transform gradient-echo sequence (3D GRASS) using a head and neck coil at 1.5 T. Optimal results were obtained with a 20-cm field of view, 512×288 matrix, flip angle of 30°, repetition time of 30 ms, and effective echo time of 4.2 ms, and acquiring 60 sections at 1.5-mm thickness without gaps. Facial nerve and intraparotid ducts have lower T1 signal intensity than glandular tissue. Signal intensity within vessels varies with saturation. Curved, orthogonal, and volumetric reconstructed images of the 3D data allow the facial nerve and its branches to be followed in most patients from the stylomastoid foramen through the posterior superior aspect of the gland to the level of the retromandibular vein, and assessment of the parotid ducts at the hilum and in the anteroinferior portion of the gland.[12] This technique is not routine in the authors' practice, because facial nerve branches are each isolated intraoperatively if a local resection is being performed. The course of the nerve is also not relevant if a total parotidectomy is necessary for treatment.

The primary role of fluorodeoxyglucose (FDG) positron emission tomography (PET) is to detect locoregional and distant metastatic disease. The standardized uptake value (SUV) on PET does not reliably distinguish between benign and malignant salivary tumors. Although high-grade tumors tend to have higher FDG uptake than low- or intermediate-grade salivary gland malignancies, benign mixed tumors and Warthin tumors may also have high FDG uptake, resulting in false-positive results (Fig. 7). FDG uptake in salivary gland malignancies has also not been shown to be useful in predicting patient survival.[13] Sensitivity of FDG-PET for detecting salivary gland primary malignant tumors has been reported to be between 75% and 100%.[14] False-negative PET results do occur, most frequently in low-grade malignancies wherein lower SUVs may be masked by physiologic FDG uptake in the salivary glands.[13] Studies have shown FDG-PET to be more accurate than conventional imaging

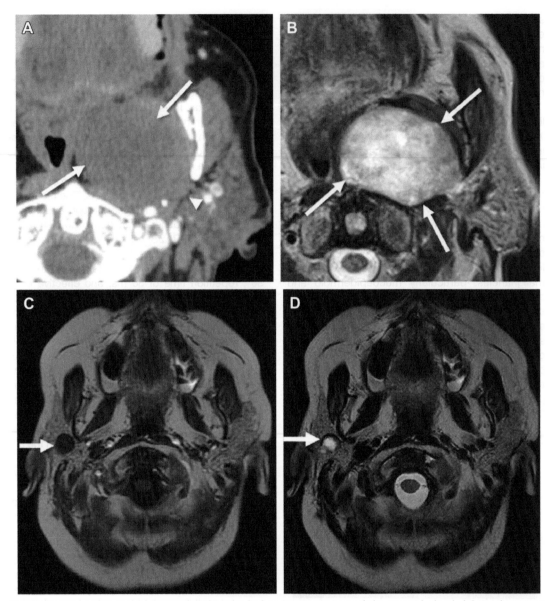

Fig. 5. Overlap in T2 signal intensities in benign and malignant lesions of the parotid gland. (*A*) Axial contrast-enhanced CT shows a well-defined hypodense mass (*arrows*) within the left parapharyngeal space. Note the cleft (*arrowhead*) between deep parotid gland and mass. (*B*) Axial T2-weighted image shows heterogeneous T2 hyperintensity (*arrow*). On surgical resection this was a benign mixed tumor. (*C*) Axial T1-weighted image in a different patient shows a 1.3-cm well-defined low T1 signal mass (*arrow*) in the right parotid gland. (*D*) Axial T2-weighed image shows marked T2 hyperintensity (*arrow*) centrally in this necrotic metastatic lymph node from lung carcinoma.

modalities in detecting locoregional and distant metastatic disease.[14] MR imaging is superior to PET in depicting perineural spread of tumor.

EPIDEMIOLOGY

A painless, enlarging mass in the major salivary glands is most likely caused by a neoplasm, a cyst, or an enlarged lymph node. In general, the rate of malignancy of salivary gland neoplasms is inversely proportional to the gland size. The rate of malignancy is approximately 15% to 32% in the parotid gland, 41% to 45% in the submandibular gland, and 70% to 90% in the sublingual and minor salivary glands.[3]

Cross-sectional imaging of salivary gland neoplasms is typically nonspecific; however, imaging patterns may suggest that a mass is either benign or low-grade malignant, or a higher-grade malignancy. Patterns of disease may help establish a differential diagnosis. Multiple parotid masses

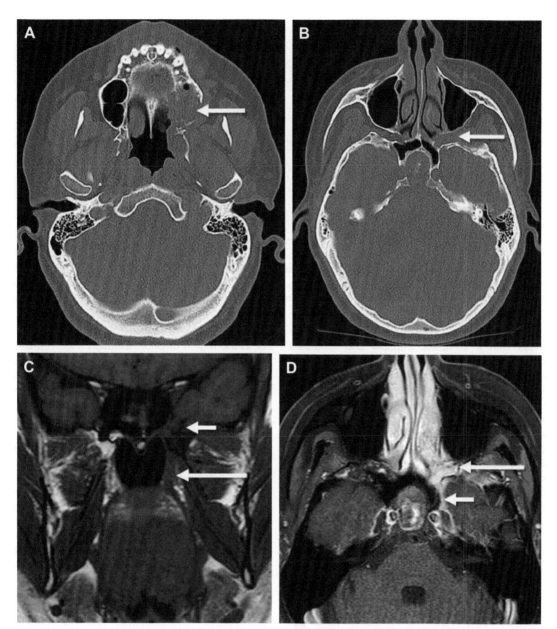

Fig. 6. Perineural tumor extension. (*A*) Axial CT bone windows shows a destructive process (*arrow*) in the left maxillary alveolar ridge in this patient with an adenoid cystic carcinoma of the palate. (*B*) Widening of the left pterygopalatine fossa (PPF) is seen (*arrow*). (*C*) Coronal T1-weighted image shows abnormal T1 hypointense soft tissue replacing the PPF (*long arrow*) and foramen rotundum (*short arrow*). (*D*) Axial postcontrast fat-saturated T1-weighted image confirms abnormal enhancement of the tissue in the PPF (*long arrow*) and foramen rotundum (*short arrow*).

may be from lymphadenopathy, Warthin tumors, Sjögren syndrome, benign lymphoepithelial lesions of HIV, lymphoma, sarcoidosis, or multiple pleomorphic adenomas (usually in the setting of prior surgery or biopsy) (Fig. 8).

Benign mixed tumor (BMT), or pleomorphic adenoma, is the most common salivary gland neoplasm, accounting for 60% to 70% of parotid tumors, with approximately 90% arising in the superficial lobe.[7] Pleomorphic adenomas are most commonly well-defined, encapsulated, solitary, T2 hyperintense, enhancing lesions. Larger lesions characteristically assume a lobular contour and are more likely to be heterogeneous in composition. Although no single imaging feature is pathognomonic for BMT, a T2 hyperintense parotid

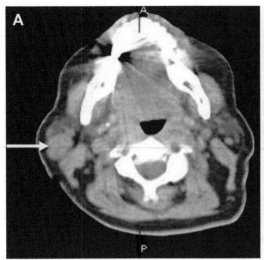
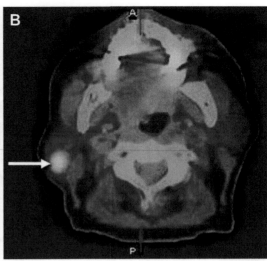

Fig. 7. Elevated FDG uptake in a benign tumor. (*A*) Axial noncontrast CT shows a mass (*arrow*) in the right parotid tail. (*B*) Fused PET-CT image shows hypermetabolism in the mass (*arrow*). On biopsy the mass represented a Warthin tumor.

mass with a complete capsule and lobulated margins is most likely to be a BMT (Fig. 9).[15] Areas of internal hemorrhage, cystic change, or calcification may be present. Dystrophic calcifications, when present, are highly suggestive of BMT.[2] Malignancy may arise in association with primary or recurrent BMT, a risk that increases with tumor duration. Carcinoma ex pleomorphic adenoma (CXPA) accounts for approximately 5% to 15% of all salivary gland malignancies. It has been estimated that malignant degeneration may eventually occur in as many as 25% of untreated BMTs.[16] Imaging features that suggest the possibility of CXPA include areas of low T2 signal and ill-defined infiltrative margins arising within a BMT

Fig. 8. Pattern of multiple parotid lesions. Axial fat-saturated T2-weighted image in a patient with HIV showing multiple solid (*arrows*) and cystic (*arrowhead*) lesions in both parotid glands, representing benign lymphoepithelial lesions.

or in the region of prior resection (Fig. 10). BMT of a deep parotid gland may be clinically silent, so CXPA is a consideration if an unusual or irregular-appearing mass presents in the deep lobe.

Warthin tumor, or papillary cystadenoma lymphomatosum, is the second most common benign tumor of the parotid gland, characteristically located in the tail of the parotid. It is the most common salivary tumor to be bilateral or multifocal. Warthin tumors maintain a well-defined margin and commonly demonstrate cyst formation; however, unlike other benign tumors, areas of low T2 signal are common.[17] Fine-needle aspiration (FNA) may yield thick black cyst contents that are characteristic of Warthin tumors. Furthermore, unlike BMTs, dystrophic calcification is not seen.[2] Other benign epithelial neoplasms of the major salivary glands include basal cell adenoma, oncocytoma, cystadenoma, and myoepithelioma.[3,18] These tumors cannot be reliably distinguished with cross-sectional imaging.

Carcinomas of the major salivary glands are composed of a diverse group of histopathologic entities, including at least 20 different histologic subtypes according to the 2005 WHO classification scheme. This classification distinguishes salivary gland carcinomas from most other head and neck cancers, which are primarily squamous cell carcinomas. According to data compiled by the Armed Forces Institute of Pathology since 1970, the most frequent malignancies of the major salivary glands are mucoepidermoid, acinic cell, adenocarcinoma not otherwise specified (NOS), adenoid cystic carcinoma, and CXPA.

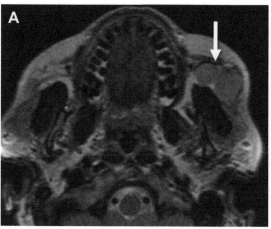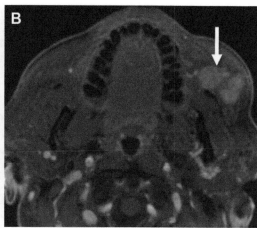

Fig. 9. Benign mixed tumor arising in accessory parotid tissue. (*A*) Axial T2-weighted image shows T2 hyperintensity (*arrow*) in this BMT. (*B*) Axial postcontrast fat-saturated T1-weighted image shows well-defined lobulated enhancing mass (*arrow*) in accessory parotid tissue superficial to the left masseter muscle.

Variability of carcinoma subtypes by demographic parameters has been noted. Squamous cell carcinoma, adenocarcinoma NOS, and salivary ductal carcinoma have higher incidence in men, whereas acinic cell and adenoid cystic carcinoma are higher in women. Except for mucoepidermoid and adenoid cystic carcinoma, which occurred with similar incidence across multiple ethnicities in the United States, all other carcinoma subtypes were more common in Caucasians compared with African Americans, Asians, and Pacific Islanders. All histologic subtypes are more frequent in people older than 50 years.[19] Ionizing radiation is the only well-established risk factor for major salivary gland carcinomas. Additional risk factors, such as viruses, tobacco, alcohol use, ultraviolet light, and occupational exposures, have been suggested to be linked with salivary gland carcinomas.[20] A positive association has been documented between smoking and Warthin tumor.[21]

Given the nonspecific imaging features of salivary malignancies, biopsy or excision is required for diagnosis. Low-grade malignancies, such as mucoepidermoid and acinic cell carcinoma, may be indistinguishable from BMT or other benign tumors on imaging (**Fig. 11**).

AJCC CANCER STAGING MANUAL, 7TH EDITION: STAGING AND CHANGES FROM PRIOR EDITION

Staging criteria for major salivary gland tumors is unchanged in the 7th edition of the *AJCC Cancer Staging Manual* (*AJCC 7th edition*); however, nomenclature has been slightly adjusted. Several factors related to prognosis and patient survival can be directly assessed radiographically, including location of origin; tumor size; extent of local spread, including facial nerve involvement or perineural extension; and lymph node or distant metastasis.

Primary tumor staging is classified based on size, extraglandular extension, and local invasion (**Tables 1** and **2**). T1 lesions are smaller than 2 cm in diameter. T2 lesions are between 2 and 4 cm in size (**Fig. 12**). T3 lesions constitute tumors

Fig. 10. Carcinoma ex pleomorphic adenoma. Axial contrast-enhanced CT shows a heterogeneously enhancing mass within the superficial left parotid gland. The mass demonstrates well-defined borders except for the posterolateral margin, consistent with extracapsular extension to the skin. A dystrophic calcification is present (*arrow*).

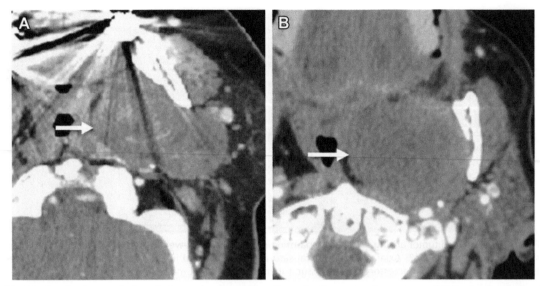

Fig. 11. Overlap in morphology between benign and malignant salivary gland neoplasms. (*A*) Contrast-enhanced CT shows a well-defined predominantly low-attenuation mass (*arrow*) in the left deep parotid lobe that was a surgically confirmed acinic cell carcinoma. (*B*) Contrast-enhanced CT in a different patient shows a similar appearing mass (*arrow*) in the same location that represented a BMT.

larger than 4 cm or those with extraglandular or extraparenchymal extension (**Fig. 13**). Locally advanced disease (T4 lesions) is stratified into moderately advanced local disease (T4a) and very advanced local disease (T4b). In the *AJCC* 6th edition, T4a and T4b tumors were referred to as resectable and unresectable lesions, respectively. Moderately advanced disease includes tumor that invades the skin (**Fig. 14**), mandible (**Fig. 15**), external auditory canal, and/or facial nerve (**Fig. 16**). Very advanced local disease describes tumor that invades the skull base and/or pterygoid plates, and/or encases the internal carotid artery (**Fig. 17**).

TRENDS IN TREATMENT AFFECTING STAGING

Preservation of the facial nerve and avoidance of iatrogenic facial nerve injury is a critical concern in planning and performing parotidectomy. Preoperative imaging reports must describe any deep lobe extension of a parotid neoplasm. MR imaging of the parotid region can be performed to demonstrate branches of the facial nerve and their anatomic relationships, but is often not routinely used in clinical practice.

Benign parotid tumors are treated with superficial parotidectomy or, in the case of deep lobe involvement, total parotidectomy with facial nerve dissection and preservation. Wide local margins are preferred, but not always possible if the mass abuts branches of the facial nerve. With optimal surgery, local control for BMT approaches 95%,

with low risk of complications. Surgery for locally recurrent disease has an increased risk of complications, particularly facial nerve injury. Postoperative radiotherapy is reserved for patients with positive margins or multifocal recurrent disease.[22] Although superficial parotidectomy is also the preferred treatment for Warthin tumors, enucleation or observation of these benign lesions may be appropriate in select cases.[23]

Treatment of salivary gland malignancies remains primarily surgical excision with wide margins. If possible, the facial nerve is spared during parotid surgery. If the facial nerve must be sacrificed because of direct neural involvement by tumor, immediate reconstruction is usually performed, if possible, using interpositional nerve grafting or segmental reanastamosis.[24] Postoperative radiation therapy is generally indicated in patients with high-grade tumors, or those with locally or regionally advanced disease (T3 or T4), recurrent tumor, or disease at high risk for locoregional recurrence, including perineural or angiolymphatic invasion or extracapsular or extraparotid spread. Neutron beam therapy is also a consideration at some centers.[25] Chemotherapy has a limited role, primarily in palliation of metastatic, recurrent, or advanced unresectable disease.[26]

Nodal spread of disease is more likely to occur with high-grade tumors, although less common than with head and neck mucosal squamous cell carcinoma.[1] Multiple studies have shown N stage to be an independent prognostic factor for survival

Table 1
AJCC 7th edition major salivary glands staging

	Primary Tumor (T)
TX	Primary tumor cannot be assessed
T0	No evidence of primary tumor
T1	Tumor 2 cm or less in greatest dimension without extraparenchymal extension*
T2	Tumor more than 2 cm but not more than 4 cm in greatest dimension without extraparenchymal extension*
T3	Tumor more than 4 cm in greatest dimension and/or tumor having extraparenchymal extension*
T4a	Moderately advanced local disease Tumor invades skin, mandible, ear canal, and/or facial nerve
T4b	Very advanced local disease Tumor invades skull base and/or pterygoid plates and/or encases carotid artery
	* Extraparenchymal extension is clinical or macroscopic evidence of invasion of soft tissues.
	Regional Lymph Nodes (N)
NX	Regional lymph nodes cannot be assessed
N0	No regional lymph node metastasis
N1	Metastasis in a single ipsilateral lymph node, 3 cm or less in greatest dimension
N2	Metastasis in a single ipsilateral lymph node, more than 3 cm but not more than 6 cm in greatest dimension; or in multiple ipsilateral lymph nodes, none more than 6 cm in greatest dimension; or in bilateral or contralateral lymph nodes, none more than 6 cm in greatest dimension
N2a	Metastasis in single ipsilateral lymph node more than 3 cm but not more than 6 cm in greatest dimension
N2b	Metastasis in multiple ipsilateral lymph nodes, none more than 6 cm in greatest dimension
N2c	Metastasis in bilateral or contralateral lymph nodes, none more than 6 cm in greatest dimension
N3	Metastasis in a lymph node more than 6 cm in greatest dimension
	Distant Metastasis (M)
M0	No distant metastasis
M1	Distant metastasis

From Greene FL, Trotti A, Fritz AG, et al, editors. AJCC cancer staging handbook. 7th edition. Chicago: American Joint Committee on Cancer; 2010. Chapter 7: Major Salivary Glands; with permission.

in salivary gland cancer.[27] The rate of lymph node metastasis is positively correlated with the extension of the primary tumor and may be as high as 53% overall.[28] Facial nerve invasion and extraglandular tumor are strongly correlated with an increased risk of nodal metastasis, which imparts a greater than 50% decrease in mean survival.[28]

Lymph node metastasis has been reported to be approximately 7% to 16% in T1 and T2 tumors, with even higher rates reported in other studies.[27] Clinically occult nodal metastases are reported to occur in 8% to 19% of cases.[25] Lymphatic spread tends to be orderly, initially involving intraglandular (parotid) and periglandular nodes, with further dissemination to upper and mid jugular chain nodes (levels II and III), followed by high posterior

triangle nodes (level VA). Retropharyngeal spread uncommonly occurs.[1]

Elective neck dissections are usually recommended for high-grade histology or T3 or T4 disease and any patients with evidence of nodal disease regardless of tumor histology.[25] Management of the clinically negative neck (N0) is more controversial. Consequently, some surgeons are more aggressive in pursuing neck dissections in treating major salivary gland cancers, particularly in patients for whom no postoperative radiation therapy is planned.[27]

PATTERNS OF DISEASE SPREAD

All salivary malignancies have the potential for perineural spread, and therefore merit attention

Table 2
Pitfalls in staging of major salivary gland cancers

Pitfall	Advice
Glandular lesion may be isodense on CT	Perform MR imaging with multiple sequences
Benign and malignant neoplasms have similar imaging appearances	FNA has an important role
Perineural tumor extension is common	Know the imaging appearance using pre-contrast T1-weighted images and fat-saturated postcontrast T1-weighted images
Metastatic submandibular lymphadenopathy difficult to differentiate from submandibular gland malignancy	Use course of facial vein to help discern
Noncontiguous involvement of the facial nerve by perineural spread from skip lesions	Evaluate the entire course of the facial nerve for skip lesions

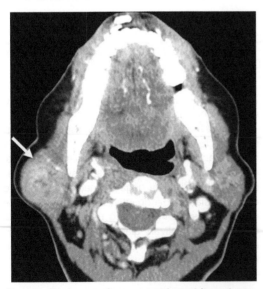

Fig. 12. T2 low-grade mucoepidermoid carcinoma. Axial contrast-enhanced CT shows heterogeneously attenuating 3-cm well-defined right superficial parotid gland mass (*arrow*).

to the skull base for retrograde perineural spread along either cranial nerve VII or the mandibular division of cranial nerve V by way of the auriculo-temporal nerve (**Fig. 18**).[29,30] Adenoid cystic carcinoma has a particular tendency toward perineural spread, even with early-stage disease.[31] Imaging findings of perineural spread include widening of neural foramen on CT and thickening of the involved nerves and replacement of fat in the neural foramen on MR imaging. Perineural spread may not always appear contiguous, and skip lesions are possible.

Distant metastases most commonly involve the lungs, followed by osseous structures and the liver. Salivary ductal carcinoma and adenoid cystic carcinoma are the most common histologic types associated with distant metastases. The risk of metastasis is best predicted by tumor size, presence of nodal disease, local extension, and tumor grade. In a retrospective study of 405 patients with major and minor salivary gland malignancies, the reported rate of distant metastases was 11% at 15 years and 24% at 40-year follow-up; 25% of patients developed distant metastases despite apparent local cure.[32]

PITFALLS IN STAGING AND DIAGNOSIS

In addition to the usual descriptions of lesion size, location, and regular or irregular margins, extraparenchymal extension of tumor upstages the mass to T3, and therefore this finding must be reported for parotid and submandibular gland neoplasms because both glands are encapsulated. Irregular border between the tumor and surrounding fibroadipose tissue or frank invasion of surrounding structures are imaging characteristics of extraglandular extension.

Compared with mucosal based lesions of other head and neck subsites, the clinical and imaging presentation of a major or minor salivary gland neoplasm is often nonspecific, with both benign and malignant tumors in the differential. Therefore, preoperative FNA is commonly performed, because both superficial and deep-seated salivary gland masses are amenable to tissue diagnosis using this technique. In fact, the salivary glands are among the most frequently aspirated sites in the head and neck. Tissue biopsy allows nonneoplastic lesions, such as reactive or inflammatory abnormalities, which can be managed medically or expectantly, to be distinguished from benign or malignant neoplastic masses. Biopsy should always be performed with image guidance, because sensitivity for malignancy in blind biopsy of salivary gland masses has been reported to be as low as 38%.[33] Most reports in the literature on

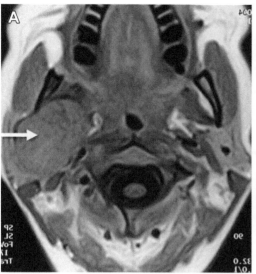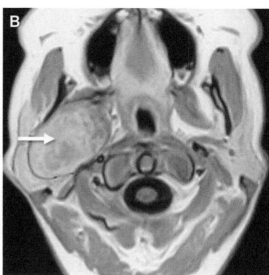

Fig. 13. T3 acinic cell carcinoma. (*A*) Axial T1-weighted image shows a 5-cm well-demarcated right parotid mass (*arrow*). (*B*) Postcontrast T1-weighted image shows fairly homogeneous enhancement in this acinic cell carcinoma (*arrow*).

the safety and efficacy of ultrasound-guided needle diagnosis are limited to the parotid and submandibular glands. This fact may be of little clinical consequence, because neoplastic masses in the sublingual and minor salivary glands are more likely to be malignant.

Tissue effects and complications have been attributed to needle biopsy, including intratumoral hemorrhage, infarction, fibrosis or granulation, and squamous metaplasia.[33] The risk of complication

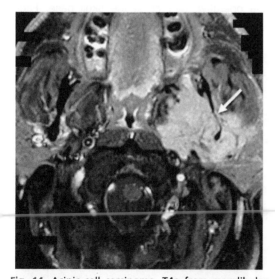

Fig. 14. Acinic cell carcinoma, T4a from mandibular involvement. Postcontrast fat-saturated T1-weighted image shows an infiltrative mass centered in the deep left parotid gland with destructive changes of the left mandible (*arrow*).

increases with needle size and the number of passes performed. The risk of vascular injury and hematoma is reported to be as high as 1% to 2% after core biopsy.[33] With FNA using a 23- or 25-gauge needle, any tissue effects will be limited in extent and will not hinder correct histopathologic diagnosis.[34]

Another criticism of FNA techniques is a higher nondiagnostic or inaccuracy rate with respect to core biopsy. Nondiagnostic or inconclusive samples have been reported to be as high as 18% after FNA.[35] Diagnostic accuracy of FNA can be maximized through onsite cytopathology assessment to confirm specimen adequacy. With appropriate expertise, the diagnostic accuracy of FNA for parotid and submandibular lesions has been reported to be 92%.[33] The nondiagnostic rate is likely to be higher in lesions that are smaller and predominantly cystic. Core needle biopsy has reported accuracy rates up to 97% in diagnosing parotid masses; however, this technique confers a higher risk of complications, such as hemorrhage, facial nerve injury, and seeding of the biopsy tract.[36] In cases showing atypical lymphoid cells on rapid assessment of aspiration samples, specimens should be sent for flow cytometry to evaluate for a monoclonal population characteristic for lymphoma.

The possibility of tumor seeding of the biopsy tract is often mentioned as a potential complication of needle biopsy. Risk of dissemination of neoplastic cells along the biopsy tract is correlated to the size of the needle bore and number of passes made. Additionally, the biopsy tract can be excised with the primary specimen. Clinically detectable tumor cell deposits after FNA are

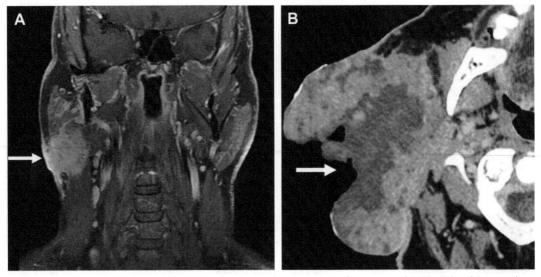

Fig. 15. T4a tumors from skin involvement. (A) Coronal postcontrast fat-saturated T1-weighted image shows a right parotid tail mass (*arrow*) that has extended to the skin surface and was visible on physical examination. (B) Axial contrast-enhanced CT shows an exophytic and ulcerated mass (*arrow*) in a different patient that has extended to the skin surface extensively.

detected at the skin puncture site in fewer than 0.009% of cases.[37]

Some advantages of FNA for salivary gland lesions are that it helps in preoperative patient counseling, especially with respect to anticipated facial nerve function; treatment planning to determine whether surgery should be urgent or a total gland resection is indicated; diagnosing lesions deemed nonsurgical (eg, lymphoma, inflammatory disease), and determining whether a neck dissection is indicated. However, the decision regarding FNA is surgeon-dependent, and it may not be requested if the mass will be excised regardless of the pathology, or if pathologic support is not available.

SURVEILLANCE PITFALLS AND APPEARANCE OF RECURRENCE

Clinical findings that are concerning for local recurrence of parotid malignancy include a mass or diffuse fullness in the operative bed, and pain in the operative bed or at the skull base. Facial paresis or paralysis in a patient with a history of

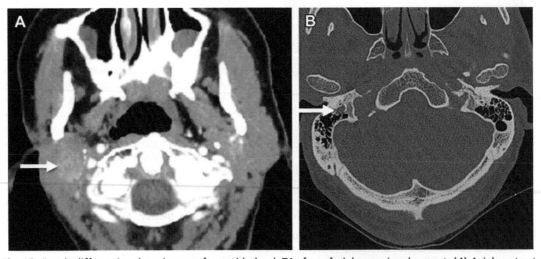

Fig. 16. Poorly differentiated carcinoma of parotid gland, T4a from facial nerve involvement. (A) Axial contrast-enhanced CT shows a 2-cm mass (*arrow*) in the right parotid gland with ill-defined margins. (B) Bone windows demonstrate enlargement of the right facial nerve canal mastoid segment (*arrow*).

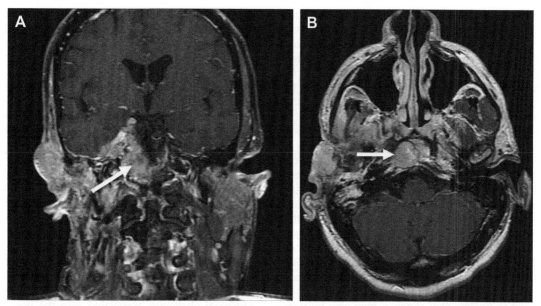

Fig. 17. Acinic cell carcinoma, T4b from skull base involvement. (*A*) Coronal postcontrast fat-saturated T1-weighed image shows extensive masticator space involvement and extension to the skull base (*arrow*) and intracranially. (*B*) Axial postcontrast T1-weighed image with abnormal expansion and enhancement in the clivus (*arrow*).

parotid malignancy must be assumed to reflect recurrent tumor, even in the absence of a clinically detectable mass. Posttreatment otalgia or periauricular pain is concerning for auriculotemporal nerve involvement.

All attempts should be made to obtain preoperative imaging before interpreting postoperative scans. After surgery, non–sharply marginated reactive enhancement and increased T2 signal may be present on MR imaging. These findings

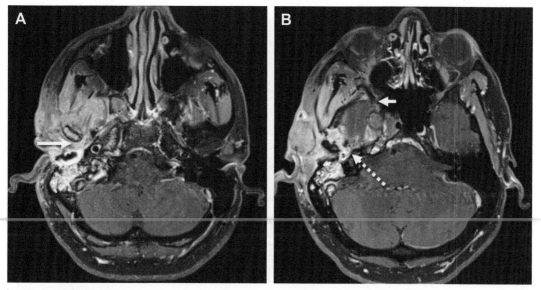

Fig. 18. Auriculotemporal nerve involvement. Axial postcontrast fat-saturated T1-weighed images from a patient with a poorly defined carcinoma. Note abnormal enhancement in the region of the right auriculotemporal nerve (*long arrow*). Perineural tumor extension has occurred along the nerve to V2 and V3 segments of the right trigeminal nerve, with tumor in the right foramen rotundum (*short arrow*) and cavernous sinus, and tumor extension along the facial nerve (*dashed arrow*).

can be misinterpreted as recurrent or residual disease, although in actuality may represent reactive postsurgical changes.[38] The location and appearance of the areas of abnormal signal intensity or attenuation must be correlated with the preoperative appearance of the tumor and the time interval from surgery when deciding whether recurrent or residual disease is likely.

Salivary malignancies may recur along a perineural distribution, especially the facial nerve. Perineural invasion may be present histopathologically, but without radiographically apparent manifestations. In other instances, subtle perineural spread may not have been appreciated on initial staging interpretation. Sialoceles are another possible imaging pitfall after salivary gland surgery (Fig. 19). Sialoceles reflect accumulation of secretions after obstruction of intraglandular ducts. Sialoceles appear as a fluid collection with or without rim enhancement. Surrounding enhancement related to postsurgical changes may also be present, complicating the appearance. Sialoceles can be misdiagnosed as abscess or tumor recurrence, particularly when surrounding enhancement or inflammatory changes are present.[38]

FUTURE DIRECTIONS AND ADVANCED IMAGING

Advanced imaging techniques have been advocated as a means to further refine the accuracy of cross-sectional imaging diagnosis. The clinical utility of these techniques is uncertain, because distinguishing whether a neoplasm is benign or low-grade versus high-grade and defining the extent of regional infiltration, perineural spread, and distant metastasis are usually sufficient for the surgeon to plan the operation and counsel the patient about the pertinent risks. Preoperative diagnosis may ultimately be most important in elderly patients and those who are poor surgical candidates, so that unnecessary surgery can be avoided.

Diffusion-weighted imaging with apparent coefficient (ADC) mapping has been used to differentiate benign and malignant salivary gland tumors.[39] Neoplasms with high ADC areas are more likely to be benign. Most malignant tumors had low or very low ADC areas constituting more than 60% of the tumor area. The problem is that this low ADC threshold does not reliably distinguish between malignancies and Warthin tumors. An additional challenge associated with the use of ADC cutoff criteria is that ADC values are affected by the strength of the diffusion gradient applied and vary between MR imaging machines.[37] ADC values can be used to evaluate for areas of malignant change within a pleomorphic adenoma, with low ADC values correlating with the hypercellular carcinomatous portions of the tumor.[40]

Dynamic contrast-enhanced MR imaging has been suggested as a way to differentiate benign from malignant disease, particularly when combined with ADC thresholds. Yabuuchi and

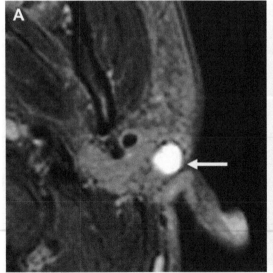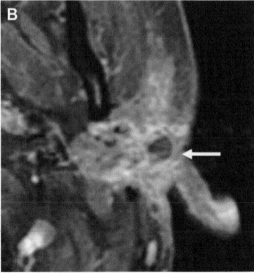

Fig. 19. Postsurgical sialocele mimicking residual tumor. (A) Axial T2-weighed image shows a well-defined markedly T2 hyperintense collection (arrow) in the postoperative bed after left superficial parotidectomy. (B) Axial postcontrast fat-saturated T1-weighed image shows nonenhancement of the area with expected surrounding postoperative changes (arrows); this should not be mistaken for an abscess or residual/recurrent tumor. (Courtesy of L. Ginsberg, MD, Anderson Cancer Center, Houston, Texas.)

colleagues[41] classified time-signal intensity curves (TIC) into 4 patterns of enhancement based on the time of peak enhancement and washout ratio. Type A (persistent pattern) shows gradual enhancement with a time to peak of longer than 120 seconds. Type B (washout pattern) has a shorter time to peak ($\leq$120 seconds) with a washout ratio of greater than 30%. Type C (plateau pattern) has a time to peak equal or less than 120 seconds and a washout ratio of less than 30%. Type D is a flat pattern, typical of predominantly cystic tumors. Histopathologically, the time to peak correlates with microvessel count, a marker for tumor vascularity, and washout ratio reflects the cellular-stromal grade of the tumor. A larger extracellular space with fibrous stromata retains contrast longer, so carcinomas that have a low cellularity-stromal grade will have a low contrast washout ratio. The persistent and flat curves show high sensitivity and specificity for benign disease. A washout curve is also typical for benign disease but not completely specific. Certain malignancies, such as acinic cell carcinoma, have a washout type TIC. A plateau curve is sensitive but demonstrates suboptimal specificity for malignant disease. Adding ADC cutoff values to tumors that demonstrate a washout or plateau TIC pattern has been proposed as a means to improve specificity in predicting benignity versus malignancy of a tumor.[42]

Proton MR spectroscopy has been evaluated for its ability to characterize salivary gland tumors, but currently has limited clinical applicability. Spectra obtained from normal parotid glands demonstrate lipids but no detectable choline (Cho) or creatine (Cr) peaks. Elevated choline, a marker of cell membrane turnover, is found in both benign and malignant tumors. An early study by King and colleagues[43] found an echo time of 136 ms to be the most successful to obtain a Cr peak for calculation of a Cho/Cr ratio. In their study, a Cho/Cr ratio greater than 2.4 had 100% positive predictive value that a salivary gland tumor was benign. Warthin tumor was likely to have a Cho/Cr ratio more than 4.5, possibly because of the larger number of lymphocytes in these tumors.

SUMMARY

Most neoplasms in other subsites in the head and neck are squamous cell carcinoma, but tumors of the salivary glands may be benign or malignant. Surgical treatment differs if the lesion is benign, and therefore preoperative FNA is important in salivary neoplasms. The role of imaging is to attempt to determine histology, predict likelihood of a lesion being malignant, and report an imaging

stage. Staging is based on size for T1 through T3 lesions and whether extraglandular extension is present. Involvement of the skull base or pterygoid plates, or the presence of pericarotid disease, upstages the lesion to T4b and must be mentioned in the radiology report.

REFERENCES

1. Greene FL, Trotti A, Fritz AG, et al, editors. AJCC cancer staging handbook. 7th edition. Chicago: American Joint Committee on Cancer; 2010.
2. Som PM, Brandwein-Gensler MS. Anatomy and pathology of the salivary glands. In: Som PM, Curtain HD, editors. Head and neck imaging. 5th edition. St Louis (MO): Elsevier Mosby; 2011. p. 2449–609.
3. Ellis GL, Auclair PL. Tumors of the salivary glands. Washington, DC: Armed Forces Institute of Pathology; 2008.
4. Standring S, editor. Grays anatomy: the anatomical base of clinical medicine. 39th edition. Edinburgh (Scotland): Elsevier Churchill Livingstone; 2005. p. 515–7, 602–4.
5. McKean ME, Lee K, McGregor IA. The distribution of lymph nodes in and around the parotid gland: an anatomical study. Br J Plast Surg 1985;38:1–5.
6. Weissman JL, Carrau RL. Anterior facial vein and submandibular gland together: Predicting the histology of submandibular masses with CT or MR imaging. Radiol 1998;208:441–6.
7. Gnepp DR, Brandwein MS, Henley JD. Salivary and lacrimal glands. In: Gnepp DR, editor. Diagnostic surgical pathology of the head and neck. 1st edition. Philadelphia: W.B. Saunders Company; 2001. p. 325–430.
8. Yousem DM, Kraut MA, Chalian AA. Major salivary gland imaging. Radiol 2000;216:19–29.
9. Sigal R, Monnet O, de Baere T, et al. Adenoid cystic carcinoma of the head and neck: evaluation with MR imaging and clinical-pathologic correlation in 27 patients. Radiology 1992;184:95–101.
10. Som PM, Biller HF. High-grade malignancies of the parotid gland: identification with MR imaging. Radiol 1989;173:823–6.
11. Christe A, Waldherr C, Hallett R, et al. MR imaging of parotid tumors: typical lesion characteristics in MR imaging improve discrimination between benign and malignant disease. AJNR Am J Neuroradiol 2011;32(7):1202–7.
12. Dailiana T, Chakeres D, Schmalbrock P, et al. High-resolution MR of the intraparotid facial nerve and parotid duct. AJNR Am J Neuroradiol 1997;18: 165–72.
13. Roh JL, Ryu CH, Choi SH, et al. Clinical utility of 18F-FDG PET for patients with salivary gland malignancies. J Nucl Med 2007;48:240–6.

14. Cermik TF, Mavi A, Acikgoz G, et al. FDG PET in detecting primary and recurrent malignant salivary gland tumors. Clin Nucl Med 2007;32:286–91.

15. Ikeda K, Katoh T, Ha-Kawa SK, et al. The usefulness of MR in establishing the diagnosis of parotid pleomorphic adenoma. AJNR Am J Neuroradiol 1996; 17:555–9.

16. Lewis JE, Olsen KD, Sebo TJ. Carcinoma ex pleomorphic adenoma: pathologic analysis of 73 cases. Hum Pathol 2001;32:596–604.

17. Ikeda M, Motoori K, Hanazawa T, et al. Warthin tumor of the parotid gland: diagnostic value of MR imaging with histopathologic correlation. AJNR Am J Neuroradiol 2004;25:1256–62.

18. Weinstein GS, Harvey RT, Zimmer W, et al. Technetium-99m pertechnetate salivary gland imaging: Its role in diagnosis of Warthin's tumor. J Nucl Med 1994;35:179–83.

19. Boukheris H, Curtis RE, Land CE, et al. Incidence of carcinoma of the major salivary glands according to the WHO classification, 1002 to 2006: a population-based study in the United States. Cancer Epidemiol Biomarkers Prev 2009;18:2899–906.

20. Horn-Ross PL, Ljung B, Morrow M. Environmental factors and the risk of salivary gland cancer. Epidemiology 1997;8:414–9.

21. Kotwall CA. Smoking as an etiologic factor in the development of Warthin's tumor of the parotid gland. Am J Surg 1992;164:646–7.

22. Mendenhall WM, Mendenhall CM, Werning JW, et al. Salivary gland pleomorphic adenoma. Am J Clin Oncol 2008;31:95–9.

23. Yoo GH, Eisele DW, Askin FB, et al. Warthin's tumor: a 40-year experience at The Johns Hopkins Hospital. Laryngoscope 1994;104:799–803.

24. Scianna JM, Petruzelli GJ. Contemporary management of tumors of the salivary glands. Curr Oncol Rep 2007;9:134–8.

25. Bell RB, Dierks EJ, Homer L, et al. Management and outcome of patients with malignant salivary gland tumors. J Oral Maxillofac Surg 2005;63:917–28.

26. Day TA, Deveikis J, Gillespie MB, et al. Salivary gland neoplasms. Curr Treatment Opin Oncol 2004;5:11–26.

27. Stennert E, Kisner D, Jungehuelsing M, et al. High incidence of lymph node metastasis in major salivary gland cancer. Arch Otolaryngol Head Neck Surg 2003;129:720–3.

28. Bhattacharyya N, Fried MP. Nodal metastasis in major salivary gland cancer. Arch Otolaryngol Head Neck Surg 2002;128:904–8.

29. Schmalfuss IM, Tart RP, Jukherji S, et al. Perineural tumor spread along the auriculotemporal nerve. Am J Neuroradiol 2002;23:303–11.

30. Ginsberg LE. Imaging of perineural tumor spread in head and neck cancer. Semin Ultrasound CT MRI 1999;20:175–86.

31. Bradley PJ. Adenoid cystic carcinoma of the head and neck: a review. Curr Opin Otolaryngol Head Neck Surg 2004;12:127–32.

32. Bradley PJ. Distant metastases from salivary glands cancer. ORL J Otorhinolaryngol Relat Spec 2001;63: 233–42.

33. Sharma G, Jung AS, Maceri DR, et al. US-guided fine-needle aspiration of major salivary gland masses and adjacent lymph nodes: accuracy and impact on clinical decision making. Radiol 2011; 259:471–8.

34. Mukunyadzi P, Bardales RH, Palmer HE, et al. Tissue effects of salivary gland fine-needle aspiration. Does this procedure preclude accurate histologic diagnosis? Anat Pathol 2000;114:741–5.

35. Cajulis RS, Gokaslan ST, Yu GH, et al. Fine needle aspiration biopsy of the salivary glands: a five-year experience with emphasis on diagnostic pitfalls. Acta Cytol 1997;41:1412–20.

36. Wan YL, Chan SC, Chen YL, et al. Ultrasonography-guided core-needle biopsy of parotid gland masses. AJNR Am J Neuroradiol 2004;25:1608–12.

37. Supriya M, Denholm S, Palmer T. Seeding of tumor cells after fine needle aspiration cytology in benign parotid tumor: a case report and literature review. Laryngoscope 2008;118:263–5.

38. Ginsberg LE. Imaging pitfalls in the postoperative head and neck. Semin Ultrasound CT MRI 2002; 23:444–59.

39. Eida S, Sumi M, Sakihama N, et al. Apparent diffusion coefficient mapping of salivary gland tumors: prediction of the benignancy and malignancy. AJNR Am J Neuroradiol 2007;28:116–21.

40. Kato H, Kanematsu M, Mizuta K, et al. Carcinoma ex pleomorphic adenoma of the parotid gland: radiographic-pathologic correlation with MR imaging including diffusion-weighted imaging. AJNR Am J Neuroradiol 2008;29:865–7.

41. Yabuuchi H, Fukuya T, Tajima T, et al. Salivary gland tumors: diagnostic value of gadolinium-enhanced dynamic MR imaging with histopathologic correlation. Radiol 2003;226:345–54.

42. Yabuuchi H, Matsuo Y, Kamitani T, et al. Parotid gland tumors: can addition of diffusion-weighted MR imaging to dynamic contrast-enhanced MR imaging improve diagnostic accuracy in characterization? Radiol 2008;249:909–16.

43. King AD, Yeung DK, Ahuja AT, et al. Salivary gland tumors at in vivo proton MR spectroscopy. Radiol 2005;237:563–9.

Pitfalls in the Staging of Cancer of Thyroid

Amit M. Saindane, MD

KEYWORDS

- Thyroid gland • Papillary thyroid carcinoma • Medullary thyroid carcinoma
- Follicular thyroid carcinoma • Anaplastic thyroid carcinoma • Extrathyroidal extension

KEY POINTS

- Thyroid cancer includes several neoplasms originating from the thyroid gland from indolent and curable histologies of differentiated thyroid carcinoma to aggressive anaplastic thyroid carcinoma.
- Differentiation of thyroid nodules is problematic on CT and MR imaging unless there is evidence of extrathyroidal extension.
- Nuclear scintigraphy is useful for staging and treatment of distant metastasis in differentiated thyroid carcinoma, and PET may have a role in aggressive cancers.
- Staging affects surgical management and subsequent therapy.

INTRODUCTION AND EPIDEMIOLOGY

The term thyroid cancer encompasses several neoplasms originating from the thyroid gland. Altogether, cancers of the thyroid gland currently have a yearly incidence of 37,000 in the United States, ranking tenth among solid organ malignancies.[1] There is a strong female predominance.[1] Papillary thyroid carcinoma (PTC) and follicular thyroid carcinoma (FTC) are tumors of the thyroid follicular cells collectively referred to as differentiated thyroid carcinoma (DTC).[2] PTC is the most common thyroid malignancy, comprising approximately 85% of cases, and often has an indolent clinical course with low mortality and high likelihood for cure. There are, however, several other subtypes of PTC based on specific histologic features. The follicular variant has the typical cellular features of nuclear grooves and Orphan Annie eye nuclei, but it predominantly has a microfollicular pattern instead of the branching papilla of typical PTC.[3] The tall cell variant of PTC histologically demonstrates cells that are twice as tall as wide and is associated with worse survival than classic PTC.[4] Similarly, insular carcinoma, which is histologically characterized by solid cell clusters with small follicles similar to pancreatic islets, has a poorer prognosis than classic PTC.[5]

FTC is often difficult to distinguish from benign follicular neoplasms on fine-needle aspiration (FNA).[6] The criteria for malignancy are capsular or vascular invasion. In contrast to PTC, spread to lymph nodes in FTC is uncommon, occurring in only 8% to 13% of cases, with typical spread via hematogenous dissemination and distant metastases in 10% to 15% of patients, even with small primary tumors. Hürthle cell carcinoma is considered a subtype of FTC and is characterized pathologically by mitochondria-rich oncocytes. It has a higher rate of lymph node metastases compared with classic FTC, rarely presents with distant metastases, but has the highest incidence of late distant metastasis.[7] Although the management of the various forms of DTC has many similarities, there are important differences in their diagnosis, treatment, and prognosis.[8] Included in the poorly-differentiated thyroid cancers is medullary thyroid

Department of Radiology and Imaging Sciences, School of Medicine, Emory University, BG-22, 1364 Clifton Road Northeast, Atlanta, GA 30322, USA
E-mail address: asainda@emory.edu

Neuroimag Clin N Am 23 (2013) 123–145
http://dx.doi.org/10.1016/j.nic.2012.08.010
1052-5149/13/$ – see front matter © 2013 Elsevier Inc. All rights reserved

carcinoma (MTC), a tumor of the thyroid parafollicular C cells that secrete calcitonin, and anaplastic thyroid carcinoma (ATC), which is thought to arise from well-differentiated thyroid cancer[9] and portends a significantly worse outcome.[8]

Thyroid nodules are commonly recognized during routine physical examination, but are also increasingly incidentally detected on various imaging examinations including ultrasonography (US), CT and MR imaging. The routine work-up of palpable and incidental thyroid nodules has been reviewed in detail.[10] In general, evaluation includes thorough physical examination of the neck, US for confirmation and characterization, which may identify other thyroid nodules or cervical lymphadenopathy, and FNA for evaluation of suspicious nodules. Appropriate diagnostic evaluation and interpretation is crucial to ensure timely treatment with patients with false-negative FNA eventually found to have higher rates of vascular and capsular invasion,[11] and with a near doubling of 30-year mortality rate when therapy was delayed by more than 1 year from diagnosis.[12]

THYROID EMBRYOLOGY AND ANATOMY

Embryologically, the thyroid gland develops as an epithelial proliferation from the floor of the pharynx in the dorsal tongue at the level of the foramen cecum. At approximately 5 weeks, fetal development the thyroid descends caudally around the hyoid bone, deep to the strap musculature, and to its expected location below the level of the laryngeal primordium, where it forms lateral lobes and isthmus.[13] The embryologic pathway from the foramen cecum to the isthmus of the thyroid is the thyroglossal duct, which subsequently involutes. Arrest of migration of part or all of the thyroid gland can result in ectopic thyroid tissue or cysts anywhere along this thyroglossal duct.

The thyroid gland resides in the lower portion of the infrahyoid neck within the visceral space (level VI), which is bounded superiorly by the hyoid bone, laterally by the carotid arteries and inferiorly by the sternal notch (**Figs. 1** and **2**). The visceral space is

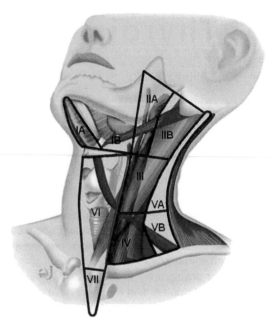

Fig. 2. The central compartment of the neck (visceral space; level VI) level VI lymph nodes lie between the carotid arteries from the level of the bottom of the body of the hyoid bone to the top of the manubrium. (*Courtesy of* Eric Jablonowski.)

encompassed by the middle layer of deep cervical fascia and also envelops the thyroid strap musculature, the parathyroid glands, larynx, hypopharynx, trachea, and esophagus. The isthmus of the thyroid gland generally lies anterior to the second to fourth tracheal rings, with the lateral thyroid lobes anterolateral to the lower thyroid cartilage, cricoid cartilage, and upper trachea. A small pyramidal lobe may be present, extending superiorly from the isthmus anterior to the thyroid cartilage, where it may connect with a thyroglossal duct remnant.

The outer surface of the thyroid gland is incompletely covered by a thin connective tissue layer in direct continuity with the stroma that defines lobules of thyroid parenchyma.[14] This discontinuous fibroadipose connective tissue layer has been described as the internal thyroid capsule. The external thyroid capsule or surgical capsule is mainly derived from the pretracheal deep cervical fascia, is adherent to the deep surface of the strap muscles, and posterolaterally continuous with the carotid sheath.[13] This external thyroid capsule is deficient in the anterior midline, so the thyroid isthmus is connected directly to the subcutaneous fat and superficial cervical fascia.[15]

The arterial supply to the thyroid gland is from the paired superior thyroidal arteries arising from the external carotid arteries and from the paired inferior thyroidal arteries arising from the

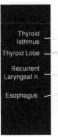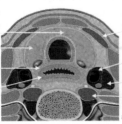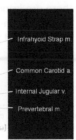

Fig. 1. Normal thyroid anatomy illustration. (*Courtesy of* Eric Jablonowski.)

thyrocervical trunks of the subclavian arteries. A rare persistent embryonic vessel called the thyroidea ima artery may arise directly from the aortic arch to supply the lower thyroid gland. Both superior and middle thyroidal veins drain the very vascular thyroid tissues via the internal jugular veins, whereas the inferior thyroidal veins drain into the brachiocephalic veins.

The lymphatic pathways in the thyroid gland are intricate and interconnected with those of the larynx, trachea, recurrent laryngeal nerve (RLN), and cervical great vessels (see **Fig. 2**). There is an extensive intrathyroidal lymphatic network that joins subcapsular lymphatic trunks, which generally drain the thyroid along the course of thyroidal veins.[16] The lymph nodes in the visceral space can be subdivided into the pretracheal, prelaryngeal (delphian), and paratracheal nodes.[17] The upper poles, isthmus, and the pyramidal lobe drain into level II and III nodal zones. The lateral aspects of the thyroid lobes drain along the middle thyroid veins into level III and IV nodal zones. The lower poles drain into the pretracheal and paratracheal lymph nodes within the level VI nodal zone, which then drain into levels IV and VII. There are also direct lymphatic communications in levels II, III, and IV, which then drain into level VII via level VI.[18] These lymphatic pathways are variable and lymphatics draining into the capsule may cross-communicate with the isthmus and the contralateral lobe.[19]

IMAGING TECHNIQUES IN THYROID CANCER
US

US has demonstrated its utility in characterizing palpable or incidentally found thyroid nodules preoperatively into groups based on benign or malignant features.[20] Based on such determination of relative risk for thyroid malignancy, US also facilitates detection of additional nonpalpable nodules, evaluation of lymph nodes in the central and lateral neck, and performance of US-guided (UG-FNA).[21,22]

A variety of US characteristics are thought to differentiate benign from malignant thyroid lesions.[20,23] Whereas smooth margins of a thyroid nodule may indicate benignity, irregular or ill-defined lesions suggest a malignant lesion. Some malignant nodules may have a cystic component, but many are solid and appear hypoechoic relative to adjacent thyroid tissue. Most benign lesions result in acoustic shadowing or enhancement. A thyroid nodule that is greater in its anteroposterior than in its transverse dimension has also been described more likely to represent a malignant instead of a benign lesion.[20] Microcalcifications are more strongly associated with malignancy compared with coarse or no calcifications. Central vascularity is more likely to be present in malignant thyroid nodules, whereas peripheral vascularity is associated with benign lesions.[20,23]

The typical US findings of metastatic lymph nodes in thyroid cancer include a homogenous hypoechoic or heterogeneous pattern, an irregular cystic appearance, the presence of internal calcification, loss of reniform shape, and increased anteroposterior diameter.[24] Cystic change is said to be highly suggestive of PTC[25] and is well-demonstrated by US. Occasionally this can appear as a cyst and thus mimic a branchial cleft cyst in younger patients (**Fig. 3**).[26] US demonstrates a high positive predictive value for lateral node metastasis, which can be increased further by UG-FNA of suspected metastasis[27]; however, there are many false negatives with US for both

A   B

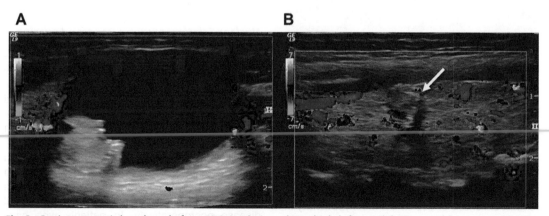

Fig. 3. Cystic metastatic lymph node from PTC simulating a branchial cleft cyst. (A) 22-year-old woman presenting with level II neck mass that on US appears cystic and compatible with a second branchial cleft cyst. (B) US of the right thyroid lobe demonstrated a 5 mm papillary microcarcinoma (*arrow*). UG-FNA revealed metastatic PTC and right neck dissection demonstrated 10 out of 41 positive lymph nodes for PTC.

central compartment and lateral lymph nodes.[28] US has additional value in the postoperative surveillance of patients treated for thyroid cancer.[29,30] Routinely, patients undergo an initial cervical US in the first year following resection of their thyroid cancer[31] with subsequent US performed according to patient's risk of locoregional recurrence.

CT

CT optimally requires the use of intravenous iodinated contrast agents to opacify normal vascular structures and to delineate abnormal enhancement. The iodine load may alter radioactive iodine uptake for 6 weeks after its administration and is, therefore, generally not ideal in initial presurgical evaluation of thyroid cancer. Characterization of thyroid nodules as benign or malignant is highly problematic on CT unless features of gross extrathyroidal extension (ETE) are present (**Fig. 4**). Both CT and MR imaging are useful tools for the evaluation of ETE into the surrounding organs such as larynx and trachea, and CT may be particularly useful in defining invasion of the cartilaginous framework of the laryngotracheal complex. Complete evaluation of cervical lymph nodes is offered by both CT and MR imaging, including retropharyngeal, deep cervical, and substernal regions. Metastatic nodes can appear as cystic masses, have multiple punctate calcifications,[32] or enhance avidly.[26] Metastatic lymph nodes may be of high attenuation even before intravenous contrast

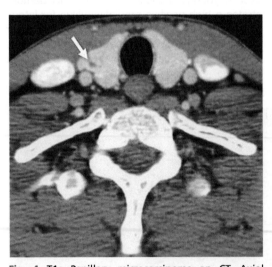

Fig. 4. T1a Papillary microcarcinoma on CT. Axial contrast-enhanced CT depicts a 4 mm hypodensity in the right thyroid lobe (*arrow*) with nonspecific features that on biopsy represented PTC. No imaging features can reliably detect microcarcinoma, emphasizing need for UG-FNA.

administration because of the presence of intranodal hemorrhage or thyroglobulin.

MR Imaging

Unlike iodinated contrast for CT, gadolinium-based contrast agents for MR imaging do not affect thyroid iodine uptake. On MR imaging, both benign thyroid nodules and malignant tumors are generally well-defined and often indistinguishable, or may be occult. Most malignant thyroid tumors demonstrate isointense signal to normal thyroid tissue on T1-weighted images and hyperintense signal on T2-weighted images, with avid enhancement[33,34] making the signal characteristics nonspecific (**Fig. 5**). Microcalcifications representing psammoma bodies are readily detected on US and sometimes on CT, but are poorly seen on MR imaging. Tumor invasion into the posterior paratracheal tissues and substernal area is better visualized on MR imaging than US because of obscuration due to the bone and lung.[2] MR imaging offers the best option for assessing soft tissue invasion, in particular when pharyngoesophageal invasion is suspected.

On MR imaging, metastatic lymph nodes can have low to intermediate signal intensity on T1-weighted and hyperintensity on T2-weighted images, or hyperintensity on both T1-weighted and T2-weighted images,[26] reflecting a high thyroglobulin content or hemorrhage (**Fig. 6**). Metastatic nodes may enhance markedly. A cystic or necrotic appearance is helpful to raise suspicion for metastasis[35] but may simulate a second branchial cleft cyst or metastasis from an oropharyngeal primary. MR imaging has been shown to be highly specific for nodal metastasis but with low sensitivity.[36] The retropharyngeal and mediastinal regions are not amenable to imaging on US, but are well-evaluated on MR imaging.[37]

Nuclear Scintigraphy and Positron Emission Tomography

Radioiodine scintigraphy provides functional information about the thyroid gland and is useful for patients with abnormal thyroid function. For focal thyroid masses, however, most nodules are hypofunctioning (cold) and the risk of malignancy in such a nodule is between 8% to 25%,[38] so radioiodine scintigraphy does not play a major role in the diagnostic workup. It is generally performed as part of postoperative radioactive iodine ablation (RAI) and may detect occult metastasis or residual disease postoperatively. In patients who have intermediate or high risk for disease recurrence, or who have elevated thyroglobulin levels, radioactive iodine scanning may be helpful in identifying

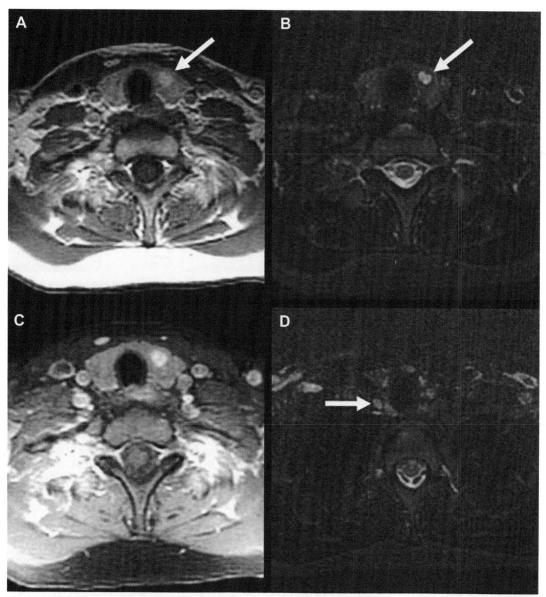

Fig. 5. T1a Papillary microcarcinoma on MR imaging. (A) Axial T1-weighted image demonstrates a slightly T1 hyperintense lesion in the left thyroid lobe (arrow). (B) Axial fat-saturated T2-weighted image demonstrates well-defined margin and T2 hyperintensity of the lesion (arrow). (C) Axial postcontrast fat-saturated T1-weighted image shows marked contrast enhancement. (D) Axial fat-saturated T2-weighted image with multiple subcentimeter level VI lymph nodes (arrow). Pathologic diagnosis was PTC.

foci of thyroid cancer.[10] This modality has low sensitivity in low-risk patients who have undergone complete resection and adjuvant radioactive iodine.[39,40] In patients with MTC, imaging with octreotide or m-iodobenzylguanidine (MIBG) may be useful.

Fluorodeoxyglucose F 18 positron-emission tomography (FDG-PET) is of limited utility for characterization of primary thyroid nodules because they may or may not be FDG-avid,[41] (Fig. 7). In the thyroglobulin-positive but radioactive iodine scan–negative patient, FDG-PET has a role in defining the location of persistent or recurrent disease but, despite a reproducible ability to detect recurrent thyroid cancer, use of FDG-PET rarely alters treatment.[42] However, it has prognostic value because the number of FDG-avid lesions and their intensity helps identify patients at highest risk for rapid disease progression and disease specific mortality.[43]

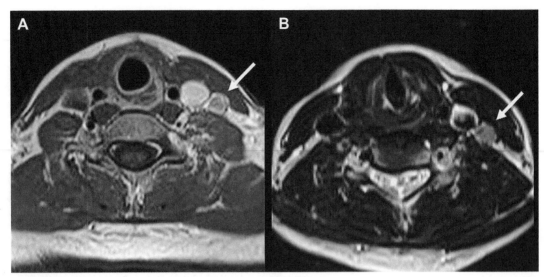

Fig. 6. Cystic lateral neck metastasis from PTC. (A) Axial T1-weighted and (B) T2-weighted images show a T1 and T2 hyperintense lymph node (arrows) in the left level III neck, which on UG-FNA was determined to be PTC.

STAGING OF DTC AND PITFALLS

The clinical and pathologic factors associated with disease recurrence and/or disease-free survival have been described.[44–46] The main clinical factors are increased age[45,46] and male gender.[12,45] Among the postoperative pathologic factors, tumor size, ETE, tumor histology, and presence of metastatic disease all have prognostic value.[45,46] Various staging systems have been proposed to stage DTC.[47] The American Joint Commission on Cancer (AJCC) scheme depends on age and a standardized TNM (tumor, node,

metastasis) classification described in Table 1. The pitfalls in staging of thyroid cancer are described in Table 2).

The primary tumor (T) classification is based on tumor size and extracapsular extension. In some cases the primary tumor is not evident on any imaging modality or even on pathologic study, representing a T0 lesion (Fig. 8). A T1 lesion is up to 2 cm in the largest dimension, a T2 primary tumor is more than 2 cm but less than 4 cm, and T3 includes an intrathyroidal lesion more than 4 cm. A T3 lesion also includes any tumor with minimal

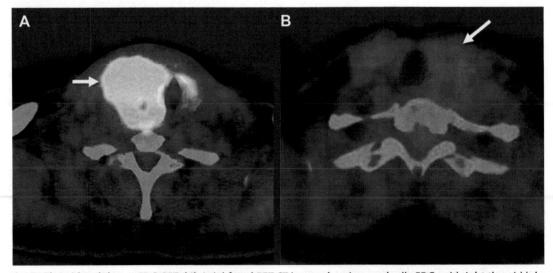

Fig. 7. Thyroid nodules on FDG-PET. (A) Axial fused PET-CT image showing markedly FDG-avid right thyroid lobe tumor (arrow). (B) Axial fused PET-CT image from a different patient showing a cystic nodule (arrow) with only mild peripheral uptake. Both were PTC on pathologic study.

Table 1	
AJCC 7 thyroid cancer staging	
Primary Tumor (T)	
TX	Primary tumor cannot be assessed
T0	No evidence of primary tumor
T1	Tumor 2 cm or less in greatest dimension limited to the thyroid
T1a	Tumor 1 cm or less, limited to the thyroid
T1b	Tumor more than 1 cm but not more than 2 cm in greatest dimension, limited to the thyroid
T2	Tumor more than 2 cm but not more than 4 cm in greatest dimension, limited to the thyroid
T3	Tumor more than 4 cm in greatest dimension limited to the thyroid, or any tumor with minimal extrathyroid extension (eg, extension to sternothyroid muscle or perithyroid soft tissues)
T4a	Moderately advanced disease Tumor of any size extending beyond the thyroid capsule to invade subcutaneous soft tissues, larynx, trachea, esophagus, or RLN
T4b	Very advanced disease Tumor invades prevertebral fascia or encases carotid artery or mediastinal vessels
All anaplastic carcinomas are considered T4 tumors	
T4a	Intrathyroidal anaplastic carcinoma
T4b	Anaplastic carcinoma with gross extrathyroid extension
Regional Lymph Nodes (N)	
NX	Regional lymph nodes cannot be assessed
N0	No regional lymph node metastasis
N1	Regional lymph node metastasis
N1a	Metastasis to level VI (pretracheal, paratracheal, and prelaryngeal/ Delphian lymph nodes)
N1b	Metastasis to unilateral, bilateral, or contralateral cervical (levels I, II, III, IVor V) or retropharyngeal or superior mediastinal lymph nodes (level VII)
Distant Metastasis (M)	
M0	No distant metastasis
M1	Distant metastasis

From Greene FL, Trotti A, Fritz AG, et al, editors. AJCC Cancer staging handbook. 7th edition. Chicago: American Joint Committee on Cancer; 2010. Chapter 7: Major Salivary Glands; with permission.

Table 2	
Pitfalls in staging of thyroid cancer	
Pitfall	**Advice**
Misdiagnosis of cystic neck mass as second branchial cleft cyst	Consider metastatic PTC (as well as oropharyngeal squamous cell carcinoma) and carefully evaluate the thyroid gland.
Misdiagnosis of thyroid nodule on PET as benign due to low FDG uptake	Evaluate incidental nodules on PET with US and UG-FNA
Misdiagnosis of thyroid nodule on CT or MR imaging as benign due to presence of multiple nodules suggestive of goiter	Evaluate any dominant nodule on CT or MR imaging with US and carefully assess for any features of ETE
Understaging due to failure to recognize ETE to the RLN	Recognize the CT/MR imaging signs of VCP and scrutinize the tracheoesophageal groove region
Upstaging to T4a: overcalling tracheal wall involvement on CT	Consider MR imaging in absence of gross intraluminal tumor to better evaluate the tracheal wall
Understaging of N stage from retropharyngeal lymph node metastasis clinically or with US	Carefully evaluate retropharyngeal lymph nodes on CT and MR imaging
Understaging of distant metastasis on neck MR imaging and CT	Evaluate the lung apices for nodules and osseous structures for lytic lesions

ETE, defined as extension to the sternothyroid muscle or perithyroid soft tissues. Tumors with further extension become T4, subdivided into T4a and T4b. T4a refers to tumors invading subcutaneous soft tissues, the larynx, trachea, esophagus, or RLN. T4b lesions are the lesions invading the prevertebral fascia or carotid artery or mediastinal vessels.

Regional lymph node spread from DTC is common. The central compartment (level VI) lymph

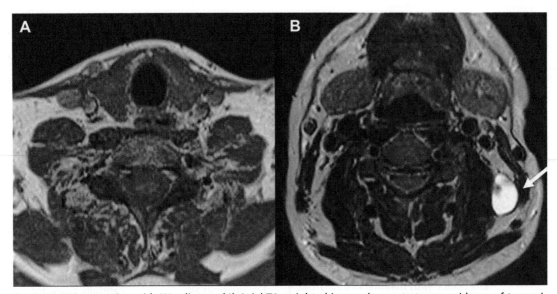

Fig. 8. T0 PTC presenting with N1a disease. (*A*) Axial T1-weighted image demonstrates no evidence of tumor in the thyroid gland. This was confirmed as no abnormality on US. (*B*) Axial T2-weighted image depicts a cystic lymph node metastasis (*arrow*) in the left level IIB station that was pathologically proven on FNA to be PTC.

nodes are the primary locations for thyroid node metastasis. The lateral cervical nodes include levels II to V, although levels II and V are less commonly involved than III and IV. Upper mediastinal (level VII) lymph node involvement is common. NX is designated when regional nodes cannot be assessed. N0 indicates no regional lymph node metastasis. N1 indicates regional lymph node metastasis, with N1a indicating metastasis to the central compartment and N1b indicating involvement of any lymph node in lateral compartment or superior mediastinum. There is no difference between ipsilateral and contralateral lymph node metastasis in staging for thyroid cancer nodal classification. M0 and M1 indicate the absence or presence of distal metastases, respectively.

Tumor Size

In DTC, primary tumor size correlates with outcome, with larger tumors more likely to present with locoregional and distant metastases.[12] Tumors less than 1 cm are rarely associated with mortality[48]; however, the risk of recurrent local disease and mortality increases linearly with tumor size. In one study, primary tumors less than 1.5 cm had 30-year cancer-specific mortality rates of 0.4% compared with 22% in tumors measuring greater than 4.5 cm.[12] The presence of underlying thyroiditis or multinodular goiter may cause difficulty in detection of small thyroid lesions (**Fig. 9**) or the presence of coexistent benign and malignant lesions (**Fig. 10**). Total thyroidectomy is the recommended surgical approach for nearly all patients with DTC. Furthermore, by surgically

removing the entire gland, total thyroidectomy facilitates the use of radioactive iodine for adjuvant therapy, serial measurement of serum thyroglobulin for surveillance, and neck US identify residual or recurrent disease. Thyroid lobectomy is an acceptable alternative for those patients with tumors less than 1 cm confined to one thyroid lobe without nodules within the contralateral lobe.[10] This more limited procedure avoids injury to structures in the contralateral neck without effect on long-term survival.[49] PTC is multifocal in 18% to 46% of cases, and can arise as independent tumors or because of intrathyroidal metastasis via the rich lymphatic network within the thyroid.[50]

ETE

About 6% to 13% of patients with DTC have ETE, which is associated with an increased incidence of local recurrence, regional and distant metastasis, and decreased survival.[51,52] The most commonly involved structures with invasive thyroid cancer are the strap muscles (53%), RLN (47%), trachea (37%), esophagus (21%), and larynx (12%).[53] Minimal extension of cancer outside the thyroid into the surrounding tissues may be found in as many as 30% of patients with PTC.[12,48] For most patients, such ETE is microscopic and only seen at histologic sectioning[48] but may be suggested on imaging (**Fig. 11**). Even the histologic interpretation of ETE can be problematic because the discontinuous pseudocapsule surrounding the gland makes involvement of surrounding fibrous and adipose tissue do not necessarily indicate

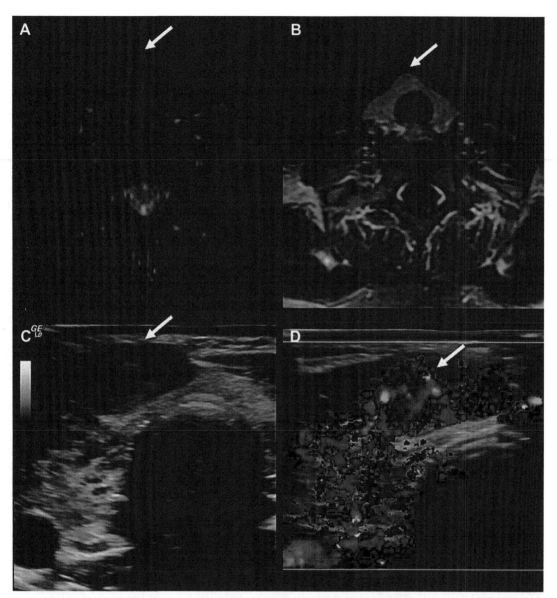

Fig. 9. T2 PTC in setting of Hashimoto's thyroiditis. Axial fat-saturated T2-weighted (*A*) postcontrast fat-saturated T1-weighted (*B*) images showing contour abnormality but no focal lesion in the isthmus of the thyroid gland (*arrow*). Grayscale (*C*) and color-Doppler (*D*) US reveal a hypoechoic mass (*arrows*) in the right aspect of the isthmus with hypervascularity of both the nodule and background thyroid gland from Hashimoto's thyroiditis.

invasion beyond the thyroid gland. Ito and colleagues[54] concluded that minimal ETE did not affect the relapse-free survival. However, some studies have shown even microscopic extension beyond the thyroid capsule may be associated with a higher risk of recurrent disease,[55] likelihood of lymph node metastases,[56] and a higher mortality rate.[12] The discordance in findings likely relates to a variable definition of minimal ETE.

Intraoperative suspicion of ETE is usually observed by adherence of the strap musculature to the external surface of the thyroid gland or adherence of the gland to the trachea, RLN, or esophageal musculature. Tumors classified as pT4 are defined by major tumor extension beyond the capsule and subcutaneous soft tissues, with invasion of larynx, trachea, esophagus, RLN, prevertebral fascia, mediastinal vessels, and carotid artery. This is associated with a high-risk of locoregional disease recurrence,[57] generally requires aggressive surgical resection,[58] and, in some cases, may benefit from external beam radiotherapy.[59]

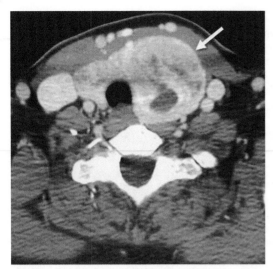

Fig. 10. T3 insular carcinoma in setting of multinodular goiter. A 4-cm dominant mass in left thyroid lobe (*arrow*) in setting of heterogeneous gland consistent with multinodular goiter. The dominant mass was biopsy proven as insular carcinoma.

Strap Muscles

The most frequently involved structure of thyroid cancer is the overlying strap musculature. Isolated strap muscle invasion has not been found to correlate with decreased survival.[53] Management of strap muscle invasion requires only wide local excision with negative margins and no significant morbidity is caused by resection of the strap

muscles. According to the AJCC 7 staging criteria, tumors with minimal ETE (invasion into sternothyroid muscle or perithyroid tissues) is classified as a pT3 tumor.

RLN

Vocal cord paralysis (VCP) on CT or MR imaging appears as ipsilateral laryngeal ventricular enlargement, internal rotation of the arytenoid, and lack of medial conversion of the vocal cord (Fig. 12). VCP is not only specifically related to RLN invasion but is also related to pressure on the nerve in the absence of invasion.[60] MR imaging has been shown to be accurate in detection of RLN invasion.[61] If the RLN is paralyzed preoperatively and found to be invaded at the time of surgery, resection of the nerve is recommended. If the RLN is functioning preoperatively, the decision to sacrifice it weighs the risk of leaving gross tumor behind against the outcome of vocal cord paralysis. Before sacrificing the RLN, however, it is critical to ensure that the opposite nerve is not directly involved with the tumor because bilateral VCP is a devastating complication that generally requires tracheostomy. When the RLN is considered to be functional in the preoperative assessment, most investigators advise preservation, if possible, because there is no survival benefit with nerve sacrifice compared with nerve preservation with postoperative RAI ablation.[62] Patients with residual microscopic disease should undergo postoperative RAI ablation or possibly external beam radiation (EBRT).

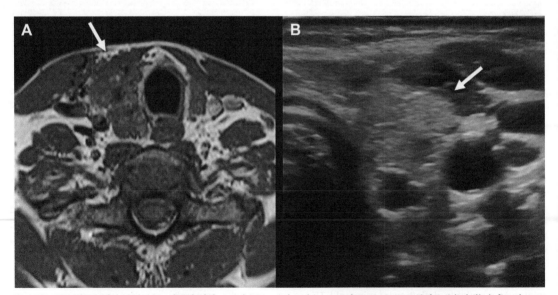

Fig. 11. Extrathyroidal extension (ETE). (*A*) Axial T1-weighted image demonstrates right-sided ill-defined mass (*arrow*) with loss of fat plane with the adjacent strap musculature. (*B*) US image in a different patient demonstrates left sided thyroid mass (*arrow*) with apparent extension in to left strap musculature.

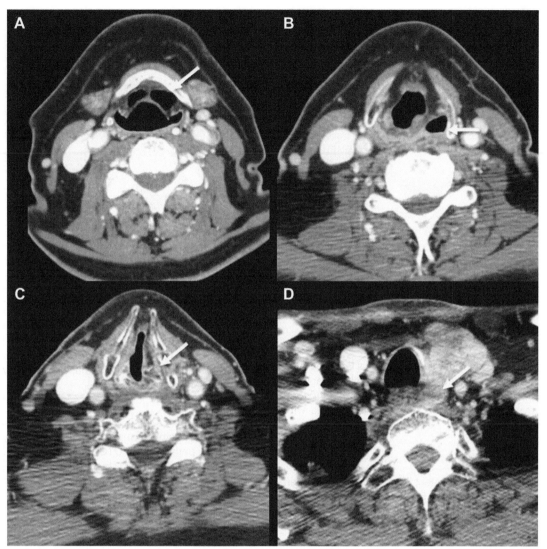

Fig. 12. RLN involvement. Axial contrast-enhanced CT images show (*A*) ipsilateral dilatation of the vallecula (*arrow*), (*B*) piriform sinus (*arrow*), (*C*) rotation of the left aretynoid cartilage (*arrow*), and paramedian location of a fatty left true vocal cord. (*D*) There is extension of left thyroid mass into the left tracheoesophageal groove (*arrow*).

Laryngotracheal Invasion

Laryngotracheal invasion (**Fig. 13**) may be subtle or clearly evident on imaging owing to gross intraluminal extension. It significantly decreases resultant survival and is an independent prognostic factor for survival in thyroid cancer, whereas the invasion of the RLN or pharyngoesophagus was not found to be a significant prognostic factor.[63] Tracheal invasion occurs in approximately one-third of invasive cases, whereas laryngeal involvement is relatively rare, occurring in approximately 12%.[53] Studies including subjects with laryngotracheal involvement have shown no

difference in survival between radical resection and shave procedures in which all gross disease is completely resected.[53,63]

The surgical options to manage intraluminal tracheal invasion include window resection or circumferential tracheal resection and reanastomosis.[64] The surgical options for management of laryngeal invasion include shave or peeling procedures, partial laryngectomy, and total laryngectomy, balancing preservation of laryngeal function, and complete resection of tumor. Laryngeal cartilage invasion without intraluminal involvement can be treated by shaving the tumor

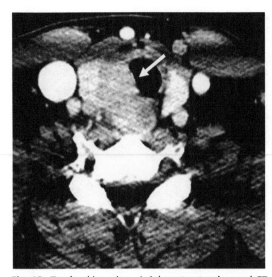

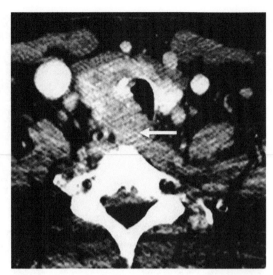

Fig. 13. Tracheal invasion. Axial contrast-enhanced CT image shows right thyroid lobe mass with gross intraluminal extension into the trachea (*arrow*). Tumor staged as T4a.

Fig. 14. Pharyngoesophageal invasion. Axial contrast-enhanced CT image demonstrates a right thyroid lobe mass (*arrow*) with invasion into the esophagus. Tumor staged as T4a.

from the underlying cartilage. Partial laryngectomy may be required with unilateral paraglottic space and hemilarynx invasion.[65] Primary total laryngectomy is rarely indicated in patients with thyroid cancer.

Pharyngoesophageal Invasion

Esophageal involvement is variable and has been reported to occur in 5% to 21% of cases with invasive disease.[53] In most cases, involvement extends to the outermost muscular layers and not the mucosa and submucosa[53] because the esophageal mucosa is relatively resistant to direct invasion of tumor.[53,66] MR imaging is preferred for preoperative evaluation of pharyngoesophageal invasion[67] (Fig. 14). In this setting, simple resection of the involved tissue with negative margins avoiding esophageal entry is sufficient. If a full-thickness defect is created for tumor exenteration, primary closure can be performed if the closure is not under tension. For more extensive resections, reconstructive options including flap reconstruction may be performed.

Prevertebral and Carotid Invasion

Involvement of the prevertebral musculature and encasement of the carotid or brachiocephalic arterial systems results in upstaging to pT4b, which portends a worse prognosis and higher likelihood of locoregional failure. True involvement of the prevertebral musculature may be difficult to differentiate

from loss of the fat plane with the muscles and may only be evident at surgery (Fig. 15).

Lymph Node Metastases

Metastases to regional lymph nodes are extremely common in patients with DTC, particularly PTC. When prophylactic neck dissections are performed, up to 50% of patients are found to have nodal metastatic disease.[68] There is, however, considerable controversy about the importance of lymph node metastasis. Studies have found no difference in survival between patients with and without lymph node metastases.[69] Other studies have found that their presence leads to an increased risk of recurrence[12] and reduced survival.[70] The crucial factor may be patient age because the presence of lymph node metastases had no effect on survival in patients aged less than 45 years, but a 46% increased risk of death in patients more than 45 years.[71] The extracapsular spread (ECS) of tumor from a lymph node is also associated with a higher risk of persistent and recurrent disease.[42]

Lymphatic metastasis from DTC is usually ipsilateral[72] and typically involves orderly progression from level VI, either laterally to levels III and IV, or inferiorly into the mediastinum (level VII). Spread into level II occurs from the superior pole of the thyroid or directly from levels III and IV. Clinical examination of the neck is relatively unreliable with reported false-positive and false-negative rates for detection of metastatic disease in nodes

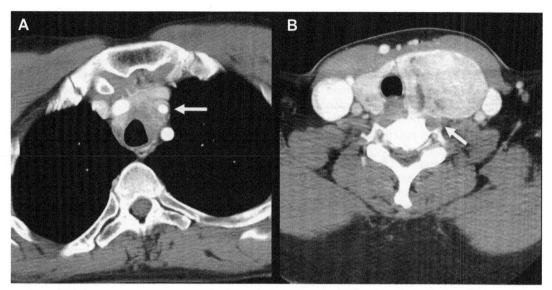

Fig. 15. Vascular encasement and prevertebral muscle involvement. (*A*) Axial contrast-enhanced CT image shows anterior mediastinal soft tissue extending from the thyroid gland to surround the left common carotid artery (*arrow*). Tumor staged as T4b. (*B*) Axial contrast-enhanced CT image in a different patient shows ill-defined margin between the left thyroid lobe mass and the prevertebral musculature (*arrow*). Tumor staged as T4b.

of 20% to 30%. Palpable cervical metastases can occur at any age and are not clearly related to the size of the primary tumor.[73] In one series, 32% of patients with papillary microcarcinoma had cervical nodal metastases at presentation.[73] Controversies surrounding the management of cervical lymph nodes relate to methods of assessment and staging, surgical management, including the extent of neck dissection, and the methods of follow-up.

Central Neck Lymph Node Metastases

Lymph node metastases frequently involve the pre-tracheal and paratracheal lymph nodes within the central compartment (level VI). The sensitivity of US, CT, and MR imaging for central compartment lymphadenopathy is low and the specificity may be decreased in the setting of coexistent thyroiditis (**Fig. 16**). In those patients with clinically evident disease in the central neck detected by palpation or ultrasound, a therapeutic lymphadenectomy of

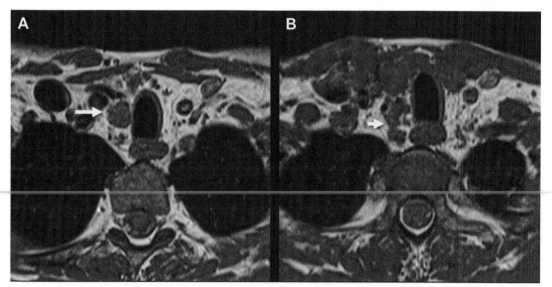

Fig. 16. Central compartment lymphadenopathy. T1-weighted images demonstrate multiple right-sided level VI lymph nodes (*long* and *short arrows*) that were surgically proven metastatic central compartment lymphadenopathy from PTC.

level VI should be performed. As stated in the current American Thyroid Association (ATA) guidelines "prophylactic central compartment neck dissection may be performed in patients with PTC with clinically uninvolved central neck lymph nodes especially for advanced primary tumors (T3 or T4)."[10] The current ATA guidelines recommend that thyroidectomy "without prophylactic central neck dissection may be appropriate for small (T1 or T2), noninvasive, clinically node-negative papillary thyroid cancers and most follicular cancer."[10] Careful intraoperative assessment of lymph nodes within the central neck compartment, however, remains advisable, and patients with documented lymph node metastases should then undergo lymph node dissection. Lymphoid tissue is present near the RLNs and inferior parathyroid glands but, despite the risk of nerve injury and hypoparathyroidism, central neck lymph node dissection remains safe in experienced hands.[74]

Lateral Neck Lymph Node Metastases

Up to 30% of patients with PTC have lateral (levels II–IV) and/or posterior (level V) cervical lymph node metastases.[75] One study of Japanese subjects undergoing prophylactic lateral neck dissection found that 67% of subjects had microscopic lymph node metastases even when no nodes were seen on preoperative US.[76] The presence of lymph node metastases was associated with higher recurrence rates but did not correlate with survival.[76] Retrospective studies have demonstrated that lymph node metastases are

most commonly found in level III.[77] This is followed by metastases in levels IV and II, with level V lymph node metastases being the least common.[78]

Complete cystic degeneration of nodes occurs predominantly in young adults and can simulate a benign cystic neck mass such as a second branchial cyst or metastatic oropharyngeal squamous cell carcinoma (Fig. 17).[79] Hypervascular metastatic lymph nodes may occasionally simulate a paraganglioma (Fig. 18). Gross ECS should be evaluated for because it is a significant negative prognostic indicator and may be an indication for more aggressive surgery including radical neck dissection (Fig. 19). Any suspicious lymph node in the lateral neck[10] should undergo FNA.[10] In the presence of histologically confirmed lymph node metastases, patients should undergo a therapeutic en bloc neck dissection of the involved levels instead of isolated node plucking because the latter is associated with increased risk of local recurrence.[10] The finding that levels IIA, III, and IV are most commonly affected supports the use of selective lateral neck dissection in the setting of metastatic DTC; however, level V has been shown to be involved with DTC in a substantial percentage of cases.[80] Radical neck dissections are almost never performed but might be considered for tumors that extensively invade the strap muscles and cannot otherwise be resected.

Mediastinal Lymph Node Metastases

Mediastinal (level VII) lymph node metastasis is thought to spread by lymph circulation from level

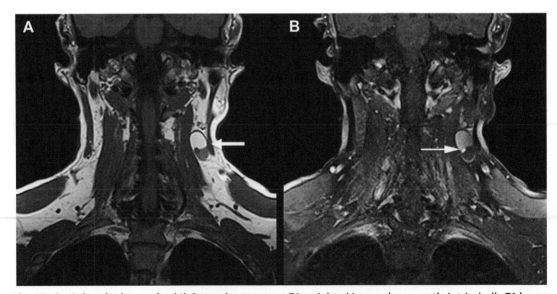

Fig. 17. Cystic lymphadenopathy. (A) Coronal precontrast T1 weighted image shows partly intrinsically T1 hyperintense left level III lymph node from PTC (arrow). (B) Coronal postcontrast fat-saturated T1-weighted image demonstrates an enhancing nodule (arrow).

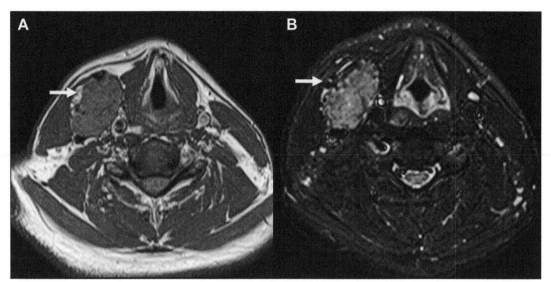

Fig. 18. Hypervascular lymphadenopathy. (*A*) Axial T1-weighted image shows intrinsic minimal T1 hyperintensity in right level III lymph node (*arrow*). (*B*) Axial T2-weighted fat-saturated image shows T2 hyperintensity with multiple peripheral flow voids (*arrow*). The pathologic condition was PTC.

VI and IV,[81] and is significantly correlated with contralateral lateral node metastasis[82]; however, metastasis may occur directly without other lymph node involvement.[75] Metastasis may be obvious on cross-sectional imaging (**Fig. 20**) but is often occult without imaging evidence. Surgical stress for patients undergoing mediastinal node dissection is greater than that for patients undergoing lateral node dissection because it requires median sternotomy; therefore, prophylactic mediastinal dissection via median sternotomy is not recommended.

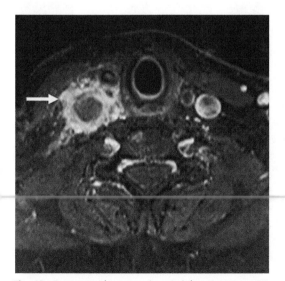

Fig. 19. Extracapsular extension. Axial postcontrast T1-weighed fat-saturated image shows extensive ill-defined margins of a right level IV lymph node (*arrow*) consistent with extracapsular extension from MTC.

Parapharyngeal and Retropharyngeal Metastases

As with mediastinal lymphadenopathy, retropharyngeal lymph nodes are not detectable by US, but can be readily seen on CT or MR imaging (**Fig. 21**). A lymphatic vessel connecting the upper pole of the thyroid gland to the retropharyngeal lymphatic system has been described in approximately 20% of patients.[83] Behind the fascia of the superior constrictor muscle is an anatomic dehiscence allowing the parapharyngeal spaces and retropharyngeal spaces to communicate freely with each other, explaining the dissemination to the parapharyngeal space through the retropharyngeal space.[84] This spread tends to occur when other levels are involved or in the neck that has previously been surgically treated.

Distant Metastases

Only 5% to 10% of patients with PTC have distant metastasis at initial presentation[85]; however the main cause of death from PTC is distant metastases (**Fig. 22**).[86] Most patients develop distant metastases in the lungs; over 50% with distant disease have lung involvement alone, 25% have bone involvement alone, 20% have both lung and bone involvement, and about 5% develop distant metastases in other sites.[85] Mortality is high with distant disease, with 50% survival at 3.5 years.[87] Survival is improved in younger patients,[87] patients with only microscopic residual disease,[85] and patients with iodine-avid tumors.[85,87] The ability to achieve a negative

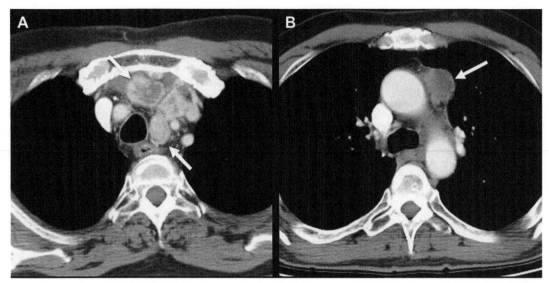

Fig. 20. Mediastinal lymphadenopathy. (*A*) Axial contrast-enhanced CT images show multiple hyperenhancing mediastinal lymph nodes from PTC (*arrows*). (*A*) Image from a different patient shows a cystic lymph node in the mediastinum from PTC (*arrow*).

posttreatment scan after multiple doses of radioiodine was associated with 92% overall 10-year survival, compared with 19% survival for patients who did not.[85]

STAGING OF MTC, ATC, AND THYROID LYMPHOMA; WITH PITFALLS

Nondifferentiated carcinomas of the thyroid gland include MTC and ATC. Lymphomas of the thyroid gland are also staged and treated differently than are DTC.

ATC

ATC is a highly aggressive malignancy with an age-adjusted annual incidence of 2 per million.[88] Most patients with ATC present in their sixth or seventh decade, with the survival for ATC measured in months with only a few survivors at more than

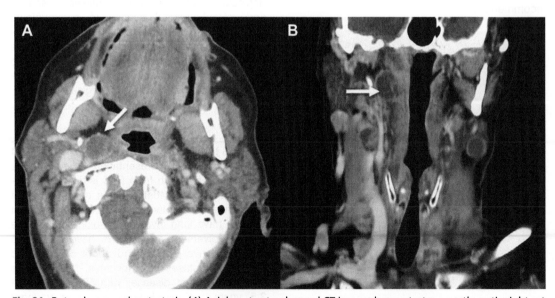

Fig. 21. Retropharyngeal metastasis. (*A*) Axial contrast-enhanced CT image demonstrates a partly cystic right retropharyngeal lymph node (*arrow*) from metastatic PTC. (*B*) Coronal reformatted contrast-enhanced CT image shows the right retropharyngeal partly cystic lymph node (*arrow*) as well as other bilateral cystic lymph node metastasis in the neck.

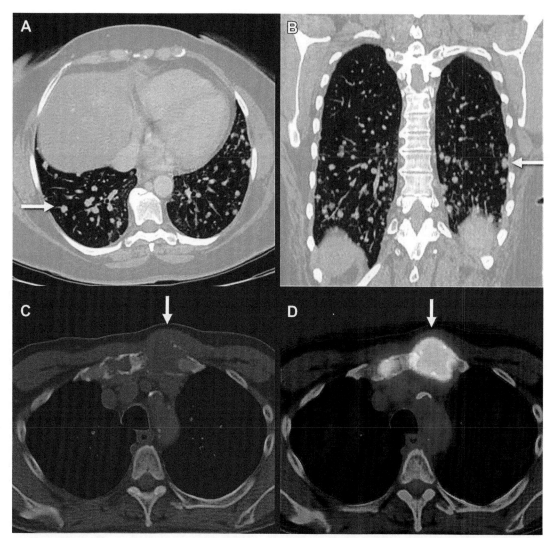

Fig. 22. Distant metastatic disease. Axial (*A*) and coronal (*B*) chest CT in lung windows demonstrating multiple lung metastases from PTC (*arrows*). Axial CT (*C*) and fused PET-CT (*D*) images showing lytic hypermetabolic metastases (*arrows*) to the sternum from PTC.

2 years.[89] Although rarely patients will have an incidentally discovered ATC at the time of surgery for a thyroid nodule, most commonly patients present with a rapidly enlarging neck mass. The mass is frequently found to be hard and fixed to surrounding structures. Local compressive and invasive symptoms occur in most patients, including dysphagia, hoarseness, dyspnea, neck pain, and sore throat.[89] Average tumor size is 6 cm at presentation. Cervical lymphadenopathy is present in as many as 40% of patients and up to half of patients present with distant metastases, most commonly to the lung, bone, and brain.[90]

All ATCs are considered T4 lesions and are subdivided into T4a and T4b, with T4a as intrathyroidal anaplastic carcinoma for which surgery can be performed and T4b referring to anaplastic carcinoma with ETE for which surgery is usually not indicated (Fig. 23). The investigation of a patient with ATC should include a CT of the neck and chest to assess the local extent of disease and invasion into surrounding structures, and a bone scan to complete a metastatic workup. MR imaging may be a helpful adjunct in determining bony and vascular involvement of the tumor.[91] PET-CT may be useful for evaluation of distant metastatic disease. Treatments include surgical resection with adjuvant chemotherapy or combination of chemotherapy and EBRT.[92]

MTC

MTC accounts for 5% to 8% of all thyroid cancers (Fig. 24). It is a poorly differentiated carcinoma

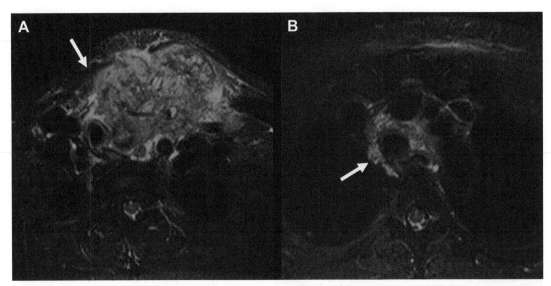

Fig. 23. Anaplastic carcinoma. Axial fat-saturated T2-weighted images showing (*A*) a large left thyroid mass with extensive ETE and mass effect on the trachea, as well as vascular invasion (*arrow*). (*B*) There is extensive mediastinal lymphadenopathy (*arrow*).

originating from the parafollicular calcitonin-secreting cells of the thyroid and has a more aggressive behavior and poorer prognosis compared with DTC. It is mainly sporadic, but a hereditary pattern in multiple endocrine neoplasia type 2 is present in 20% to 30% of cases.

US often shows echogenic foci within the lesion, representing calcium surrounded by amyloid.[93] On MR imaging, medullary carcinoma is usually well-

defined but can have irregular margins. The tumor demonstrates early lymph node metastases and distant metastases outside the neck may occur in the liver, lungs, bones and, less frequently, brain and skin. The primary treatment of both hereditary and sporadic forms of MTC is total thyroidectomy and surgical removal of all neoplastic tissue present in the neck. Medullary carcinoma does not concentrate radioiodine, so RAI is not

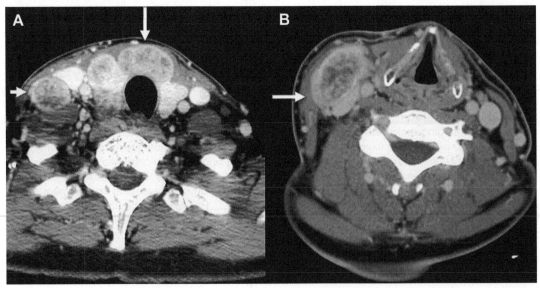

Fig. 24. Medullary carcinoma. Axial contrast-enhanced CT images show (*A*) extensive involvement of the thyroid isthmus (*arrow*) and right lobe, and right level III/IV lymphadenopathy (*short arrow*). (*B*) A level III lymph node demonstrates evidence of ECS (*arrow*).

indicated. Postoperative EBRT to the neck and the mediastinum may be used as adjuvant treatment. Metastatic lesions may be difficult to detect by US, CT, or MR imaging. ^{131}I- MIBG, ^{111}In-octreotide, or ^{99m}Tc-dimercaptosuccinic acid scintigraphy and FDG-PET are reported to be useful. Sensitivity of FDG-PET is reportedly 78%.[94] Measurements of serum calcitonin and carcinoembryonic antigen are critical in the postsurgical follow-up of patients with MTC because they reflect the presence of persistent or recurrent disease.

Thyroid Lymphoma

Thyroid lymphoma (TL) accounts for 1% to 5% of all thyroid neoplasms, less than 2% of extranodal lymphomas,[95] and tends to occur in elderly female patients. Hashimoto's thyroiditis is a risk factor for TL. There are two histologic subtypes, the diffuse large B-cell lymphoma, and the mucosa-associated lymphoid tissue (MALT) lymphoma. The most common presentation is a rapidly enlarging neck mass. TL often has a diffusely infiltrative appearance on imaging instead of a focal mass lesion (**Fig. 25**). Once the diagnosis of a TL

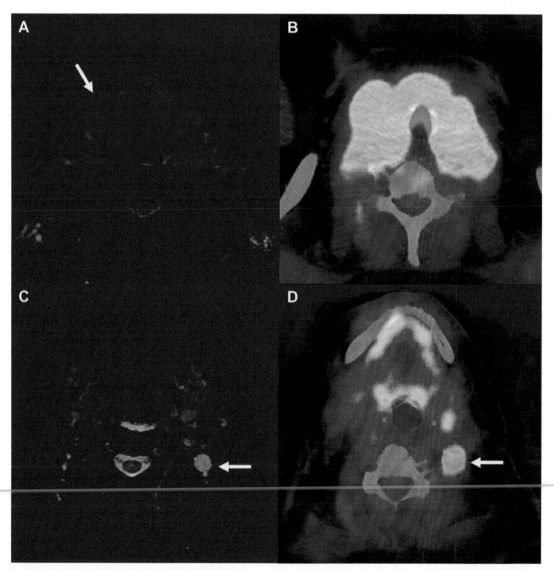

Fig. 25. TL. (*A*) Axial fat-saturated T2-weighted image shows homogeneous mass-like enlargement of the thyroid gland (*arrow*). (*B*) Axial fused PET-CT image shows diffuse extensive FDG uptake in the gland. (*C*) Axial fat-saturated T2-weighted image shows an abnormal rounded left level II lymph node (*arrow*). (*D*) Axial fused PET-CT image shows high FDG uptake within the lymph node (*arrow*).

has been established, the proper staging based on the AJCC classification should be determined: stage IE, disease localized within the thyroid; IIE, disease localized to the thyroid and regional lymph node basins; IIIE, disease involvement on both sides of the diaphragm; and IVE, disseminated disease. Poor prognostic indicators for TL include tumor size greater than 10 cm, advanced stage (greater than stage IE), the presence of compressive symptoms, mediastinal involvement, and rapid tumor growth.[91] Patients presenting with MALT lymphoma are generally diagnosed at a earlier stage (stage IE, IIE) and have a better prognosis than those with diffuse or mixed large cell lymphomas. The treatment of TL depends on the histologic subtype. TLs are both radiation and chemosensitive and are best treated with multimodality therapy consisting of chemotherapy as well as EBRT.

SUMMARY

Thyroid cancer includes several neoplasms originating from the thyroid gland ranging from indolent and highly curable histologies of DTC to highly aggressive ATC. Differentiation of benign and malignant thyroid nodules is highly problematic on CT and MR imaging unless there is evidence of ETE, and often requires correlation with US and UG-FNA. Staging of the primary site in DTC is based on primary tumor size and degree of ETE; specifically, involvement of the subcutaneous soft tissues, larynx, trachea, esophagus, RLN, and prevertebral muscles, and encasement of vascular structures, for which CT and MR imaging are valuable. Evaluation of regional lymph nodes is often performed clinically or with US; however, the retropharyngeal and mediastinal lymph nodes are better evaluated by CT and MR imaging. Nuclear scintigraphy is useful for staging and in treatment of distant metastasis in DTC. PET may have a role in more aggressive cancers such as ATC. Accurate staging, particularly evaluation of ETE and nodal disease, affects surgical management and subsequent therapy.

REFERENCES

1. Jemal A, Siegel R, Ward E, et al. Cancer statistics, 2009. CA Cancer J Clin 2009;59(4):225–49.
2. Davies L, Welch HG. Increasing incidence of thyroid cancer in the United States, 1973–2002. JAMA 2006;295(18):2164–7.
3. Chem KT, Rosai J. Follicular variant of thyroid papillary carcinoma: a clinicopathologic study of six cases. Am J Surg Pathol 1977;1(2):123–30.
4. Leung AK, Chow SM, Law SC. Clinical features and outcome of the tall cell variant of papillary thyroid carcinoma. Laryngoscope 2008;118(1):32–8.
5. Volante M, Collini P, Nikiforov YE, et al. Poorly differentiated thyroid carcinoma: the Turin proposal for the use of uniform diagnostic criteria and an algorithmic diagnostic approach. Am J Surg Pathol 2007;31(8):1256–64.
6. Mazzaferri EL. Thyroid cancer in thyroid nodules: finding a needle in the haystack. Am J Med 1992; 93(4):359–62.
7. Slough CM, Randolph GW. Workup of well-differentiated thyroid carcinoma. Cancer Control 2006; 13(2):99–105.
8. Hundahl SA, Fleming ID, Fremgen AM, et al. A National Cancer Data Base report on 53,856 cases of thyroid carcinoma treated in the U.S., 1985-1995 [see comments]. Cancer 1998;83(12):2638–48.
9. Smallridge RC, Marlow LA, Copland JA. Anaplastic thyroid cancer: molecular pathogenesis and emerging therapies. Endocr Relat Cancer 2009;16(1): 17–44.
10. Cooper DS, Doherty GM, Haugen BR, et al. Revised American Thyroid Association management guidelines for patients with thyroid nodules and differentiated thyroid cancer. Thyroid 2009;19(11):1167–214.
11. Yeh MW, Demircan O, Ituarte P, et al. False-negative fine-needle aspiration cytology results delay treatment and adversely affect outcome in patients with thyroid carcinoma. Thyroid 2004;14(3):207–15.
12. Mazzaferri EL, Jhiang SM. Long-term impact of initial surgical and medical therapy on papillary and follicular thyroid cancer. Am J Med 1994; 97(5):418–28.
13. De Felice M, Di Lauro R. Thyroid development and its disorders: genetics and molecular mechanisms. Endocr Rev 2004;25(5):722–46.
14. Bliss RD, Gauger PG, Delbridge LW. Surgeon's approach to the thyroid gland: surgical anatomy and the importance of technique. World J Surg 2000;24(8):891–7.
15. Stewart WB, Rizzolo LL. Embryology and surgical anatomy of the thyroid and parathyroid glands. In: Oertli D, Udelsman R, editors. Surgery of the thyroid and parathyroid glands. New York: Springer; 2007. p. 13–20.
16. Shaha AR. Management of the neck in thyroid cancer. Otolaryngol Clin North Am 1998;31(5):823–31.
17. Roh JL, Park JY, Park CI. Total thyroidectomy plus neck dissection in differentiated papillary thyroid carcinoma patients: pattern of nodal metastasis, morbidity, recurrence, and postoperative levels of serum parathyroid hormone. Ann Surg 2007; 245(4):604–10.
18. Watkinson JC, Franklyn JA, Olliff JF. Detection and surgical treatment of cervical lymph nodes in differentiated thyroid cancer. Thyroid 2006;16(2):187–94.

19. Rubello D, Pelizzo MR, Al-Nahhas A, et al. The role of sentinel lymph node biopsy in patients with differentiated thyroid carcinoma. Eur J Surg Oncol 2006; 32(9):917–21.

20. Kim EK, Park CS, Chung WY, et al. New sonographic criteria for recommending fine-needle aspiration biopsy of nonpalpable solid nodules of the thyroid. AJR Am J Roentgenol 2002;178(3):687–91.

21. Marqusee E, Benson CB, Frates MC, et al. Usefulness of ultrasonography in the management of nodular thyroid disease. Ann Intern Med 2000; 133(9):696–700.

22. Kouvaraki MA, Shapiro SE, Fornage BD, et al. Role of preoperative ultrasonography in the surgical management of patients with thyroid cancer. Surgery 2003;134(6):946–54 [discussion: 954–5].

23. Papini E, Guglielmi R, Bianchini A, et al. Risk of malignancy in nonpalpable thyroid nodules: predictive value of ultrasound and color-Doppler features. J Clin Endocrinol Metab 2002;87(5):1941–6.

24. Antonelli A, Miccoli P, Ferdeghini M, et al. Role of neck ultrasonography in the follow-up of patients operated on for thyroid cancer. Thyroid 1995;5(1):25–8.

25. Kessler A, Rappaport Y, Blank A, et al. Cystic appearance of cervical lymph nodes is characteristic of metastatic papillary thyroid carcinoma. J Clin Ultrasound 2003;31(1):21–5.

26. Som PM, Brandwein M, Lidov M, et al. The varied presentations of papillary thyroid carcinoma cervical nodal disease: CT and MR findings. AJNR Am J Neuroradiol 1994;15(6):1123–8.

27. Ito Y, Tomoda C, Uruno T, et al. Papillary microcarcinoma of the thyroid: how should it be treated? World J Surg 2004;28(11):1115–21.

28. Ito Y, Tomoda C, Uruno T, et al. Clinical significance of metastasis to the central compartment from papillary microcarcinoma of the thyroid. World J Surg 2006;30(1):91–9.

29. Milas M, Stephen A, Berber E, et al. Ultrasonography for the endocrine surgeon: a valuable clinical tool that enhances diagnostic and therapeutic outcomes. Surgery 2005;138(6):1193–200 [discussion: 1200–1].

30. Solorzano CC, Carneiro DM, Ramirez M, et al. Surgeon-performed ultrasound in the management of thyroid malignancy. Am Surg 2004;70(7):576–80 [discussion: 580–2].

31. Tuttle RM, Leboeuf R. Follow up approaches in thyroid cancer: a risk adapted paradigm. Endocrinol Metab Clin North Am 2008;37(2):419–35, ix–x.

32. Weber AL, Randolph G, Aksoy FG. The thyroid and parathyroid glands. CT and MR imaging and correlation with pathology and clinical findings. Radiol Clin North Am 2000;38(5):1105–29.

33. Nakahara H, Noguchi S, Murakami N, et al. Gadolinium-enhanced MR imaging of thyroid and parathyroid masses. Radiology 1997;202(3):765–72.

34. Mihailovic J, Stefanovic L, Prvulovic M. Magnetic resonance imaging in diagnostic algorithm of solitary cold thyroid nodules. J BUON 2006;11(3):341–6.

35. Gross ND, Weissman JL, Talbot JM, et al. MRI detection of cervical metastasis from differentiated thyroid carcinoma. Laryngoscope 2001;111(11 Pt 1): 1905–9.

36. Takashima S, Sone S, Takayama F, et al. Papillary thyroid carcinoma: MR diagnosis of lymph node metastasis. AJNR Am J Neuroradiol 1998;19(3): 509–13.

37. Otsuki N, Nishikawa T, Iwae S, et al. Retropharyngeal node metastasis from papillary thyroid carcinoma. Head Neck 2007;29(5):508–11.

38. Price DC. Radioisotopic evaluation of the thyroid and the parathyroids. Radiol Clin North Am 1993; 31(5):991–1015.

39. Torlontano M, Crocetti U, Augello G, et al. Comparative evaluation of recombinant human thyrotropin-stimulated thyroglobulin levels, 131I whole-body scintigraphy, and neck ultrasonography in the follow-up of patients with papillary thyroid microcarcinoma who have not undergone radioiodine therapy. J Clin Endocrinol Metab 2006;91(1):60–3.

40. Pacini F, Capezzone M, Elisei R, et al. Diagnostic 131-iodine whole-body scan may be avoided in thyroid cancer patients who have undetectable stimulated serum Tg levels after initial treatment. J Clin Endocrinol Metab 2002;87(4):1499–501.

41. Mitchell JC, Grant F, Evenson AR, et al. Preoperative evaluation of thyroid nodules with 18FDG-PET/CT. Surgery 2005;138(6):1166–74 [discussion: 1174–5].

42. Leboulleux S, Schroeder PR, Busaidy NL, et al. Assessment of the incremental value of recombinant thyrotropin stimulation before 2-[18F]-Fluoro-2-deoxy-D-glucose positron emission tomography/computed tomography imaging to localize residual differentiated thyroid cancer. J Clin Endocrinol Metab 2009;94(4):1310–6.

43. Robbins RJ, Wan Q, Grewal RK, et al. Real-time prognosis for metastatic thyroid carcinoma based on 2-[18F]fluoro-2-deoxy-D-glucose-positron emission tomography scanning. J Clin Endocrinol Metab 2006;91(2):498–505.

44. Sherman SI, Brierley JD, Sperling M, et al. Prospective multicenter study of thyroiscarcinoma treatment: initial analysis of staging and outcome. National Thyroid Cancer Treatment Cooperative Study Registry Group. Cancer 1998;83(5):1012–21.

45. Ito Y, Higashiyama T, Takamura Y, et al. Risk factors for recurrence to the lymph node in papillary thyroid carcinoma patients without preoperatively detectable lateral node metastasis: validity of prophylactic modified radical neck dissection. World J Surg 2007;31(11):2085–91.

46. Chew MH, Chan G, Siddiqui MM, et al. Risk-stratified management of well-differentiated thyroid

cancers: a review of experience from a single institution, 1990–2003. World J Surg 2008;32(3):386–94.

47. Zeiger MA, Dackiw AP. Follicular thyroid lesions, elements that affect both diagnosis and prognosis. J Surg Oncol 2005;89(3):108–13.

48. Mazzaferri EL. Management of low-risk differentiated thyroid cancer. Endocr Pract 2007;13(5): 498–512.

49. Bilimoria KY, Bentrem DJ, Ko CY, et al. Extent of surgery affects survival for papillary thyroid cancer. Ann Surg 2007;246(3):375–81 [discussion: 381–4].

50. Shattuck TM, Westra WH, Ladenson PW, et al. Independent clonal origins of distinct tumor foci in multifocal papillary thyroid carcinoma. N Engl J Med 2005;352(23):2406–12.

51. Andersen PE, Kinsella J, Loree TR, et al. Differentiated carcinoma of the thyroid with extrathyroidal extension. Am J Surg 1995;170(5):467–70.

52. Hay ID, McConahey WM, Goellner JR. Managing patients with papillary thyroid carcinoma: insights gained from the Mayo Clinic's experience of treating 2,512 consecutive patients during 1940 through 2000. Trans Am Clin Climatol Assoc 2002;113: 241–60.

53. McCaffrey TV, Bergstralh EJ, Hay ID. Locally invasive papillary thyroid carcinoma: 1940–1990. Head Neck 1994;16(2):165–72.

54. Ito Y, Tomoda C, Uruno T, et al. Minimal extrathyroid extension does not affect the relapse-free survival of patients with papillary thyroid carcinoma measuring 4 cm or less over the age of 45 years. Surg Today 2006;36(1):12–8.

55. Jukkola A, Bloigu R, Ebeling T, et al. Prognostic factors in differentiated thyroid carcinomas and their implications for current staging classifications. Endocr Relat Cancer 2004;11(3):571–9.

56. Lee SH, Lee SS, Jin SM, et al. Predictive factors for central compartment lymph node metastasis in thyroid papillary microcarcinoma. Laryngoscope 2008;118(4):659–62.

57. Gemsenjager E, Heitz PU, Seifert B, et al. Differentiated thyroid carcinoma. Follow-up of 264 patients from one institution for up to 25 years. Swiss Med Wkly 2001;131(11–12):157–63.

58. McCaffrey JC. Evaluation and treatment of aerodigestive tract invasion by well-differentiated thyroid carcinoma. Cancer Control 2000;7(3):246–52.

59. Brierley J, Tsang R, Panzarella T, et al. Prognostic factors and the effect of treatment with radioactive iodine and external beam radiation on patients with differentiated thyroid cancer seen at a single institution over 40 years. Clin Endocrinol (Oxf) 2005;63(4): 418–27.

60. Chiang FY, Wang LF, Huang YF, et al. Recurrent laryngeal nerve palsy after thyroidectomy with routine identification of the recurrent laryngeal nerve. Surgery 2005;137(3):342–7.

61. Takashima S, Takayama F, Wang J, et al. Using MR imaging to predict invasion of the recurrent laryngeal nerve by thyroid carcinoma. AJR Am J Roentgenol 2003;180(3):837–42.

62. Falk SA, McCaffrey TV. Management of the recurrent laryngeal nerve in suspected and proven thyroid cancer. Otolaryngol Head Neck Surg 1995;113(1): 42–8.

63. Czaja JM, McCaffrey TV. The surgical management of laryngotracheal invasion by well-differentiated papillary thyroid carcinoma. Arch Otolaryngol Head Neck Surg 1997;123(5):484–90.

64. Friedman M. Surgical management of thyroid carcinoma with laryngotracheal invasion. Otolaryngol Clin North Am 1990;23(3):495–507.

65. McCaffrey JC. Aerodigestive tract invasion by well-differentiated thyroid carcinoma: diagnosis, management, prognosis, and biology. Laryngoscope 2006;116(1):1–11.

66. Grillo HC, Suen HC, Mathisen DJ, et al. Resectional management of thyroid carcinoma invading the airway. Ann Thorac Surg 1992;54(1):3–9 [discussion: 9–10].

67. Wang J, Takashima S, Matsushita T, et al. Esophageal invasion by thyroid carcinomas: prediction using magnetic resonance imaging. J Comput Assist Tomogr 2003;27(1):18–25.

68. Bonnet S, Hartl D, Leboulleux S, et al. Prophylactic lymph node dissection for papillary thyroid cancer less than 2 cm: implications for radioiodine treatment. J Clin Endocrinol Metab 2009;94(4):1162–7.

69. Bhattacharyya N. A population-based analysis of survival factors in differentiated and medullary thyroid carcinoma. Otolaryngol Head Neck Surg 2003;128(1):115–23.

70. Podnos YD, Smith D, Wagman LD, et al. The implication of lymph node metastasis on survival in patients with well-differentiated thyroid cancer. Am Surg 2005;71(9):731–4.

71. Zaydfudim V, Feurer ID, Griffin MR, et al. The impact of lymph node involvement on survival in patients with papillary and follicular thyroid carcinoma. Surgery 2008;144(6):1070–7 [discussion: 1077–8].

72. Qubain SW, Nakano S, Baba M, et al. Distribution of lymph node micrometastasis in pN0 well-differentiated thyroid carcinoma. Surgery 2002; 131(3):249–56.

73. Hay ID, Grant CS, van Heerden JA, et al. Papillary thyroid microcarcinoma: a study of 535 cases observed in a 50-year period. Surgery 1992; 112(6):1139–46 [discussion: 1146–7].

74. White ML, Gauger PG, Doherty GM. Central lymph node dissection in differentiated thyroid cancer. World J Surg 2007;31(5):895–904.

75. Machens A, Hinze R, Thomusch O, et al. Pattern of nodal metastasis for primary and reoperative thyroid cancer. World J Surg 2002;26(1):22–8.

76. Wada N, Suganuma N, Nakayama H, et al. Microscopic regional lymph node status in papillary thyroid carcinoma with and without lymphadenopathy and its relation to outcomes. Langenbecks Arch Surg 2007;392(4):417–22.

77. Kupferman ME, Patterson M, Mandel SJ, et al. Patterns of lateral neck metastasis in papillary thyroid carcinoma. Arch Otolaryngol Head Neck Surg 2004;130(7):857–60.

78. Caron NR, Tan YY, Ogilvie JB, et al. Selective modified radical neck dissection for papillary thyroid cancer-is level I, II and V dissection always necessary? World J Surg 2006;30(5):833–40.

79. Wunderbaldinger P, Harisinghani MG, Hahn PF, et al. Cystic lymph node metastases in papillary thyroid carcinoma. AJR Am J Roentgenol 2002; 178(3):693–7.

80. Farrag T, Lin F, Brownlee N, et al. Is routine dissection of level II-B and V-A necessary in patients with papillary thyroid cancer undergoing lateral neck dissection for FNA-confirmed metastases in other levels. World J Surg 2009;33(8):1680–3.

81. Sisson GA, Edison BD, Bytell DE. Transsternal radical neck dissection. Postoperative complications and management. Arch Otolaryngol 1975;101(1):46–9.

82. Sugenoya A, Asanuma K, Shingu K, et al. Clinical evaluation of upper mediastinal dissection for differentiated thyroid carcinoma. Surgery 1993;113(5): 541–4.

83. Rouviere H. Anatomie Humaine descriptive et topographique: vo. 3 Membres, systeme nerveux central. 10th edition. Paris: Masson Et.Cie Editeurs; 1967.

84. Sirotnak JJ, Loree TR, Penetrante R. Papillary carcinoma of the thyroid metastatic to the parapharyngeal space. Ear Nose Throat J 1997;76(5):342–4.

85. Durante C, Haddy N, Baudin E, et al. Long-term outcome of 444 patients with distant metastases from papillary and follicular thyroid carcinoma: benefits and limits of radioiodine therapy. J Clin Endocrinol Metab 2006;91(8):2892–9.

86. Mazzaferri EL. Thyroid carcinoma: papillary and follicular. In: Mazzaferri EL, Samaan N, editors. Endocrine tumors. Cambridge (MA): Blackwell Scientific Publications Inc; 1993. p. 278.e333.

87. Sampson E, Brierley JD, Le LW, et al. Clinical management and outcome of papillary and follicular (differentiated) thyroid cancer presenting with distant metastasis at diagnosis. Cancer 2007; 110(7):1451–6.

88. Ain KB. Anaplastic thyroid carcinoma: a therapeutic challenge. Semin Surg Oncol 1999;16(1):64–9.

89. Rosen IB, Asa SL, Brierley JD. Anaplastic carcinoma of the thyroid gland. In: Clark OH, Duh QY, Kebebew E, editors. Textbook of endocrine surgery. Philadelphia: Elsevier Saunders; 2005. p. 159–67.

90. McIver B, Hay ID, Giuffrida DF, et al. Anaplastic thyroid carcinoma: a 50-year experience at a single institution. Surgery 2001;130(6):1028–34.

91. Pasieka JL. Hashimoto's disease and thyroid lymphoma: role of the surgeon. World J Surg 2000; 24(8):966–70.

92. Kebebew E, Greenspan FS, Clark OH, et al. Anaplastic thyroid carcinoma. Treatment outcome and prognostic factors. Cancer 2005;103(7): 1330–5.

93. Gorman B, Charboneau JW, James EM, et al. Medullary thyroid carcinoma: role of high-resolution US. Radiology 1987;162(1 Pt 1):147–50.

94. Diehl M, Risse JH, Brandt-Mainz K, et al. Fluorine-18 fluorodeoxyglucose positron emission tomography in medullary thyroid cancer: results of a multicentre study. Eur J Nucl Med 2001;28(11):1671–6.

95. Honing ML, Seldenrijk CA, de Maat CE. Primary thyroid lymphoma. Neth J Med 1998;52(2):75–8.

Pitfalls in the Staging of Cervical Lymph Node Metastasis

Amit M. Saindane, MD

KEYWORDS

- Lymph nodes • Ultrasound • Computed tomography • Magnetic resonance imaging
- Positron emission tomography • Fine-needle aspiration

KEY POINTS

- Lymph nodes status is one or the most important predictors of prognosis in head and neck squamous cell carcinoma, making accurate staging critical.
- The physical examination of the neck is highly inaccurate.
- Imaging by CT, MR imaging, ultrasound (US), and positron emission tomography-CT (PET-CT) improve accuracy of staging, but all have limitations, particularly detection of small metastatic lymph nodes harboring microscopic metastatic disease.
- This article reviews the classification of cervical lymph nodes, findings that suggest metastatic involvement of lymph nodes, and the evidence for staging using CT, MR imaging, US, and PET-CT.

INTRODUCTION

Head and neck squamous cell carcinoma (HNSCC) comprises most head and neck malignancies.[1] Regardless of the primary tumor site, the presence of a single metastatic lymph node in HNSCC reduces the 5-year survival rate by approximately 50%. The presence of bilateral metastatic lymph nodes in the neck reduces the survival rate to about 25% of that of patients without nodal metastasis.[2,3] Cervical lymph node metastases influence not only the risk of local recurrence but also the risk of distant metastases,[4,5] making lymph node status one of the most important predictors of prognosis in HNSCC.[6,7]

It takes an estimated one billion malignant cells to create a 1 mm^3 mass.[8] Although such tumors can be readily identified under microscopy, such minute foci of metastatic disease are not visible on gross inspection and cannot be reliably detected by any current imaging technique. Depending on the primary tumor site, lymph node metastasis will be histopathologically present in as high as 32%[9,10] of patients with HNSCC. The inaccuracy of the physical examination for detection of metastatic cervical lymph nodes has been documented in several studies.[11,12] The false-negative and false-positive rates of the physical examination are 15% to 20% and 30% to 50%, respectively,[12] so the treatment of patients with a clinically negative neck stage of N0 remains controversial (Fig. 1).

Up to 32% of patients with clinically negative lymph nodes who are not treated will develop lymph node metastasis in the neck, leading to a poorer outcome,[9,10,13] making undertreatment of the N0 neck undesirable. Given the relatively high risk of clinically occult cervical lymph node metastasis, most head and neck surgeons promote elective treatment of the neck.[14,15] About 75% of elective neck dissections, however, prove to be free of tumor at histopathologic examination.[14,15] Although neck dissections have low complication rates in experienced hands, there is still considerable morbidity and mortality to both neck dissection and radiation therapy to the neck.[14,16,17] Radiation therapy and chemotherapy

Department of Radiology and Imaging Sciences, Emory University School of Medicine, BG-22, 1364 Clifton Road Northeast, Atlanta, GA 30322, USA
E-mail address: asainda@emory.edu

Neuroimag Clin N Am 23 (2013) 147–166
http://dx.doi.org/10.1016/j.nic.2012.08.011
1052-5149/13/$ – see front matter © 2013 Elsevier Inc. All rights reserved.

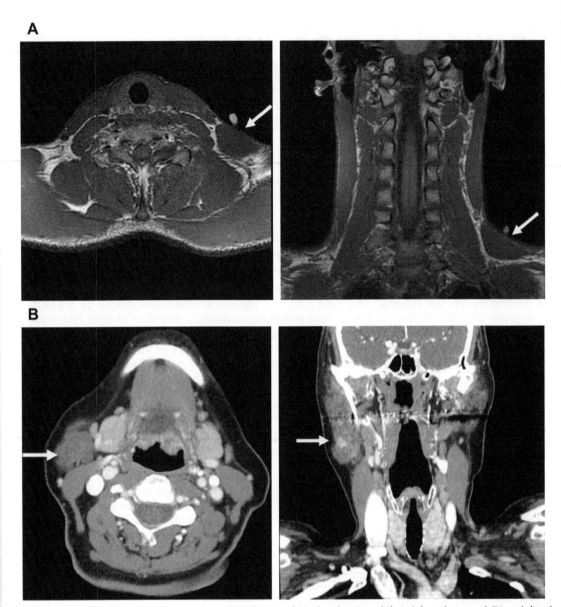

Fig. 1. Pitfalls (false-postives) in nodal staging due to clinical palpation. (*A*) Axial and coronal T1-weighted images demonstrate a palpable left level VB mass (*arrow*) to be a levator claviculae muscle. (*B*) Axial and coronal reformatted CE-CT images show a prominent right parotid tail mass (*arrow*) misinterpreted clinically as a right IIA palpable mass.

are frequently used concurrently in the treatment of primaries such as oropharyngeal HNSCC to avoid the morbidity of surgical resection,[18,19] but both of these treatments can also have severe local adverse effects and systemic toxicities. Furthermore, the use of radiation therapy precludes its future use for management of second head and neck primary cancers that occur in up to 25% of these patients.[20,21] For these reasons, overtreatment of a high percentage of necks that are ultimately negative for metastatic lymph nodes is also not optimal.

So, what is the role of imaging in the staging of lymph nodes if we cannot identify and categorically exclude micrometastases, and the treatment of the neck by surgical dissection or radiation therapy may already be decided based on standard management of the primary tumor and the head and neck surgeon's practice preferences? A major role of imaging lymph nodes in the staging of HNSCC is to guide decisions for unexpected lymph node metastasis present in the contralateral neck and detection of ipsilateral metastatic lymph nodes where they may not be suspected and may not

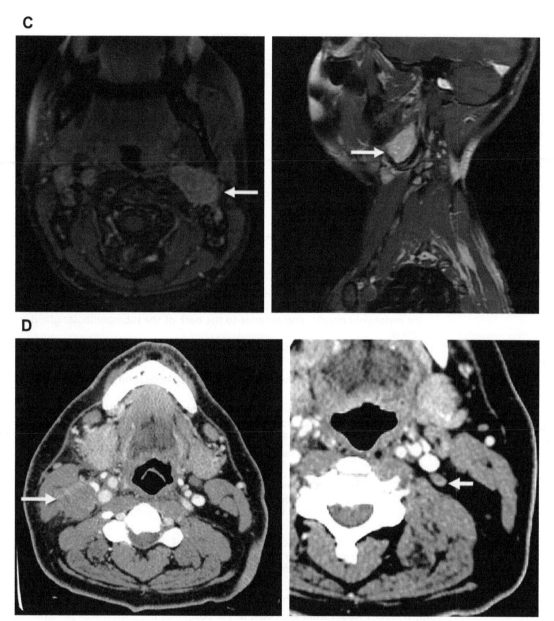

Fig. 1. (*C*) Axial and sagittal postcontrast fat-saturated T1-weighted images showing bilateral palpable carotid body tumors (*arrow*) in the level II stations. (*D*) Axial CE-CT image on left shows a clinically-palpated right level II metastatic lymph node (*arrow*) from a right oral cavity primary. Image on right shows a nonpalpable centrally necrotic left IIB lymph node (*short arrow*) deep to the sternocleidomastoid muscle that upstaged the patient to N2C disease. Multiple metastatic lymph nodes were present in the bilateral neck at selective neck dissection.

otherwise be treated. In a patient with a left-sided primary tumor site who will be undergoing surgical resection of the primary and left-sided neck dissection, the detection of even a single metastatic contralateral neck lymph node on imaging alters the management substantially. Most standard neck dissections for HNSCC do not address lymph nodes in level V, some do not include level I, IIB, or IV, and retropharyngeal lymph nodes are not routinely addressed surgically. Therefore, the detection of metastatic lymph nodes in these locations also affects the extent of surgical management. Even when treatment is nonsurgical, the planning of radiation therapy is influenced by presence and location of metastatic lymph nodes on imaging. The preoperative detection of extracapsular spread (ECS) from lymph nodes and any resultant carotid arterial encasement affects whether or not surgery is performed at all, planning of the type of neck dissection performed (radical vs selective), and whether or not preoperative chemotherapy is used. Therefore, accurate assessment of lymph node status by imaging is critical for the management of HNSCC.

CERVICAL LYMPH NODE CLASSIFICATION

The imaging-based classification of lymph nodes in the neck has been described in detail previously by Som and colleagues[22] The anatomic boundaries and locations of the lymph nodes in the neck are listed in **Table 1** and depicted in **Fig. 2**. This nodal scheme is universally accepted and used, and should be incorporated into cross-sectional neck imaging interpretations by the radiologist.

CT STAGING OF CERVICAL LYMPH NODE METASTASES AND PITFALLS

CT is commonly the imaging modality used for staging the primary site of HNSCC and is, therefore, used to stage the lymph nodes in the neck. CT has improved the accuracy of nodal staging over physical examination, allowing for evaluation of retropharyngeal, tracheoesophageal, and lymph nodes deep to the sternocleidomastoid muscle, decreasing the error rate of palpation by 7.5% to 19%.[23–26] CT

Table 1
Imaging-based nodal classification

Level	Description
I	The submental and submandibular nodes, located above the hyoid bone, below the mylohyoid muscle, and anterior to the back of the submandibular gland (SMGs)
IA	The submental nodes. These lie between the medial margins of the anterior bellies of the digastric muscles.
IB	The submandibular nodes. These lie lateral to the IA nodes and anterior to the back of the SMGs
II	The upper internal jugular nodes, lying from the skull base to the bottom of the body of the hyoid bone, posterior to the back of the SMG, and anterior to the back of the sternocleidomastiod muscle (SCM)
IIA	The level II nodes anterior, medial, lateral, and immediately posterior to the internal jugular vein (IJV)
IIB	The level II nodes posterior to the IJV separated by a fat plane
III	The midjugular nodes, located from the bottom of the body of the hyoid bone to the level of the bottom of the cricoid arch. These lie anterior to the back of the SCM.
IV	The low jugular nodes, located from the bottom of the cricoid arch to the level of the clavicle. These lie anterior to the back of the SCM and the posterolateral margin of the anterior scalene muscle.
V	The posterior triangle nodes, located posterior to the back of the SCM from the skull base to the level of the clavicles.
VA	Upper level V nodes from skull base to the bottom of the cricoid arch posterior to the SCM.
VB	Lower level V nodes from the bottom of the cricoid arch to the level of the clavicles as seen on axial images. These are posterior to a line connecting the back of the SCM and the posterolateral margin of the anterior scalene muscle.
VI	The visceral nodes, located between the carotid arteries from the level of the bottom of the body of the hyoid bone to the top of the manubrium.
VII	The superior mediastinal nodes, located between the carotid arteries below the level of the manubrium and above the level of the innominate vein.
Supraclavicular	These are located caudal to the level of the clavicle on axial images and lateral to the carotid arteries on each side of the neck.
Retropharyngeal	These are located within 2 cm of the skull base and medial to the internal carotid arteries.

Adapted from Som PM, Curtin HD, Mancuso AA. The new imaging-based classification for describing the location of lymph nodes in the neck with particular regard to cervical lymph nodes in relation to cancer of the larynx. ORL J Otorhinolaryngol Relat Spec 2000;62(4):186–98.

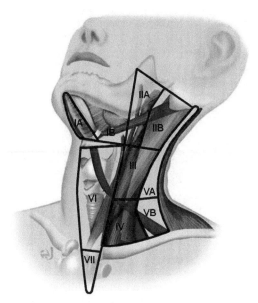

Fig. 2. Lymph node stations in the neck. (*Courtesy of* E. Jablonowski.)

criteria for assessing nodal metastases are nodal size, shape, presence of central necrosis, and grouping of nodes in an expected draining nodal station for a specific primary tumor (**Table 2**).[4,27,28]

Lymph Node Size

A multicenter study of nodal size in 100 neck dissections for HNSCC showed that 46% of metastatic nodes were less than 10 mm and 22% of metastatic nodes were between 10 and 15 mm in diameter.[29] Another pathologic analysis of 750 lymph nodes in subjects with HNSCC demonstrated that most normal nodes are less than 5 mm in diameter but that metastatic nodes vary in size without having any peak in size distribution.[30] Many different size criteria for metastatic nodes have been proposed for CT and MR imaging.[31,32] Some investigators consider any node greater than 10 mm as abnormal,[33] whereas other investigators[4,34] have used varying size criteria according to the location of lymph nodes.[28] Frequently used criteria for the greatest transaxial nodal diameter (long axis) is 15 mm for level I and II lymph nodes and 10 mm for all other cervical nodes.[35] Using these criteria, lymph nodes that exceed these dimensions are metastatic about 80% of the time. Other studies have found slightly different size criteria, with different balances of sensitivity and specificity.[4] Regardless of the size criteria used, there will always be borderline sized nodes without evidence of necrosis that remain indeterminate (**Fig. 3**).

Table 2 Pitfalls in staging of lymph nodes	
Pitfall	**Advice**
Understaging of HNSCC due to reliance on clinical palpation	CT, MR imaging, US, and PET-CT all can detect nonpalpable deep and small lymph nodes
Understaging of clustered small lymph nodes	Clustered nonnecrotic lymph nodes not meeting size-criteria are still suspicious for nodal metastasis when in the primary drainage pathway for the primary site
Misdiagnosis of necrotic infectious lymphadenitis as metastatic disease	Always consider the clinical context and use UG-FNA to troubleshoot, when needed
Overdiagnosis of a hilar fat as necrosis on thick-section CT images	For small lymph nodes review the thinnest image dataset obtained and use pixel analysis to identify fat density
Misdiagnosis of the thoracic duct as a cystic level IV lymph node	Consider a prominent thoracic duct when dealing with a left level IV lymph node and use coronal reformatted images to identify the characteristic location at the junction of the IJV and subclavian vein
Overdiagnosis of ECS	Review the medical record for any recent biopsy or local infection that may falsely result in the appearance of ECS
Understaging of small necrotic lymph nodes on PET	Use CE-CT for attenuation correction for PET to identify small necrotic or cystic hypometabolic metastatic lymph nodes

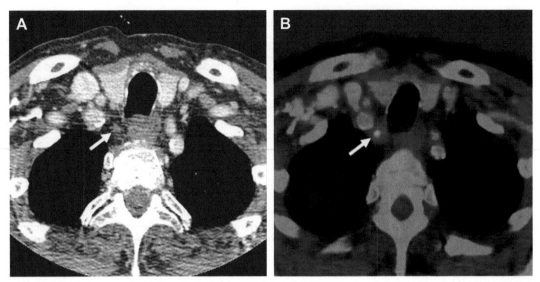

Fig. 3. Pitfall of size criteria for lymph nodes on CT. (*A*) Axial CE-CT image from a patient with T4b posterior hypopharyngeal wall primary shows a nonnecrotic subcentimeter right paratracheal lymph node (*arrow*). (*B*) Fused axial FDG-PET-CE-CT image shows the lymph node is hypermetabolic with SUV of 3.9 (*arrow*).

Nodal Shape and Grouping

The addition of nodal shape as a criterion to nodal size only minimally improves the sensitivity of CT diagnosis. This criterion is based on the pathologic observation that reactive lymph nodes are generally kidney-bean shaped, whereas most metastatic nodes are spherical. If a lymph node is borderline pathologic by size criteria but is spherical, it is slightly more likely to truly contain metastatic tumor. Nodal grouping refers to three or more contiguous and confluent lymph nodes, each of which has a maximal diameter of 8 to 15 mm. Such a grouping in the lymphatic drainage chain of the tumor is highly suggestive of metastatic lymph node involvement (**Fig. 4**).[4,28] Close and colleagues[25] evaluated 61 subjects with HNSCC by CT and reported that the presence of multiple otherwise benign looking nodes in a high

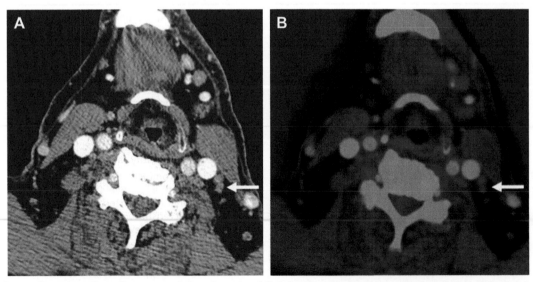

Fig. 4. Clustering of small nonnecrotic lymph nodes. (*A*) Axial CE-CT image in a patient with T4b left alveolar ridge squamous cell carcinoma (SCC) show a cluster of three nonnecrotic subcentimeter left level IIA and IIB lymph nodes (*arrow*). (*B*) Fused axial FDG-PET-CE-CT image shows no evidence of hypermetabolism (*arrow*). Neck dissection demonstrated metastatic SCC.

risk lymphatic station correctly predicted metastases in 61%.

Central Necrosis

The most accurate CT finding for the presence of metastatic lymphadenopathy from HNSCC is central necrosis.[4,36] Tumor cells initially replace the medulla of the node, which later undergoes necrosis, so the medullary region of lymph nodes contain tumor cells as well as necrotic tissue, both of which result in central low attention on CT in contrast to the cortical portions of the node that enhance with iodinated contrast material.[4,27] In a large clinical series, however, 74% of metastatic nodes contained central necrosis on pathologic study, whereas central necrosis was seen in only 32% of metastatic lymph nodes on imaging.[4] Therefore, a homogeneous appearance of lymph nodes on CT or MR imaging does not exclude the presence of nodal metastasis. Particularly, the percentage of central nodal necrosis is greatly reduced in smaller nodes.[33,37] Contrast-enhanced CT (CE-CT) is considered to be the best imaging modality for identification of necrosis, with a sensitivity of 74% and a specificity of 94% reported for areas of necrosis larger than 3 mm.[4]

Both lipid metaplasia and infection resulting in nodal abscess formation can simulate necrosis due to metastasis on CT (**Fig. 5**). Lipid metaplasia or fatty degeneration can rarely occur in lymph nodes after severe inflammatory disease or after radiation therapy. In most cases, such fat is peripheral,

corresponding to the hilum instead of central, but this may be difficult to determine on CT. The lower attenuation of fat compared with necrosis may also be difficult to differentiate for small nodes due to partial volume effects (**Fig. 6**). A node with abscess formation is almost always accompanied by corresponding signs and symptoms of infection. Such a lymph node can have central low attenuation and irregular enhancing margins, all of which simulate a metastatic node. Evaluation for associated adjacent cellulitis to assist in diagnosis may be problematic in a patient who has been incompletely treated with antibiotics, or recently postsurgical or postradiation therapy.

Cystic lymph nodes are frequently seen in the setting of human papilloma virus–positive oropharyngeal carcinoma. When located in level II, these may be mistaken for second branchial cleft cyst (**Fig. 7**) or a cystic nerve sheath tumor (**Fig. 8**) leading to misdiagnosis. When located in left level IV, the thoracic duct as it enters the confluence of the left internal jugular vein and subclavian vein may simulate a cystic lymph node, potentially leading to a false positive for metastatic lymphadenopathy (**Fig. 9**).

ECS

Extension of metastatic tumor beyond the lymph node capsule, or ECS is the best prognostic factor for local treatment failure in the neck and an indicator of reduction of survival rate by an additional 50%.[2,3,38,39] Postoperative radiation therapy is

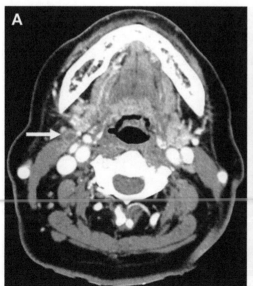
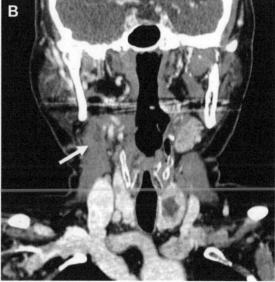

Fig. 5. Infection mimicking a centrally-necrotic lymph node. Axial (A) and coronal reformatted (B) CE-CT images in a 71-year-old male show a 1 cm peripherally enhancing centrally necrotic right level IIA lymph node (*arrows*). UG-FNA demonstrated acid-fast bacilli diagnostic of tuberculous adenitis.

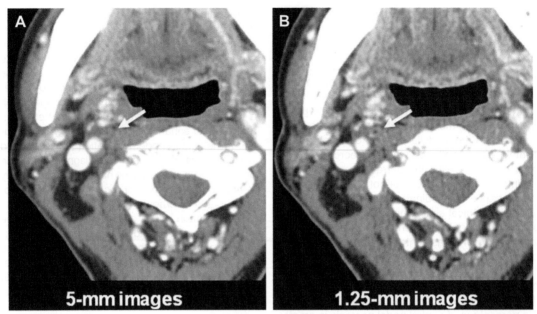

Fig. 6. Effect of slice thickness on a nodal fatty hilum. Axial CE-CT image on at 5-mm thick sections (*A*) demonstrates what appears to be central necrosis and ill-defined margins of a subcentimeter right level IIA lymph node (*arrow*). 1.25 mm reconstructions (*B*) reveal that partial-volume effects obscured the fat-density hilum and well-defined margins of the lymph node (*arrow*).

usually indicated for treatment of the neck if ECS is demonstrated by histology. Studies have also established histologically-identified ECS as a major determinant of whether a patient would benefit from adjuvant chemotherapy[40] because patients with distant metastasis have higher rates of ECS.[41]

On CT, ECS is diagnosed when there is enhancement of the nodal periphery with poorly defined

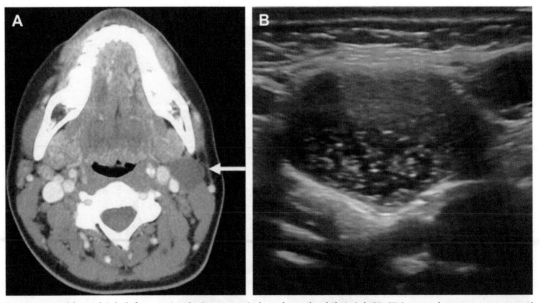

Fig. 7. Second branchial cleft cyst simulating a cystic lymph node. (*A*) Axial CE-CT image demonstrates a cystic appearing node (*arrow*) at the angle of the mandible without enhancing nodularity. (*B*) US image shows multiple echogenic foci in the lesion. UG-FNA demonstrated chronic inflammation and cholesterol crystals, confirmed at surgical excision to represent a second branchial cleft cyst.

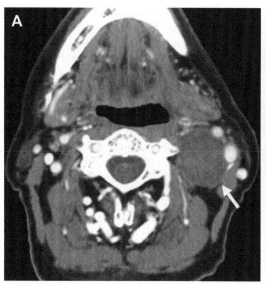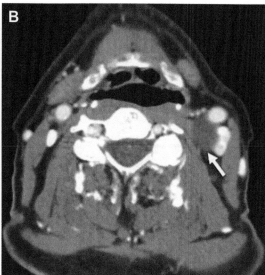

Fig. 8. Cystic nerve sheath tumor simulating cystic lymphadenopathy. (*A, B*) axial CE-CT images show a minimally enhancing cystic appearing mass (*arrows*) in the left level II neck displacing the internal carotid artery and internal jugular vein laterally. At surgical excision this represented a cystic nerve sheath tumor.

margins, infiltration of adjacent fat or muscle planes, and capsular contour irregularity.[42,43] These criteria are accurate only if the patient has not recently had surgery, irradiation, or an active infection in the area.[27,28,44] (Fig. 10). Although it was initially believed that ECS occurred only in lymph nodes larger than 3 cm in greatest diameter, studies correlating CT and histologic findings have shown that such extension actually occurs in 23% of nodes less than 1 cm in greatest diameter, in 53% of nodes 2 to 3 cm in greatest diameter, and

in 74% of nodes greater than 3 cm in greatest diameter.[39,45] Woolgar and colleagues[46] reported histologic evidence of ECS in 16% of HNSCC subjects staged as N0 by CT.

Carotid Encasement

The common or internal carotid artery is invaded in up to 5% to 10% of cervical lymph node metastasis of HNSCC,[47] placing the patient at risk of life-threatening hemorrhage from rupture. Surgical

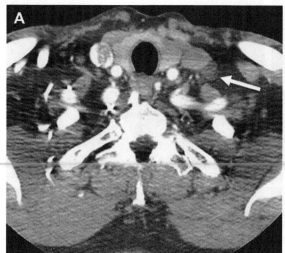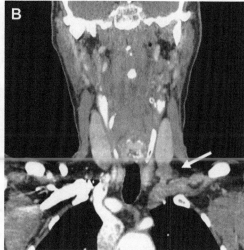

Fig. 9. Thoracic duct appearing as cystic level IV lymphadenopathy. Axial (*A*) and coronal reformatted (*B*) CE-CT images show a cystic mass (*arrows*) in the left level IV neck at the confluence of the left internal jugular vein and left subclavian vein representing the thoracic duct.

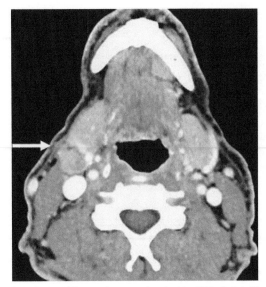

Fig. 10. Postbiopsy changes simulating ECS. Axial CE-CT image from a patient with unknown primary with recent FNA of a right level II lymph node showing ill-defined borders of the node (*arrow*), particularly laterally where the FNA was performed. Cytology demonstrated SCC, however, the post-biopsy findings are indeterminate for ECS.

dissection of tumor abutting the carotid artery can be performed as long as there is not invasion of the vessel adventitia.[48] Rarely in cases with arterial invasion, en bloc resection of the artery and reconstruction may be performed resulting in better

regional control of the disease.[48,49] If the carotid artery is removed but not reconstructed, the risk for developing a stroke is nearly 30%.[49,50] Because tumor adherence to the vessel adventitia is all that is required oncologically to prevent surgical resection or rarely sacrifice of the artery, presurgical identification of carotid encasement is crucial.

Even if the carotid artery appears almost entirely encased by tumor on CT or MR images, in some cases the surgeon finds the arterial adventitia to be free of tumor. Conversely, where just a margin of the tumor abuts the carotid artery, the adventitia may be involved at surgery (**Fig. 11**).[34] Deformation of the contour of the carotid artery is a highly specific indicator of massive invasion of the carotid artery.[51,52] Pons and colleagues[52] found that only 1 of 17 subjects with greater than 180° of circumferential involvement of the carotid were resectable at surgery. Interestingly, in this study the size of lymphadenopathy was not a significant indicator of carotid invasion. Surgical resection is generally not attempted if the affected area is encased by more than 270°[53–55] and, in general, the greater the amount of arterial circumference that is in contact with tumor, the more likely it is that tumor has invaded the arterial wall.[27]

MR IMAGING

Despite the superior contrast resolution of MR imaging over CT, conventional MR imaging has added little to the ability to differentiate benign

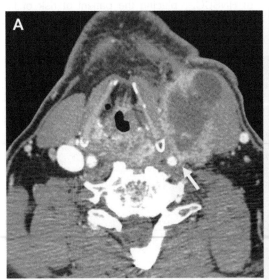

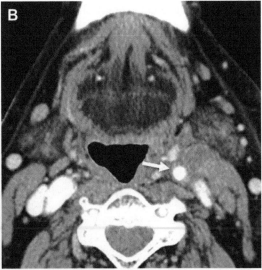

Fig. 11. Indeterminate cases of carotid arterial encasement. (*A*) CE-CT image in a patient with necrotic lymphadenopathy from a hypopharyngeal primary results in approximately 180° of contact with the common carotid artery (*arrow*). There was no evidence of carotid adventitial invasion at surgery. (*B*) CE-CT image shows necrotic lymphadenopathy resulting in near-circumferential abnormal soft tissue around the left common carotid artery (*arrow*). There was no evidence of carotid adventitial invasion at surgery.

from malignant lymph nodes in HNSCC. Signal intensity of metastatic nodes does not differ consistently from that of normal nodes on T1-weighted and T2-weighted images. Even measurement of T1 and T2 relaxation times of metastatic and normal lymph nodes has demonstrated substantial overlap.[56,57] Most reactive lymph nodes have a homogeneously low signal intensity on T1-weighted images and high signal intensity on T2-weighted images. However, non-necrotic and even some necrotic metastatic nodes can have these same signal intensities, making dependence on signal intensities on MR imaging unreliable.[56,57] If lymph nodes have tumor necrosis, they usually have a heterogeneous MR imaging appearance on both T1-weighted and T2-weighted studies. So, purely based on signal intensity, the most reliable MR imaging appearance suggestive of nodal metastasis is signal heterogeneity on T2-weighted images.[56,58]

As on CT, commonly used size-cutoff point on MR imaging is a short axial diameter of 10 mm or long axis of 10 to 15 mm based on location, but multiple size thresholds have been described.[33,59] The challenge remains the detection of metastases in small lymph nodes. de Bondt and colleagues[60] demonstrated that in addition to the nodal size, use of criteria such as border irregularity and heterogeneity on T2-weighted images resulted in a better diagnostic performance of MR imaging for the detection of cervical lymph node metastases in HNSCC. Earlier comparisons of MR imaging with CT resulted in poorer performance of MR imaging.[43,56,57] However, these were likely contributed by limitations of slice thickness and fat saturation techniques. Subsequent studies have shown that MR imaging and CT are probably equivalent for staging of lymph nodes in the neck, including detection of features such as central necrosis[37] and ECS, where the accuracy, sensitivity and specificity were, respectively, 73%, 65%, and 93% for CT, and 80%, 78%, and 86% for MR imaging.[61] Another article found the use of CT for the identification of ECS has a sensitivity of 81% and a specificity of 72%, compared with 57% to 77% and 57% to 72%, respectively, for MR imaging.[32] As with CT, greater than 270° of circumferential involvement of the carotid artery by nodal disease on MR imaging is highly suggestive of unresectability for patients with HNSCC, but false positives with apparent complete encasement of carotid artery without tumor invasion have been described.[55]

Several studies have reported on the ability of diffusion-weighted imaging (DWI) to differentiate metastatic from benign lymph nodes in HNSCC.[62–65] Metastatic lymph nodes have consistently been described to have a significantly lower

apparent diffusion coefficient (ADC) compared with benign lymph nodes. This significantly lower ADC is attributed to densely-packed enlarged tumor cells in comparison to normal small lymphoid cells that are organized in germinal centers and vessel-like sinusoids.[63] Overall, when compared with conventional MR imaging, the additional value of DWI lies mainly in the detection and differentiation of subcentimeter nodal metastases.[62,63]

US

Ultrasound (US) has greater spatial resolution and better capacity to characterize the architectural changes of lymph nodes in the neck than CT or MR imaging.[66–68] The ability to perform US-guided fine-needle aspiration (UG-FNA) for cytology in indeterminate cases also provides US a potential advantage over CT and MR imaging in staging cervical lymph nodes. However, there are some definite disadvantages of US in assessment of cervical nodal status, including operator dependence with a steep learning curve and the lack of sufficient penetration to assess deep lymph nodes (retropharyngeal and mediastinal) that may critically affect staging (Fig. 12).

A high-frequency transducer is used in the diagnosis of cervical lymph node metastases, with the focus, gain, and depth optimized.[69] Metastatic lymph nodes are typically hypoechoic relative to skeletal muscle but this is nonspecific, with multiple inflammatory, infectious, and other neoplastic causes demonstrating similar echogenicity.[70] Most normal lymph nodes have an echogenic hilum related to interfaces between lymphatic sinuses as they converge on the medulla.[71] In 458 lymph nodes in subjects with HNSCC, Yuasa and colleagues[72] found the echogenic hilum absent in 90% of metastatic lymph nodes, but also absent in 44% of benign nodes. Therefore, if the echogenic hilum is present then it is highly likely to be benign; however if it is absent it may or may not be metastatic.

As with other modalities, the difficulty in staging lymph nodes in the neck with US comes in assessing small nodes without malignant features. The reported sensitivity of US for detecting lymph node metastases ranges from 63% to 97%, whereas the reported specificity ranges from 74% to 100%.[73] van den Brekel and colleagues[74] used US to measure the minimum axial diameter of nodes from a series of 184 surgically treated subjects with HNSCC, approximately half of which clinically had N0 disease, the size criteria giving the optimal compromise between sensitivity and specificity in the N0 subgroup was 6 mm (7 mm for level II), resulting in an 80% sensitivity and 59% specificity. The same cutoff in the N-all

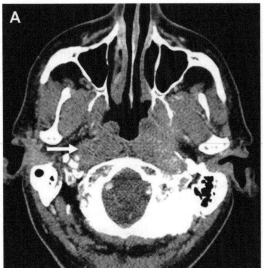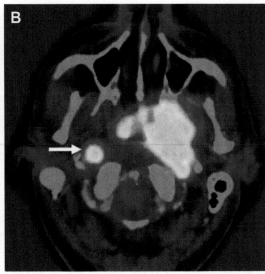

Fig. 12. Metastatic retropharyngeal lymph nodes on CT and CT-PET. (*A*) CE-CT shows a centrally necrotic right retropharyngeal lymph node (*arrow*) from a left nasopharyngeal primary. (*B*) Fused PET-CE-CT shows abnormal FDG uptake in the node (*arrow*). US of this region is impossible due to the depth and lack of an acoustic window, which would result in understaging if this were the only imaging modality used.

(any clinical evidence of lymph node metastasis) subgroup for detection of occult metastases had a sensitivity of 91% and specificity of 52%.

Normal lymph nodes are usually elliptical with a maximal longitudinal to transverse (L/T) dimension ratio of greater than 2, whereas metastatic nodes tend to be rounder. Using an L/T ratio of greater than 2 achieves approximately a 95% sensitivity for detection of abnormal lymph nodes,[75] however, this includes benign and malignant causes for lymphadenopathy. King and colleagues[37] in 27 subjects with N-all HNSCC showed sensitivity of both MR imaging (93%) and CT (91%) was significantly better for necrosis than US (77%) but the specificity of all three techniques was similar, ranging from 89% to 93%. None of the modalities could reliably detect necrotic areas of 3 mm. Steinkamp and colleagues[76] examined 110 subjects with N-all HNSCC for ECS with US and reported a sensitivity of 79% with a specificity of 82%, which was comparable to CT and MR imaging. There is no literature on the detection of ECS by US in N0 HNSCC, although it is unlikely to be very sensitive in small nodes.

Power Doppler is the modality of choice for the assessment of a vascular pattern in cervical lymph nodes because it is most suitable for the detection of weak signal, does not alias, it is not angle-dependent, and gain can be increased without filling the image with noise. Major vascular patterns that have been described include avascularity, a hilar pattern where vessels radiate out from the hilum into the node, and other patterns, such as vascular displacement due to a focal intranodal lesion and a peripheral pattern due to neovascularization where vessels enter the node via the capsule away from the hilum. Avascularity is not a good discriminator of metastatic from benign nodes in HNSCC.[77,78] A hilar pattern is highly specific for benign lymph nodes, whereas a nonhilar pattern is highly specific for metastatic involvement.[77,79,80] Overall, the presence of a normal hilum and normal hilar blood flow indicate nonmetastatic nodes, whereas obliteration of the nodal hilum and loss of normal hilar blood flow are predictive of metastatic nodes.[68,81]

The usefulness of ultrasound as an imaging modality in evaluation of cervical lymphadenopathy is further improved by its high sensitivity (98%) and specificity (95%) when combined with FNA and cytologic analysis.[82] For UG-FNA, there is an inverse relationship between nodal size and the ability to obtain sufficient material with most nondiagnostic samples being taken from nodes less than 5 mm in size.[83–85] US-FNA is 100% specific for nodal metastases in HNSCC,[83,86] however, the reported sensitivity in N0 HNSCC ranges from 42% to 73%, depending on the criteria used to select nodes for aspiration. In contrast to CT, MR imaging, and diagnostic US, this is also affected by more operator-dependent factors affecting the rate of false-negative aspirates and nondiagnostic samples.

POSITRON EMISSION TOMOGRAPHY-CT

Positron emission tomography (PET) using fluoro-deoxyglucose F 18 (FDG-18) has been successfully applied to the evaluation of mucosal HNSCC,[87–89] as well as thyroid and salivary gland malignancies.[90–92] FDG, a glucose analog, is a marker of tumor viability reflecting that malignant lymph nodes having higher glucose use than normal nodes.[93] Integrated PET-CT units have improved the accuracy of PET image interpretation,[94] using attenuation correction from the CT

imaging and semiquantitative analysis expressed as the maximum standardized uptake value (max-SUV), corrected for the injected radioactivity and patient body weight. In general, hypermetabolic lesions with strong focal uptake (maxSUV $\geq$2.5) are considered malignant.

Although FDG-PET-CT rarely adds additional useful information regarding the initial T staging of a known primary site,[95] it has applications for detection of regional lymph node metastasis, distant metastases, identification of an unknown primary site, monitoring treatment response, and

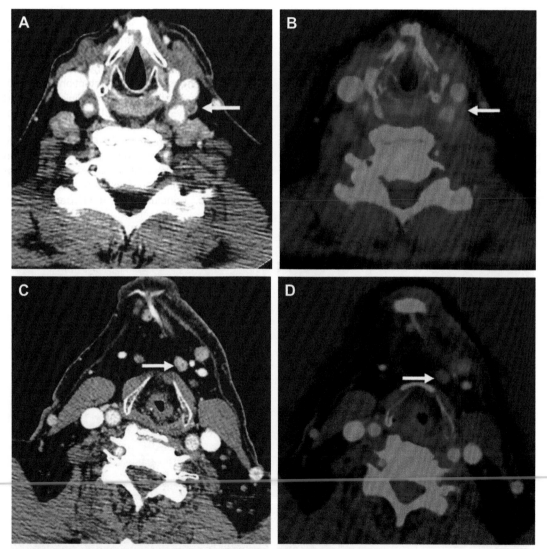

Fig. 13. Small necrotic lymph nodes on CE-CT negative on PET. (*A*) CE-CT image from a patient with T4b left oral cavity SCC showing a 7 mm centrally necrotic left level III lymph node (*arrow*). (*B*) Fused PET-CE-CT shows no significant abnormal FDG uptake (*arrow*). (*C*) Different patient with left oral cavity primary and CE-CT showing a tiny focus of necrosis within a left IB lymph node (*arrow*). (*D*) Fused PET-CE-CT image shows no abnormal FDG uptake (*arrow*).

long-term surveillance for recurrence and metastases.[96,97] For highly hypermetabolic nodal metastases, PET-CT has the potential to detect small metastatic deposits in normal-sized nodes.[98] However, PET and PET-CT have definite limitations. Although the spatial resolution of the technique is 4 to 5 mm,[99] the smallest detectable lymph node metastatic deposits is generally 8 to 10 mm, translating into a lower sensitivity for PET-CT in diagnosis of lymph nodes less than 10 mm (Fig. 13).[100,101] Nodal necrosis may cause false-negative findings on PET because of the low glycolytic activity of the necrotic material (Fig. 14).[102] For this reason, it has been found that CE-CT and PET-CE-CT perform equally and better than nonenhanced PET-CT in detecting cystic lymph node metastasis in oropharyngeal squamous cell carcinoma (SCC).[103] Finally, false-positive PET results may be caused by inflammatory and infectious processes in benign lymph nodes (Fig. 15).[89,104,105]

Several recent studies have demonstrated high sensitivity and specificity for PET-CT in the detection of cervical lymph node metastases in HNSCC. These ranged from 84% to 92% for sensitivity and from 95% to 99% for specificity.[106–108] FDG-PET has a higher sensitivity and specificity than CT or MR imaging for detection of lymph node metastases in head and neck cancer.[34,87,109] Adams and colleagues[87] compared PET with CT, MR imaging, and US in lymph node staging in 60 subjects with HNSCC. PET showed the highest sensitivity (90%) and specificity (94%) for the detection of cervical nodal metastasis on a node-by-node basis; sensitivities and specificities for conventional imaging modalities were 72% to 82% and 79% to 85%. Lonneux,[92] in a prospective, multicenter study showed that FDG-PET was significantly more accurate than conventional staging, improving staging accuracy in 20% of subjects with HNSCC and modified the management of 13.7% of subjects.

Clinical N0 disease still represents a dilemma for all imaging modalities. Studies have[110,111] concluded that PET-CT is not accurate enough for detection of occult nodal disease and would not help the surgeon if the study is negative. False-negative findings were attributed to the presence of microscopic metastases not detected by PET-CT, or by proximity of nodal metastases to the primary tumor obscuring their detection. In a study by Richard and colleagues[112] for clinically staged N0 neck, the negative predictive value (NPV) of PET-CT was 89% leading the investigators to conclude that, at present, PET-CT cannot reliably predict the need for surgical neck dissection in patients with a clinically N0 neck.[113,114] Fig. 16 illustrates a case with a nonpalpable, normal-sized, nonnecrotic, nonclustered, nonhypermetabolic

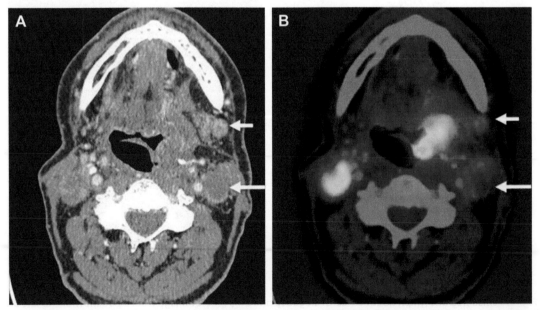

Fig. 14. Large necrotic lymph nodes on CE-CT negative on PET. (A) CE-CT image shows multiple necrotic bilateral lymph nodes (short and long arrows) in a patient with an oropharyngeal primary. (B) Fused PET-CE-CT shows abnormal FDG uptake in a solid right level II lymph node (SUV of 11.6) and at the primary site (SUV of 12.5) but not at large left level IB and IIA necrotic lymph nodes (short and long arrows).

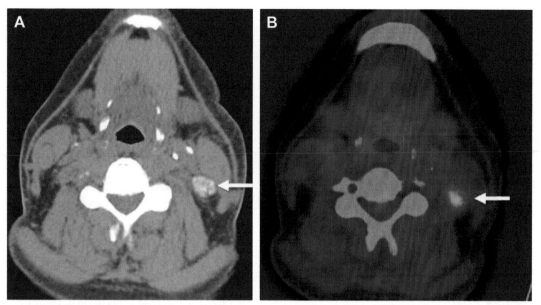

Fig. 15. A false positive for metastatic lymphadenopathy due to sarcoidosis. (A) Axial noncontrast CT image from a patient with left glossotonsillar sulcus SCC shows a partially calcified 2 cm left level III lymph node (arrow). (B) Fused PET-CT image shows elevated FDG uptake (arrow; SUV of 3.9). Biopsy of the lymph node revealed noncaseating granulomas of sarcoidosis.

lymph node in the neck that was proven at neck dissection to have metastatic involvement. The author recommends performing a fully diagnostic quality CE-CT for attenuation correction for PET examinations in HNSCC and that, in general, all patients with HNSCC (except T1 oral tongue lesions) should undergo PET-CE-CT for initial staging.

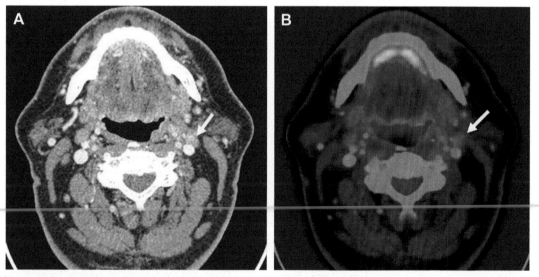

Fig. 16. False-negative contrast-enhanced CT-PET examination. (A) CE-CT image on left in a patient with left tonsillar SCC shows subcentimeter, nonnecrotic, nonclustered left level II lymph node (arrow). (B) PET-CE-CT of the lymph node (arrow) demonstrates no abnormal FDG uptake. Transoral robotic surgery and left selective neck dissection (levels II through IV) showed positive metastatic SCC in 7 of 28 lymph nodes in IIA, IIB, and III stations.

SUMMARY

Lymph node status is one of the most important predictors of prognosis in HNSCC, making accurate staging critical. The physical examination of the neck is highly inaccurate. Imaging by CT, MR imaging, US, and PET-CT improve accuracy of staging but all have limitations, particularly detection of small metastatic lymph nodes harboring microscopic metastatic disease. Size criteria, nodal shape and clustering, central necrosis, and findings of ECS and vascular encasement are means of suggesting metastatic involvement on CT and MR imaging. US features, including echogenicity, size, morphology, and pattern of Doppler flow, help differentiate benign from malignant nodes, aided by UG-FNA for indeterminate cases. PET-CT is extremely useful for staging the lymph nodes and for detection of distant metastasis, particularly when performed with a diagnostic quality CE-CT.

REFERENCES

1. van de Velde C. Oncologie. Zesde Herziene Oncologie 2001; p.1326–39.
2. Farr HW, Goldfarb PM, Farr CM. Epidermoid carcinoma of the mouth and pharynx at Memorial Sloan-Kettering Cancer Center, 1965 to 1969. Am J Surg 1980;140(4):563–7.
3. Spiro RH. The management of neck nodes in head and neck cancer: a surgeon's view. Bull N Y Acad Med 1985;61(7):629–37.
4. van den Brekel MW, Stel HV, Castelijns JA, et al. Cervical lymph node metastasis: assessment of radiologic criteria. Radiology 1990;177(2):379–84.
5. van den Brekel MW, Bartelink H, Snow GB. The value of staging of neck nodes in patients treated with radiotherapy. Radiother Oncol 1994;32(3):193–6.
6. Foote RL, Olsen KD, Davis DL, et al. Base of tongue carcinoma: patterns of failure and predictors of recurrence after surgery alone. Head Neck 1993;15(4):300–7.
7. Leemans CR, Tiwari R, Nauta JJ, et al. Recurrence at the primary site in head and neck cancer and the significance of neck lymph node metastases as a prognostic factor. Cancer 1994;73(1):187–90.
8. Tannock IF. Principles of cell proliferation: cell kinetics. In: Dc Vita VT Jr, editor. Principles and practice of oncology. 2nd edition. Philadelphia: Lippincott; 1988. p. 3–13.
9. Ali S, Tiwari RM, Snow GB. False-positive and false-negative neck nodes. Head Neck Surg 1985;8(2):78–82.
10. Sako K, Pradier RN, Marchetta FC, et al. Fallibility of palpation in the diagnosis of metastases to cervical nodes. Surg Gynecol Obstet 1964;118:989–90.
11. Lindberg R. Distribution of cervical lymph node metastases from squamous cell carcinoma of the upper respiratory and digestive tracts. Cancer 1972;29(6):1446–9.
12. Johnson JT. A surgeon looks at cervical lymph nodes. Radiology 1990;175(3):607–10.
13. Jesse RH, Barkley HT Jr, Lindberg RD, et al. Cancer of the oral cavity. Is elective neck dissection beneficial? Am J Surg 1970;120(4):505–8.
14. Byers RM, Wolf PF, Ballantyne AJ. Rationale for elective modified neck dissection. Head Neck Surg 1988;10(3):160–7.
15. Chow JM, Levin BC, Krivit JS, et al. Radiotherapy or surgery for subclinical cervical node metastases. Arch Otolaryngol Head Neck Surg 1989; 115(8):981–4.
16. Ferlito A, Rinaldo A, Robbins KT, et al. Changing concepts in the surgical management of the cervical node metastasis. Oral Oncol 2003;39(5): 429–35.
17. Olsen KD, Caruso M, Foote RL, et al. Primary head and neck cancer. Histopathologic predictors of recurrence after neck dissection in patients with lymph node involvement. Arch Otolaryngol Head Neck Surg 1994;120(12):1370–4.
18. Holsinger FC, McWhorter AJ, Menard M, et al. Transoral lateral oropharyngectomy for squamous cell carcinoma of the tonsillar region: I. Technique, complications, and functional results. Arch Otolaryngol Head Neck Surg 2005;131(7): 583–91.
19. Walvekar RR, Li RJ, Gooding WE, et al. Role of surgery in limited (T1-2, N0-1) cancers of the oropharynx. Laryngoscope 2008;118(12):2129–34.
20. Sturgis EM, Cinciripini PM. Trends in head and neck cancer incidence in relation to smoking prevalence: an emerging epidemic of human papillomavirus-associated cancers? Cancer 2007; 110(7):1429–35.
21. Galati LT, Myers EN, Johnson JT. Primary surgery as treatment for early squamous cell carcinoma of the tonsil. Head Neck 2000;22(3):294–6.
22. Som PM, Curtin HD, Mancuso AA. The new imaging-based classification for describing the location of lymph nodes in the neck with particular regard to cervical lymph nodes in relation to cancer of the larynx. ORL J Otorhinolaryngol Relat Spec 2000;62(4):186–98.
23. Friedman M, Shelton VK, Mafee M, et al. Metastatic neck disease. Evaluation by computed tomography. Arch Otolaryngol 1984;110(7):443–7.
24. Stevens MH, Harnsberger HR, Mancuso AA, et al. Computed tomography of cervical lymph nodes. Staging and management of head and neck cancer. Arch Otolaryngol 1985;111(11):735–9.
25. Close LG, Merkel M, Vuitch MF, et al. Computed tomographic evaluation of regional lymph node

involvement in cancer of the oral cavity and oropharynx. Head Neck 1989;11(4):309–17.

26. Mancuso AA, Maceri D, Rice D, et al. CT of cervical lymph node cancer. AJR Am J Roentgenol 1981; 136(2):381–5.

27. Som PM. Lymph nodes of the neck. Radiology 1987;165(3):593–600.

28. Mancuso AA, Harnsberger HR, Muraki AS, et al. Computed tomography of cervical and retropharyngeal lymph nodes: normal anatomy, variants of normal, and applications in staging head and neck cancer. Part II: pathology. Radiology 1983; 148(3):715–23.

29. Friedman M, Roberts N, Kirshenbaum GL, et al. Nodal size of metastatic squamous cell carcinoma of the neck. Laryngoscope 1993;103(8):854–6.

30. Don DM, Anzai Y, Lufkin RB, et al. Evaluation of cervical lymph node metastases in squamous cell carcinoma of the head and neck. Laryngoscope 1995;105(7 Pt 1):669–74.

31. Castelijns JA, van den Brekel MW. Detection of lymph node metastases in the neck: radiologic criteria. AJNR Am J Neuroradiol 2001;22(1):3–4.

32. Steinkamp HJ, Hosten N, Richter C, et al. Enlarged cervical lymph nodes at helical CT. Radiology 1994;191(3):795–8.

33. Curtin HD, Ishwaran H, Mancuso AA, et al. Comparison of CT and MR imaging in staging of neck metastases. Radiology 1998;207(1):123–30.

34. Som PM. Detection of metastasis in cervical lymph nodes: CT and MR criteria and differential diagnosis. AJR Am J Roentgenol 1992;158(5):961–9.

35. Sakai O, Curtin HD, Romo LV, et al. Lymph node pathology. Benign proliferative, lymphoma, and metastatic disease. Radiol Clin North Am 2000; 38(5):979–98, x.

36. Steinkamp HJ, van der Hoeck E, Bock JC, et al. The extracapsular spread of cervical lymph node metastases: the diagnostic value of computed tomography. Rofo 1999;170(5):457–62 [in German].

37. King AD, Tse GM, Ahuja AT, et al. Necrosis in metastatic neck nodes: diagnostic accuracy of CT, MR imaging, and US. Radiology 2004;230(3):720–6.

38. Batsakis JG. Squamous cell carcinoma of the oral cavity and the oropharynx. In: Tumors of the head and neck. Clinical and pathological considerations. 2nd edition. Baltimore: Williams & Wilkins; 1979. p. 240–50.

39. Snyderman NL, Johnson JT, Schramm VL, et al. Extracapsular spread of carcinoma in cervical lymph nodes. Cancer 1985;56:1597–9.

40. Cooper JS, Pajak TF, Forastiere AA, et al. Postoperative concurrent radiotherapy and chemotherapy for high-risk squamous-cell carcinoma of the head and neck. N Engl J Med 2004;350(19):1937–44.

41. Alvi A, Johnson JT. Extracapsular spread in the clinically negative neck (N0): implications and

outcome. Otolaryngol Head Neck Surg 1996; 114(1):65–70.

42. van den Brekel MW, van der Waal I, Meijer CJ, et al. The incidence of micrometastases in neck dissection specimens obtained from elective neck dissections. Laryngoscope 1996;106(8):987–91.

43. Yousem DM, Som PM, Hackney DB, et al. Central nodal necrosis and extracapsular neoplastic spread in cervical lymph nodes: MR imaging versus CT. Radiology 1992;182(3):753–9.

44. Reede DL, Bergeron RT. Computed tomography of cervical lymph nodes. In: Clouse ME, Wallace S, editors. Lymphatic imaging: lymphography, computed tomography, and scintigraphy. 2nd edition. Baltimore: Williams & Wilkins; 1985. p. 472–95.

45. Snow GB, Annyas AA, van Slooten EA, et al. Prognostic factors of neck node metastasis. Clin Otolaryngol Allied Sci 1982;7(3):185–92.

46. Woolgar JA, Rogers SN, Lowe D, et al. Cervical lymph node metastasis in oral cancer: the importance of even microscopic extracapsular spread. Oral Oncol 2003;39(2):130–7.

47. Németh Z, Dömötör G, Tálos M. Resection and replacement of the carotid artery in metastatic head and neck cancer. Int J Oral Maxillofac Surg 2003;32(6):645–50.

48. Pons Y, Ukkola-Pons E, Clement P, et al. Carotid artery resection and reconstruction with superficial femoral artery transplantation: a case report. Head Neck Oncol 2009;1:19.

49. Ozer E, Agrawal A, Ozer HG, et al. The impact of surgery in the management of the head and neck carcinoma involving the carotid artery. Laryngoscope 2008;118(10):1771–4.

50. Miao B, Lu Y, Pan X, et al. Carotid artery resection and reconstruction with expanded polytetrafluoroethylene for head and neck cancer. Laryngoscope 2008;118(12):2135–8.

51. Yu Q, Wang P, Shi H, et al. Carotid artery and jugular vein invasion of oral-maxillofacial and neck malignant tumors: diagnostic value of computed tomography. Oral Surg Oral Med Oral Pathol Oral Radiol Endod 2003;96(3):368–72.

52. Pons Y, Ukkola-Pons E, Clement P, et al. Relevance of 5 different imaging signs in the evaluation of carotid artery invasion by cervical lymphadenopathy in head and neck squamous cell carcinoma. Oral Surg Oral Med Oral Pathol Oral Radiol Endod 2010;109(5):775–8.

53. Yoo GH, Hocwald E, Korkmaz H, et al. Assessment of carotid artery invasion in patients with head and neck cancer. Laryngoscope 2000;110(3 Pt 1):386–90.

54. Mack MG, Rieger J, Baghi M, et al. Cervical lymph nodes. Eur J Radiol 2008;66(3):493–500.

55. Yousem DM, Hatabu H, Hurst RW, et al. Carotid artery invasion by head and neck masses: prediction with MR imaging. Radiology 1995;195(3):715–20.

56. Dooms GC, Hricak H, Crooks LE, et al. Magnetic resonance imaging of the lymph nodes: comparison with CT. Radiology 1984;153(3):719–28.

57. Dooms GC, Hricak H, Moseley ME, et al. Characterization of lymphadenopathy by magnetic resonance relaxation times: preliminary results. Radiology 1985;155(3):691–7.

58. Dillon WP, Mills CM, Kjos B, et al. Magnetic resonance imaging of the nasopharynx. Radiology 1984;152(3):731–8.

59. van den Brekel MW, Castelijns JA, Stel HV, et al. Modern imaging techniques and ultrasound-guided aspiration cytology for the assessment of neck node metastases: a prospective comparative study. Eur Arch Otorhinolaryngol 1993;250(1):11–7.

60. de Bondt RB, Nelemans PJ, Bakers F, et al. Morphological MRI criteria improve the detection of lymph node metastases in head and neck squamous cell carcinoma: multivariate logistic regression analysis of MRI features of cervical lymph nodes. Eur Radiol 2009;19(3):626–33.

61. King AD, Tse GM, Yuen EH, et al. Comparison of CT and MR imaging for the detection of extranodal neoplastic spread in metastatic neck nodes. Eur J Radiol 2004;52(3):264–70.

62. de Bondt RB, Hoeberigs MC, Nelemans PJ, et al. Diagnostic accuracy and additional value of diffusion-weighted imaging for discrimination of malignant cervical lymph nodes in head and neck squamous cell carcinoma. Neuroradiology 2009;51(3):183–92.

63. Vandecaveye V, De Keyzer F, Vander Poorten V, et al. Head and neck squamous cell carcinoma: value of diffusion-weighted MR imaging for nodal staging. Radiology 2009;251(1):134–46.

64. Perrone A, Guerrisi P, Izzo L, et al. Diffusion-weighted MRI in cervical lymph nodes: differentiation between benign and malignant lesions. Eur J Radiol 2011;77(2):281–6.

65. Holzapfel K, Duetsch S, Fauser C, et al. Value of diffusion-weighted MR imaging in the differentiation between benign and malignant cervical lymph nodes. Eur J Radiol 2009;72(3):381–7.

66. Sumi M, Ohki M, Nakamura T. Comparison of sonography and CT for differentiating benign from malignant cervical lymph nodes in patients with squamous cell carcinoma of the head and neck. AJR Am J Roentgenol 2001;176(4):1019–24.

67. Vassallo P, Wernecke K, Roos N, et al. Differentiation of benign from malignant superficial lymphadenopathy: the role of high-resolution US. Radiology 1992;183(1):215–20.

68. Yonetsu K, Sumi M, Izumi M, et al. Contribution of doppler sonography blood flow information to the diagnosis of metastatic cervical nodes in patients with head and neck cancer: assessment in relation to anatomic levels of the neck. AJNR Am J Neuroradiol 2001;22(1):163–9.

69. Furukawa Mk, Furukawa M, MF. Ultrasonography covered within the field of otolaryngology head and neck surgery. Tokyo (Japan): Ishiyaku; 1999.

70. Ahuja A, Ying M. An overview of neck node sonography. Invest Radiol 2002;37(6):333–42.

71. Rubaltelli L, Proto E, Salmaso R, et al. Sonography of abnormal lymph nodes in vitro: correlation of sonographic and histologic findings. AJR Am J Roentgenol 1990;155(6):1241–4.

72. Yuasa K, Kawazu T, Nagata T, et al. Computed tomography and ultrasonography of metastatic cervical lymph nodes in oral squamous cell carcinoma. Dentomaxillofac Radiol 2000;29(4):238–44.

73. de Bondt RB, Nelemans PJ, Hofman PA, et al. Detection of lymph node metastases in head and neck cancer: a meta-analysis comparing US, USgFNAC, CT and MR imaging. Eur J Radiol 2007;64(2):266–72.

74. van den Brekel MW, Castelijns JA, Snow GB. The size of lymph nodes in the neck on sonograms as a radiologic criterion for metastasis: how reliable is it? AJNR Am J Neuroradiol 1998;19(4):695–700.

75. Steinkamp HJ, Cornehl M, Hosten N, et al. Cervical lymphadenopathy: ratio of long- to short-axis diameter as a predictor of malignancy. Br J Radiol 1995;68(807):266–70.

76. Steinkamp HJ, Beck A, Werk M, et al. Extracapsular spread of cervical lymph node metastases: diagnostic relevance of ultrasound examinations. Ultraschall Med 2003;24(5):323–30.

77. Sakaguchi T, Yamashita Y, Katahira K, et al. Differential diagnosis of small round cervical lymph nodes: comparison of power Doppler US with contrast-enhanced CT and pathologic results. Radiat Med 2001;19(3):119–25.

78. Ariji Y, Kimura Y, Hayashi N, et al. Power Doppler sonography of cervical lymph nodes in patients with head and neck cancer. AJNR Am J Neuroradiol 1998;19(2):303–7.

79. Eida S, Sumi M, Yonetsu K, et al. Combination of helical CT and Doppler sonography in the follow-up of patients with clinical N0 stage neck disease and oral cancer. AJNR Am J Neuroradiol 2003;24(3):312–8.

80. Ahuja A, Ying M. Sonographic evaluation of cervical lymphadenopathy: is power Doppler sonography routinely indicated? Ultrasound Med Biol 2003;29(3):353–9.

81. Chikui T, Yonetsu K, Nakamura T. Multivariate feature analysis of sonographic findings of metastatic cervical lymph nodes: contribution of blood flow features revealed by power Doppler sonography for predicting metastasis. AJNR Am J Neuroradiol 2000;21(3):561–7.

82. Baatenburg de Jong RJ, Rongen RJ, Verwoerd CD, et al. Ultrasound-guided fine-needle aspiration biopsy of neck nodes. Arch Otolaryngol Head Neck Surg 1991;117(4):402–4.

83. van den Brekel MW, Castelijns JA, Stel HV, et al. Occult metastatic neck disease: detection with US and US-guided fine-needle aspiration cytology. Radiology 1991;180(2):457–61.

84. van den Brekel MW, Castelijns JA, Reitsma LC, et al. Outcome of observing the N0 neck using ultrasonographic-guided cytology for follow-up. Arch Otolaryngol Head Neck Surg 1999;125(2):153–6.

85. Castelijns JA, van den Brekel MW. Imaging of lymphadenopathy in the neck. Eur Radiol 2002; 12(4):727–38.

86. Righi PD, Kopecky KK, Caldemeyer KS, et al. Comparison of ultrasound-fine needle aspiration and computed tomography in patients undergoing elective neck dissection. Head Neck 1997;19(7): 604–10.

87. Adams S, Baum RP, Stuckensen T, et al. Prospective comparison of 18F-FDG PET with conventional imaging modalities (CT, MRI, US) in lymph node staging of head and neck cancer. Eur J Nucl Med 1998;25(9):1255–60.

88. Braams JW, Pruim J, Freling NJ, et al. Detection of lymph node metastases of squamous-cell cancer of the head and neck with FDG-PET and MRI. J Nucl Med 1995;36(2):211–6.

89. Laubenbacher C, Saumweber D, Wagner-Manslau C, et al. Comparison of fluorine-18-fluorodeoxyglucose PET, MRI and endoscopy for staging head and neck squamous-cell carcinomas. J Nucl Med 1995;36(10):1747–57.

90. Hain SF. Positron emission tomography in cancer of the head and neck. Br J Oral Maxillofac Surg 2005; 43(1):1–6.

91. Zimmer LA, Branstetter BF, Nayak JV, et al. Current use of 18F-fluorodeoxyglucose positron emission tomography and combined positron emission tomography and computed tomography in squamous cell carcinoma of the head and neck. Laryngoscope 2005;115(11):2029–34.

92. Lonneux M. Current applications and future developments of positron emission tomography in head and neck cancer. Cancer Radiother 2005;9(1):8–15 [in French].

93. Haberkorn U, Strauss LG, Reisser C, et al. Glucose uptake, perfusion, and cell proliferation in head and neck tumors: relation of positron emission tomography to flow cytometry. J Nucl Med 1991; 32(8):1548–55.

94. Schoder H, Yeung HW, Gonen M, et al. Head and neck cancer: clinical usefulness and accuracy of PET/CT image fusion. Radiology 2004; 231(1):65–72.

95. Quon A, Fischbein NJ, McDougall IR, et al. Clinical role of 18F-FDG PET/CT in the management of squamous cell carcinoma of the head and neck and thyroid carcinoma. J Nucl Med 2007; 48(Suppl 1):58S–67S.

96. Schwartz DL, Rajendran J, Yueh B, et al. Staging of head and neck squamous cell cancer with extended-field FDG-PET. Arch Otolaryngol Head Neck Surg 2003;129(11):1173–8.

97. Stuckensen T, Kovacs AF, Adams S, et al. Staging of the neck in patients with oral cavity squamous cell carcinomas: a prospective comparison of PET, ultrasound, CT and MRI. J Craniomaxillofac Surg 2000;28(6):319–24.

98. Jabour BA, Choi Y, Hoh CK, et al. Extracranial head and neck: PET imaging with 2-[F-18]fluoro-2-deoxy-D-glucose and MR imaging correlation. Radiology 1993;186(1):27–35.

99. Yamazaki Y, Saitoh M, Notani K, et al. Assessment of cervical lymph node metastases using FDG-PET in patients with head and neck cancer. Ann Nucl Med 2008;22(3):177–84.

100. Stoeckli SJ, Steinert H, Pfaltz M, et al. Is there a role for positron emission tomography with 18F-fluorodeoxyglucose in the initial staging of nodal negative oral and oropharyngeal squamous cell carcinoma. Head Neck 2002;24(4): 345–9.

101. Hyde NC, Prvulovich E, Newman L, et al. A new approach to pre-treatment assessment of the N0 neck in oral squamous cell carcinoma: the role of sentinel node biopsy and positron emission tomography. Oral Oncol 2003;39(4):350–60.

102. Kau RJ, Alexiou C, Laubenbacher C, et al. Lymph node detection of head and neck squamous cell carcinomas by positron emission tomography with fluorodeoxyglucose F 18 in a routine clinical setting. Arch Otolaryngol Head Neck Surg 1999; 125(12):1322–8.

103. Haerle SK, Strobel K, Ahmad N, et al. Contrast-enhanced (1)F-FDG-PET/CT for the assessment of necrotic lymph node metastases. Head Neck 2011;33(3):324–9.

104. Di Martino E, Nowak B, Hassan HA, et al. Diagnosis and staging of head and neck cancer: a comparison of modern imaging modalities (positron emission tomography, computed tomography, color-coded duplex sonography) with panendoscopic and histopathologic findings. Arch Otolaryngol Head Neck Surg 2000;126(12):1457–61.

105. Paulus P, Sambon A, Vivegnis D, et al. 18FDG-PET for the assessment of primary head and neck tumors: clinical, computed tomography, and histopathological correlation in 38 patients. Laryngoscope 1998;108(10):1578–83.

106. Murakami R, Uozumi H, Hirai T, et al. Impact of FDG-PET/CT imaging on nodal staging for head-and-neck squamous cell carcinoma. Int J Radiat Oncol Biol Phys 2007;68(2):377–82.

107. Gordin A, Golz A, Keidar Z, et al. The role of FDG-PET/CT imaging in head and neck malignant conditions: impact on diagnostic accuracy and

patient care. Otolaryngol Head Neck Surg 2007; 137(1):130–7.

108. Jeong HS, Baek CH, Son YI, et al. Use of integrated 18F-FDG PET/CT to improve the accuracy of initial cervical nodal evaluation in patients with head and neck squamous cell carcinoma. Head Neck 2007;29(3):203–10.

109. Feinmesser R, Freeman JL, Noyek AM, et al. Metastatic neck disease. A clinical/radiographic/pathologic correlative study. Arch Otolaryngol Head Neck Surg 1987;113(12):1307–10.

110. Ferlito A, Rinaldo A. Level I dissection for laryngeal and hypopharyngeal cancer: is it indicated? J Laryngol Otol 1998;112(5):438–40.

111. Gregor RT, Oei SS, Hilgers FJ, et al. Management of cervical metastases in supraglottic cancer. Ann Otol Rhinol Laryngol 1996;105(11):845–50.

112. Richard C, Prevot N, Timoshenko AP, et al. Preoperative combined 18-fluorodeoxyglucose positron emission tomography and computed tomography imaging in head and neck cancer: does it really improve initial N staging? Acta Otolaryngol 2010; 130(12):1421–4.

113. Schoder H, Carlson DL, Kraus DH, et al. 18F-FDG PET/CT for detecting nodal metastases in patients with oral cancer staged N0 by clinical examination and CT/MRI. J Nucl Med 2006; 47(5):755–62.

114. Gourin CG, Boyce BJ, Williams HT, et al. Revisiting the role of positron-emission tomography/computed tomography in determining the need for planned neck dissection following chemoradiation for advanced head and neck cancer. Laryngoscope 2009;119(11):2150–5.

Pitfalls in Image Guided Tissue Sampling in the Head and Neck

Gamaliel Lorenzo, MD*, Amit M. Saindane, MD

KEYWORDS

- Ultrasound-guided fine-needle aspiration • Computed tomography-guided fine-needle aspiration
- Ultrasonography • Computed tomography • Magnetic resonance imaging
- Positron emission tomography • Fine-needle aspiration

KEY POINTS

- The ability to easily and accurately establish a histologic diagnosis from the soft tissues of the neck using image guidance is becoming increasingly important.
- Definite histologic characterization of deep and nonpalpable targets often requires image-guided tissue sampling.
- Patient management frequently depends on accurate characterization of suspicious or indeterminate findings in the neck to determine initial stage malignancy or the presence or absence of residual, progressive, or recurrent malignancy.
- This article reviews the technique and relative advantages for tissue sampling guided by ultrasonography and computed tomography.

INTRODUCTION

The ability to easily and accurately establish a histologic diagnosis in the soft tissues of the neck using image guidance is becoming increasingly important. Improved sensitivity afforded by advances in computed tomography (CT), magnetic resonance (MR) imaging, ultrasonography (US), and CT-positron emission tomography (PET) for diagnosis, staging, and surveillance now depict subclinical, small, and deep lesions that are inaccessible by palpation-guided (PG) histologic sampling. For example, CT-PET is increasingly being used for staging and surveillance of head and neck squamous cell carcinoma (HNSCC), sometimes resulting in indeterminate standardized uptake values for fluorodeoxyglucose (FDG) uptake in lymph nodes. Postoperative infection or posttreatment inflammatory changes can result in false-positive FDG uptake in the setting of recent surgery or radiation therapy,[1–3] and small or necrotic lymph nodes can lead to false-negative FDG uptake.[4] US is commonly used in initial staging and for routine surveillance of patients with papillary thyroid carcinoma (PTC), resulting in detection of new, enlarging, or mildly hypervascular lymph nodes, which may be suspicious for but not diagnostic of PTC.

Although mucosal lesions in the head and neck are readily biopsied under direct clinical inspection or endoscopically, the definite histologic characterization of submucosal or deep primary sites and nonpalpable lymph nodes often requires image-guided tissue sampling. Patient management frequently depends on accurate characterization of suspicious or indeterminate findings in the neck to determine initial stage or presence or absence of residual, progressive, or recurrent malignancy. These factors have made the ability to perform image-guided tissue sampling in the head and neck a critical skill.

Options for Tissue Sampling in the Head and Neck

There are several options for tissue sampling of nonmucosal lesions in the head and neck, including PG fine-needle aspiration (PG-FNA),

Department of Radiology and Imaging Sciences, Emory University School of Medicine, BG, 1364 Clifton Road Northeast, Atlanta, GA 30322, USA
* Corresponding author.
E-mail address: GLorenzo@salud.unm.edu

Neuroimag Clin N Am 23 (2013) 167–178
http://dx.doi.org/10.1016/j.nic.2012.08.012

US-guided FNA (UG-FNA), core biopsy, CT-guided FNA (CTG-FNA) or core biopsy and open surgical biopsy. Frequently, masses found on imaging studies are deep and nonpalpable, precluding the simplest and most inexpensive option, PG-FNA. UG-FNA has many desirable features for tissue sampling in the head and neck, making it ideal for evaluating nodal disease. CTG-FNA is extremely useful for lesions within the deep face and skull base that are too deep or do not have an adequate sonographic window for UG-FNA. Surgical excision should be reserved for cases in which image-guided biopsy is inconclusive or in which performing image-guided biopsy would not affect the decision to perform surgery.

Observation with repeat US, CT, MR imaging, or CT-PET is also a reasonable alternative to tissue sampling in certain circumstances, but despite considerably increased cost, short-interval follow-up examinations may not be definitive to exclude malignancy. Before initiating chemotherapy or radiation therapy regimens or performing potentially risky surgical procedures, referring services may desire a tissue diagnosis of malignancy regardless of the follow-up examination results, mandating image-guided tissue sampling. The small percentage of nondiagnostic image-guided FNAs/biopsies can be repeated at a fraction of the cost of follow-up imaging, if needed.

UG-FNA: TECHNIQUE AND PITFALLS
Rationale for and Advantages of UG-FNA

There are multiple advantages of UG-FNA in the neck over PG-FNA and CTG-FNA. In experienced hands, UG-FNA is safe and simple to perform. Although a lesion may be palpable, its depth relative to the neck musculature and relationship to surrounding vascular structures may be unknown, precluding safe PG tissue sampling if previous imaging is not available documenting the location of the lesion. In the neck, lymph nodes are typically in close relation to the carotid arterial system or internal jugular veins. UG-FNA allows for precise targeting of small nodes with a larger safety margin, because the needle tip can be imaged in real time, and adjacent vascular structures can be clearly delineated using color Doppler techniques, allowing safe sampling of even small targets (Fig. 1). Targets for aspiration may be heterogeneous in composition and contain cystic or necrotic spaces. Under US guidance, the needle can be precisely positioned to a specific abnormal area of a mass such as solid or cystic portions to maximize yield depending on the suspected diagnosis (Fig. 2), and areas of

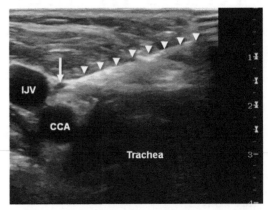

Fig. 1. Safe and precise tissue sampling adjacent to vascular structures using UG-FNA. Transverse US image showing successful needle targeting of a 3-mm nodule (*arrow*) adjacent to the internal jugular vein (IJV) and common carotid artery (CCA).

hypervascularity including hilar vascularity (Fig. 3) can be avoided to decrease the likelihood of aspirating purely bloody or blood-diluted samples. UG-FNA has shown improved sensitivity and specificity over CT and MR imaging for staging the N0 neck in HNSCC,[5–7] and for detecting neck recurrence after previous treatment.[8]

The UG-FNA procedure itself can be performed quickly and with minimal setup time. With an experienced technologist, much of the preparation, including equipment setup, target measurement, and initial optimization of the US acquisition parameters, can be standardized and completed before the radiologist's involvement in the procedure. Compared with CTG-FNA, there is less time spent bringing the patient in and out of the CT gantry and repositioning the needle. Particularly, if the first pass is nondiagnostic, the setup time for a second pass is typically shorter for UG-FNA than CTG-FNA, unless a larger introducer needle has been used during CT guidance.

With CT guidance, a portion of the procedure is performed blind, with safeguards in place for the length of needle throw during positioning before aspiration. Unless iodinated intravenous (IV) contrast material is used for the CTG-FNA, a complex solid and cystic mass may have fairly uniform attenuation under CT, so solid elements may not always be visible and adjacent vasculature may have similar attenuation. In contrast to CTG-FNA, there is no ionizing radiation used in UG-FNA, which is particularly problematic when repeated thin-collimation CT imaging is used in the same location. Although radiation is not a critical issue for patients with known malignancy and who have undergone or will undergo radiation therapy, it is generally favorable to try to limit

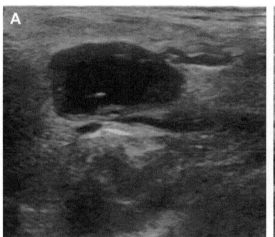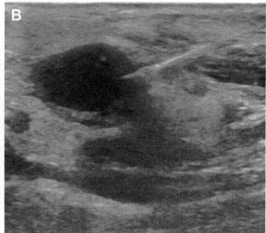

Fig. 2. UG-FNA of heterogeneous lesions. Transverse US images through the right parotid gland. (*A*) A heterogeneous centrally cystic and peripherally solid mass. (*B*) The needle is targeting the solid wall of the lesion.

exposure whenever possible, particularly in the pediatric population or in younger patients, who are less likely to have a malignant diagnosis. The lack of need for IV placement, renal function testing, and injection of iodinated contrast material if vascular visualization is required is also an advantage of UG-FNA. In general, we reserve CTG-FNA for deep targets with no sonographic window for UG-FNA (masticator space, parapharyngeal space, retropharyngeal space, pterygopalatine fossa, and deep lobe of the parotid gland).

Advantages of a Neuroradiologist-Run UG-FNA Service

There is great variability in who performs UG-FNA in the neck, ranging from the neuroradiologist/head and neck radiologist, body radiologist, head and neck surgeon, and cytopathologist. This situation is often dictated by local referral patterns and personal expertise in the technique. However,

there are many potential advantages of having a neuroradiologist perform this procedure. Thorough knowledge of the neck imaging anatomy, normal and abnormal appearance of the postoperative/postradiotherapy neck, and specific patterns of nodal spread for various head and neck malignancies is a major advantage over a body radiologist.

The neuroradiologist often interprets the imaging that may recommend FNA, leading to familiarity with the case and deliberation on the advantages and disadvantages of UG-FNA, CTG-FNA, and follow-up. At institutions with multidisciplinary tumor boards, cases requiring FNA for pathologic diagnosis often have the imaging presented by the neuroradiologist/head and neck radiologist at tumor board, so there is familiarity with the specific question to be answered by UG-FNA, which is important in complex cases with more than 1 potential target. There is also an automatic trigger for radiologic-pathologic

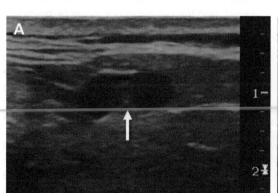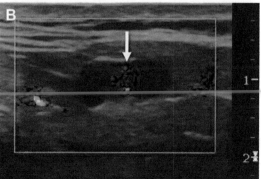

Fig. 3. Avoidance of the hilar vascularity on UG-FNA. Longitudinal US images through the left neck. (*A*) Note a hypoechoic but normal reniform appearance to a lymph node with echogenic hilum (*arrow*). (*B*) Doppler US image shows normal flow in the hilum (*arrow*), which should be avoided when performing UG-FNA.

discordance, so that mismatches can be discussed and further passes/alternative targets selected during the UG-FNA. Compared with surgical and cytopathologic colleagues, we are familiar with the imaging anatomy on multiple modalities and may already have skill sets from other image-guided procedures, including CTG-FNA.

Important to the success of a UG-FNA service is the presence of a dedicated US technologist with familiarity with setup of UG procedures. Also critical is the presence of an on-site cytopathologist. At our institution, all image-guided FNAs are performed with a cytopathologist present so that the appropriate number of needle passes are performed to obtain an adequate tissue sample for diagnosis. This process leads to immediate feedback on whether or not the procedure is being performed properly, and nondiagnostic passes can lead to adjustments in technique and sampling of different areas to achieve the highest possible yield, without performing additional unnecessary passes. For example, Fig. 4 shows a case of metastatic lymphadenopathy from melanoma that resulted in several nondiagnostic bloody passes through an obviously abnormal hypervascular lymph node. Attention was paid to an adjacent node with less vascularity, yielding melanoma on the first pass. In practices in which an on-site cytopathologist cannot be present, learning to properly smear and stain slides from a specimen is a desirable skill for the neuroradiologist performing UG-FNA. Maintaining a record of diagnostic yield and following up final pathologic diagnosis on each case, and troubleshooting nondiagnostic UG-FNAs, are critical to ongoing improvement with the technique.

Whether or Not to Perform UG-FNA

Knowledge of the disease processes involving the head and neck, as well as the advantages and disadvantages of UG-FNA versus CTG-FNA, is a major benefit of a neuroradiologist determining how a lesion should be sampled. The choice of US or CT guidance depends on a variety of factors. In general, the size, depth, and location of a lesion influence the choice of technique. Most lesions less than 3 cm from the skin surface on cross-sectional imaging are accessible with UG-FNA and a standard 3.8-cm (1.5-in) 23-gauge needle, because after compression of the skin by the transducer, this results in a depth less than 2 cm and an oblique needle trajectory less than 4 cm, leaving sufficient needle length for sampling. Fig. 5 depicts the general area accessible by UG-FNA with a standard 3.8-cm (1.5-in) needle. Deeper areas can be reached with a longer needle if required, although the resolution of the lower frequency of US needed to penetrate deeper may prohibit adequate needle and target visualization. On occasion, cases are referred for findings reported as indeterminate on CT or MR imaging, which the authors on review believe are probably benign. These cases are scheduled for an UG-FNA but may be converted to a diagnostic neck US examination without FNA if the neuroradiologist feels it has a benign sonographic appearance.

Patient Scheduling and Procedure Consent

We review all cases for potential UG-FNA before scheduling. During this process, the indication, past medical history, and all recent imaging are reviewed. We do not routinely obtain laboratory studies on patients for UG-FNA, no IV line is placed, and the patient is not made nil-by-mouth for the procedure. When the patient arrives to our preprocedure/postprocedure care area (PPCA), the neuroradiologist performing the procedure introduces themselves to the patient, reviews the reason for the UG-FNA, describes the procedure in detail, and discusses risks, benefits, and alternatives. Bleeding and infection are mentioned as the primary risks, although we have had no complications from either. We discuss that the chance of a nondiagnostic procedure is approximately 5% to 10% from the group's experience, and mention that repeat UG-FNA or surgical biopsy may be required if that occurs. We describe that it typically takes 3 passes with the needle, but may take a few more or less. We mention that although we may get

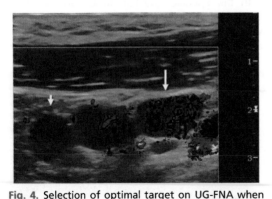

Fig. 4. Selection of optimal target on UG-FNA when multiple available. Longitudinal US image through the right neck, showing 3 hypoechoic lymph nodes. The lymph node on the right (*large arrow*) shows markedly increased Doppler flow and yielded only blood during multiple passes. The lymph node on the left (*small arrow*) was then sampled, yielding metastatic melanoma.

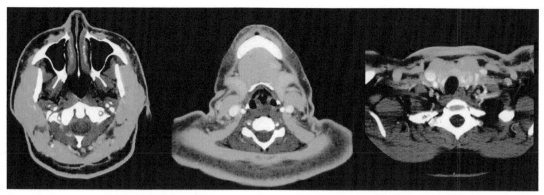

Fig. 5. Regions accessible by UG-FNA. Axial contrast-enhanced CT images showing the areas accessible by UG-FNA with a standard 3.8-cm (1.5-in) needle, yielding a depth of approximately 3 cm. Deeper lesions with a sonographic window for access may be sampled with a longer needle.

an immediate result, the final diagnosis may take time for the cytopathologist to review, and on rare occasions may change from the immediate diagnosis.

Equipment and FNA Procedure

Generally, we review the relevant previous in-house or outside imaging with the US technologist to guide target localization. The manufacturer of the particular US equipment used is not as critical as use of the appropriate transducer and familiarity with the technique. We use a linear high-frequency (8–12 MHz) transducer with a small footplate. When performing a UG-FNA, the highest possible frequency should be used to achieve optimal resolution, with sufficient depth of penetration to visualize structures deep to the target. In deep lesions, a curved lower frequency transducer may be required along with echogenic needle tip. Our setup for FNA is an inexpensive tray that contains all the elements needed for the procedure. These elements consist of sterile skin cleanser, drape, towels, US probe cover with sterile gel, 5-cm^3 syringes, 23-G needles, an 18-G drawing needle, gauze, and a band-aid (Fig. 6). A 4-mL to 1-mL mixture of 2% lidocaine and 8.4% sodium bicarbonate is used for local anesthesia.

Before the neuroradiologist enters the US room, the US technologist identifies the target, optimizes parameters (including the depth, frequency, and gain), makes measurements in 3 dimensions, and captures images. The neuroradiologist rescans the patient to ensure that the target corresponds to the abnormality in question, then marks the skin at the intended needle entry point. In general, the target should be in the center or side of the screen closer to the needle, but this depends on intervening vascular structures and target depth. When using color Doppler imaging to plan the

trajectory, it is important to use the correct gain, because the Doppler signal can be artifactually diminished by insufficient gain (Fig. 7).

Proper positioning is critical for successful UG-FNA. This positioning involves adjusting the bed height, lowering the bed railings, and positioning the patient, bed, and US monitor such that there is a direct line of sight between the needle, the transducer, and the monitor and a comfortable balanced posture is maintained by the neuroradiologist during FNA. The handedness of the operator influences the position for FNA. Generally, we perform most FNAs with the patient in the supine position, facing away from the direction of needle entry, but FNAs are sometimes better performed with the patient in a decubitus position (for lateral targets), prone (for posterior targets), or supine with head extended and a sheet rolled under the shoulders (for submandibular/submental targets). Most often, we perform the FNA with the transducer in the transverse plane

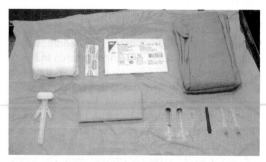

Fig. 6. Typical tray for UG-FNA, with sterile skin cleanser, drape, towels, US probe cover with sterile gel, 5-cm^3 syringes, 23-G needles, an 18-G drawing needle, gauze, and a band-aid. A 4-mL to 1-mL mixture of 2% lidocaine and 8.4% sodium bicarbonate is used for local anesthesia.

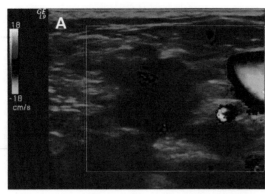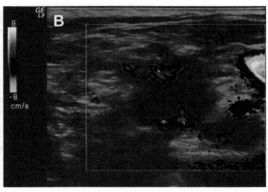

Fig. 7. Effect of Doppler gain on apparent vascularity for UG-FNA planning. (*A*) Transverse Doppler US images of the neck show a hypoechoic ill-defined mass. Because correct gain has been chosen, the less vascular regions of the mass can be targeted. (*B*) Same mass, improperly low gain resulting in an apparently low-vascularity target.

to allow visualization of the adjacent carotid and jugular vasculature in relation to the needle throughout the course of the procedure.

Using the usual sterile technique, the neuroradiologist cleans the skin, places the sterile drape and towels on the patient to allow the transducer to rest on the patient when not in use during the procedure, and places the sterile cover on the transducer. Five milliliters of 4:1 bicarbonate-buffered lidocaine is drawn into the syringe using the 18-G needle, and subsequently replaced with a 23-G to be used for local anesthesia. The target is localized with US using the sterile covered probe and sterile gel. Once the optimal approach has been chosen, the skin at the margin of the US probe footplate and immediate subcutaneous tissues are anesthetized generously. The target is again localized with the transducer, the needle advanced to the edge of the lesion under US guidance, and a tract of the buffered local anesthetic deposited as the needle is slowly retracted. In our experience, this process is almost always completely painless if performed correctly, and is the foundation for a successful procedure.

Any gel should be removed from the edge of the transducer and skin where the needle enters, because this results in gel artifact within the aspirated sample. A 23-G needle is attached to a 5-cm³ syringe and the plunger retracted by a few millimeters to remove the vacuum. The edge of the transducer is often lifted slightly to allow the needle to enter the skin a few millimeters under the transducer, so that the entry point and entire course of the needle can be seen. The fundamental skill in targeting a lesion with US is keeping either the needle or the transducer fixed, but not moving both. In general, it is best to keep the transducer firmly planted, while making small adjustments with the needle. If the initial positioning

under the transducer is correct, the entire path of the needle is visible on US as the target is reached. If the initial entry point is suboptimal, this should be readjusted close to the skin surface or through another puncture site within the anesthetized skin, because improper needle positioning becomes increasingly difficult to correct as the needle gets deeper. The entire process should occur while observing the monitor, and not the needle. Once the target is entered, small rapid motions should be used while using gentle suction with the syringe to aspirate cells from the target. Again, this should be performed while continuously viewing the monitor. Periodically, the needle hub should be quickly inspected for any material to suggest that a sufficient sample has been aspirated for analysis. Suction should be removed, and the needle withdrawn for cytologic analysis. Gentle pressure with sterile gauze resolves any bleeding at the needle entry site.

If a specimen is being reviewed by a cytopathologist, then the remainder of the procedure is guided by whether or not the individual passes are deemed sufficient. If lymphoma is a consideration, a separate pass and specimen processing may be needed for flow cytometry. If infection is a consideration, placement into an appropriate specimen container for culture is required. At a site without a cytopathologist physically present at the FNA, it may be helpful to familiarize yourself with the smearing and staining process. Slide preparation is not a replacement for dedicated cytologic examination, but may be useful to determine whether or not a target has been sampled. After completion of FNA, the skin is cleaned and a band-aid placed. We typically observe the patient in the PPCA for 30 minutes for any bleeding or increasing discomfort and then discharge the patient if there are no concerns.

SPECIAL CIRCUMSTANCES AND PITFALLS
Thyroid Bed and Relation to Trachea

When evaluating targets close to the trachea, such as within the thyroid bed after thyroidectomy, generally a steep approach to the target with sufficient visualization of the shadowing trachea is desirable. The patient should be instructed on suspending their swallowing and breathing during the critical portion of the tissue sampling, as opposed to taking a deep inspiration and holding their breath, which may suddenly change the position of the needle or target. The patient should also be informed that if the trachea is inadvertently entered, it is not dangerous but that they may get a sensation to cough. If the needle is seen entering the trachea on US, and the patient appears as if they will cough, quickly withdraw the needle.

Parotid and Submandibular Gland

Although hypointense lesions may stand out against the generally highly echogenic background of the parotid and submandibular gland, the needle is often difficult to see as it is traversing the gland (**Fig. 8**), particularly for deeper lesions with a longer required needle path length. Consider a needle trajectory from outside the gland for entry into an intraglandular mass (**Fig. 9**), or use of an echogenic tip needle. Even if accessible by UG-FNA, deep parotid and parapharyngeal space lesions are probably best biopsied under CTG with some degree of sedation, because they are often painful.

Esophagus

When collapsed, the esophagus can look like a mass within the thyroid fossa on CT and MR imaging, and can be hypermetabolic on FDG-PET in the setting of mucosal inflammation. For example, **Fig. 10** shows a patient who was referred for a UG-FNA of a large hypermetabolic mass in the left thyroid fossa after hemithyroidectomy. On US of the area in question, there was a leftward displaced echogenic mass, with the appearance of a normal esophagus displaced into the left thyroid fossa. When the patient was asked to swallow, a peristaltic wave was noted.

Carotid Arterial System and Internal Jugular Vein

For nodes deep to or along the trajectory of the carotid arterial system and internal jugular veins, there are various options. First, the jugular vein can often be displaced or completely compressed from the trajectory of the needle using gentle pressure on transducer (**Fig. 11**). Confirmation of any potential intervening vasculature with color Doppler US imaging is often helpful. Injection of a few milliliters of sterile saline into the space between the carotid artery and jugular vein is an alternative if venous compression is not successful, although it risks further posteriorly displacing any target between the 2 vessels. If positioning into a lateral decubitus position does not allow for a far lateral approach deep to the vasculature using US, CTG-FNA may be required.

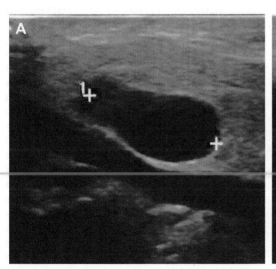
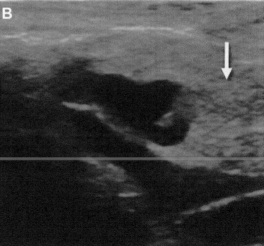

Fig. 8. Echogenic parotid gland precluding needle visualization. (*A*) Transverse US images through the parotid gland, showing a cystic mass. (*B*) Note the needle entering the mass, but the needle path within the gland (*arrow*) is difficult to discern because of the highly echogenic gland parenchyma.

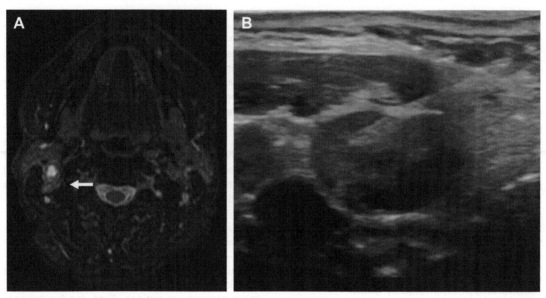

Fig. 9. Avoidance of the echogenic parotid gland on UG-FNA. (*A*) Axial T2-weighted fat-saturated MR image shows a subcentimeter hyperintense lesion (*arrow*) in the deep lobe of the right parotid gland. (*B*) Transverse US image shows needle path partly through the sternocleidomastoid muscle to avoid the echogenic parotid gland and aid in visualization of the needle throughout the procedure.

Vagus Nerve

With a high-frequency transducer, the vagus nerve can frequently be seen coursing between the common carotid artery and internal jugular vein. This situation should be noted when planning the UG-FNA, and the needle entry site and needle trajectory should be adjusted to avoid the structure. **Fig. 12** describes a case in which the most

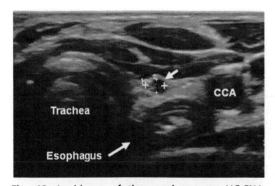

Fig. 10. Avoidance of the esophagus on UG-FNA. Transverse US image in a patient status after total thyroidectomy with report of a large hypermetabolic mass in the left thyroid fossa on CT-PET. Real-time sonography showed displacement of the esophagus into the left thyroid fossa, with peristalsis noted during patient swallowing. An incidental 3-mm benign-appearing nodule was present in the left thyroid fossa. CCA, common carotid artery.

direct trajectory that was initially planned was altered to avoid the vagus nerve.

Nerve Sheath Tumors

Nerve sheath tumors may mimic lymphadenopathy on imaging. These tumors are often extremely painful and preclude adequate sampling, compounded by their frequently fibrous and hypocellular nature (**Fig. 13**). If this diagnosis is a consideration, patients should be instructed that they may feel intense pain as the needle enters the mass, and coached on not moving suddenly as the needle is safely withdrawn. The sudden intense pain, in our experience, is virtually diagnostic of a schwannoma or neurofibroma. These lesions may be safely followed or may require excision for histologic diagnosis.

Supraclavicular Fossa

FNA in this region frequently requires a transverse approach, with the transducer parallel to and against the clavicle. If the target is underneath or below the clavicle, this requires angling the transducer and needle in concert slightly toward the feet. It is important to remember the close relationship of the supraclavicular fossa to the subclavian vasculature and lung apices, and appreciate the limitations of the UG-FNA technique in this area, particularly for deep lesions (**Fig. 14**).

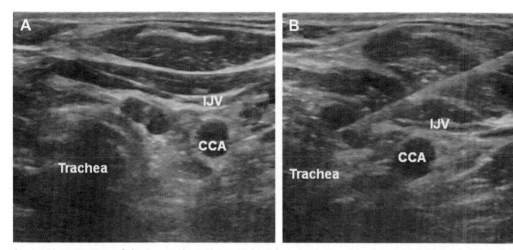

Fig. 11. Compression of the internal jugular vein (IJV) for access to a target. Transverse US images show a 1-cm mass adjacent to the trachea. A large IJV was noted to be along the trajectory of the needle, but with compression the IJV could be displaced and the needle safely guided into the lesion (*arrow*). CCA, common carotid artery.

Suspected Infection Versus Malignancy

Postoperatively, the differential diagnosis of a lesion in the neck may include abscess, necrotic malignant lymphadenopathy, or recurrent primary tumor. Because both may coexist, it is prudent to send specimens for culture as well as cell block even if cytology suggests only 1 diagnosis. **Fig. 15** describes a case of a patient with drainage from postauricular surgery for squamous cell carcinoma, with the lesion decreasing in size. The presumptive diagnosis was an abscess; however,

cytology showed recurrent HNSCC, presumably in the setting of resolving postoperative infection.

CTG-FNA AND CORE BIOPSY: TECHNIQUE AND PITFALLS

CTG-FNA and core biopsy are safe and reliable techniques for obtaining cytologic and core tissue samples in the head and neck, avoiding open surgical biopsy. This technique is most useful in regions of the deep face, where US guidance is not possible because of inadequate sonographic windows from bone or air-containing structures.[9,10] CTG-FNA has an overall low complication rate in the head and neck,[10–12] with complications

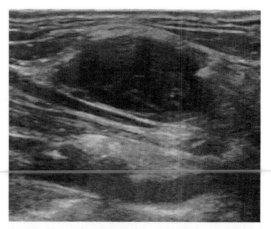

Fig. 12. Avoidance of the vagus nerve on UG-FNA. Transverse US image shows a mass posterior to the internal jugular vein (IJV) and common carotid artery (CCA). The shortest needle trajectory is between the IJV and CCA; however, the vagus nerve (*arrow*) is noted. An alternative path posterior to the CCA was chosen.

Fig. 13. Nerve sheath tumor on UG-FNA. Longitudinal US image showing a hypoechoic mass. The patient showed intense pain when the needle contacted the surface of the mass, precluding any tissue sampling. Follow-up imaging showed stability in the presumed nerve sheath tumor.

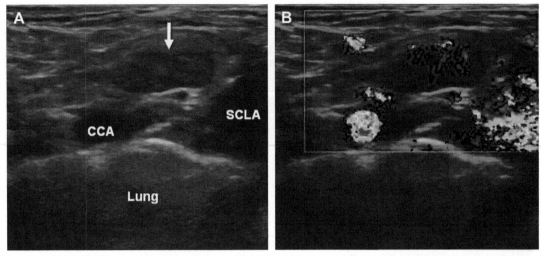

Fig. 14. Pitfalls of UG-FNA in the supraclavicular fossa. (*A, B*) Transverse images of the supraclavicular fossa, with transducer parallel to and contacting the clavicles with caudal angulation of the transducer. Heterogeneous nodule in this location is bounded posteriorly by the common carotid artery (CCA), subclavian artery (SCLA), and the lung apex.

including local pain, vasovagal reaction, cellulitis, and minor bleeding.[13] There are rare reports of hemorrhage after CTG biopsy.[14] Consideration should be taken that CTG techniques expose the patient to radiographic radiation repeatedly to the same anatomic region, particularly if CT fluoroscopy is used, with the largest contribution to the peak absorbed dose because of positioning of sampling instrumentation.[15]

Conscious sedation may be used for patient comfort, and general anesthesia is particularly useful when performing the procedure in children or in patients with an uncontrollable movement disorder. The use of iodinated contrast is often useful to map out important adjacent vascular structures that are critical to avoid during needle positioning. A wide variety of CTG approaches are used for sampling deep spaces and masses that are difficult to reach, including retromandibular, paramaxillary, transoral, subzygomatic, submastoid, and posterior approaches.[16–18] The specifics of the setup and performance of the technique have been described in detail elsewhere.[19] The use of a coaxial technique may be helpful in avoiding multiple skin punctures and avoiding the need to reposition the sampling needle after each pass.[9,20] Various biopsy guns are available for obtaining core samples of tissues

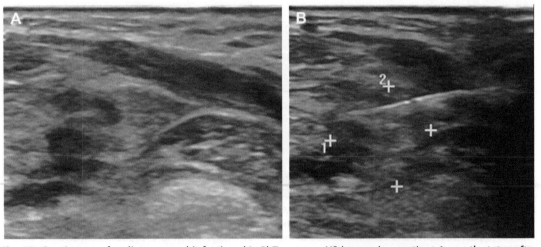

Fig. 15. Coexistence of malignancy and infection. (*A, B*) Transverse US images in a patient 1 month status after recent surgery for squamous cell carcinoma of the postauricular region and decreasing swelling and redness in the high neck after antibiotic initiation show ill-defined hypodensity and muscular edema. UG-FNA showed metastatic squamous cell carcinoma in the setting of a resolving postoperative infection.

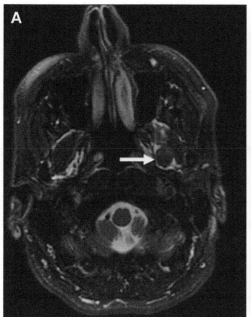
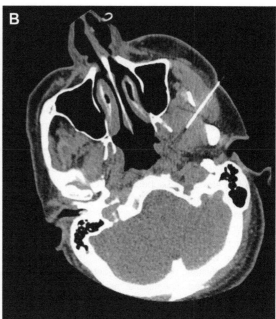

Fig. 16. Fibrous mass presenting difficulty to CTG-FNA and CTG core biopsy. (*A*) Axial T2-weighted fat-saturated MR image showing a 1-cm hypointense lesion (*arrow*) in the left masticator space. (*B*) CTG-FNA shows core biopsy needle at the edge of the lesion; the lesion was fibrous, and it was difficult to aspirate or core an adequate sample in this presumed V3 schwannoma.

for analysis, if needed. The overall diagnostic yield of CTG sampling is reported to be 80% to 91% in the literature,[10,11,21] with usefulness for diagnosis of both malignant and benign causes such as paragangliomas and schwannomas,[19] although tumors that are hypervascular (**Fig. 16**) or fibrous

(**Fig. 17**) may have diminished diagnostic yield for CTG-FNA and CTG core biopsy.

SUMMARY

Image-guided tissue sampling is becoming increasingly important for management of head and neck cancers. UG-FNA is safe, effective, and has many advantages compared with PG-FNA and CTG-FNA. The technique of UG-FNA is highly operator and experience dependent; however, understanding the complex anatomy, disease processes, and patterns of nodal spread in the head and neck make this technique ideally suited for the neuroradiologist. Proper technique, particularly optimal patient positioning, effective local anesthesia, and transducer-needle manipulation, as well as recognition of pitfalls, is critical to successful UG-FNA. CTG-FNA is valuable for tissue sampling from deep lesions and for those without a sonographic window for UG-FNA.

Fig. 17. Hypervascular mass presenting difficulty with CTG-FNA. Axial CT images from CTG-FNA show a large mass (*arrow*) within the left carotid space. Repeated FNA samples yielded only blood in this presumed paraganglioma.

REFERENCES

1. Laubenbacher C, Saumweber D, Wagner-Manslau C, et al. Comparison of fluorine-18-fluorodeoxyglucose PET, MRI and endoscopy for staging head and neck squamous-cell carcinomas. J Nucl Med 1995; 36(10):1747–57.

2. Di Martino E, Nowak B, Hassan HA, et al. Diagnosis and staging of head and neck cancer: a comparison of modern imaging modalities (positron emission tomography, computed tomography, color-coded duplex sonography) with panendoscopic and histopathologic findings. Arch Otolaryngol Head Neck Surg 2000;126(12):1457–61.

3. Paulus P, Sambon A, Vivegnis D, et al. 18FDG-PET for the assessment of primary head and neck tumors: clinical, computed tomography, and histopathological correlation in 38 patients. Laryngoscope 1998;108(10):1578–83.

4. Kau RJ, Alexiou C, Laubenbacher C, et al. Lymph node detection of head and neck squamous cell carcinomas by positron emission tomography with fluorodeoxyglucose F 18 in a routine clinical setting. Arch Otolaryngol Head Neck Surg 1999;125(12):1322–8.

5. van den Brekel MW, Castelijns JA, Stel HV, et al. Occult metastatic neck disease: detection with US and US-guided fine-needle aspiration cytology. Radiology 1991;180(2):457–61.

6. Takes RP, Knegt P, Manni JJ, et al. Regional metastasis in head and neck squamous cell carcinoma: revised value of US with US-guided FNAB. Radiology 1996;198(3):819–23.

7. Righi PD, Kopecky KK, Caldemeyer KS, et al. Comparison of ultrasound-fine needle aspiration and computed tomography in patients undergoing elective neck dissection. Head Neck 1997;19(7):604–10.

8. Westhofen M. Ultrasound B-scans in the follow-up of head and neck tumors. Head Neck Surg 1987;9(5):272–8.

9. Robbins KT, van Sonnenberg E, Casola G. Image-guided needle biopsy of inaccessible head and neck lesions. Arch Otolaryngol Head Neck Surg 1990;116(8):957–61.

10. DelGaudio JM, Dillard DG, Albritton FD, et al. Computed tomography-guided needle biopsy of head and neck lesions. Arch Otolaryngol Head Neck Surg 2000;126(3):366–70.

11. Sherman PM, Yousem DM, Loevner LA. CT-guided aspirations in the head and neck: assessment of the first 216 cases. AJNR Am J Neuroradiol 2004;25(9):1603–7.

12. Gatenby RA, Mulhern CB, Richter MP, et al. CT-guided biopsy for the detection and staging of tumors of the head and neck. AJNR Am J Neuroradiol 1984;5(3):287–90.

13. Charboneau JW, Reading CC, Welch TJ. CT and sonographically guided needle biopsy: current techniques and new innovations. AJR Am J Roentgenol 1990;154(1):1–10.

14. Walker AT, Chaloupka JC, Putman CM, et al. Sentinel transoral hemorrhage from a pseudoaneurysm of the internal maxillary artery: a complication of CT-guided biopsy of the masticator space. AJNR Am J Neuroradiol 1996;17(2):377–81.

15. Tsalafoutas IA, Tsapaki V, Triantopoulou C, et al. CT-guided interventional procedures without CT fluoroscopy assistance: patient effective dose and absorbed dose considerations. AJR Am J Roentgenol 2007;188(6):1479–84.

16. Gupta S. Approaches for percutaneous needle placement for various head and neck procedures. Neuroimaging Clin North Am 2009;19(2):149–60.

17. Gupta S, Henningsen JA, Wallace MJ, et al. Percutaneous biopsy of head and neck lesions with CT guidance: various approaches and relevant anatomic and technical considerations. Radiographics 2007;27(2):371–90.

18. Gupta S, Madoff DC. Image-guided percutaneous needle biopsy in cancer diagnosis and staging. Tech Vasc Interv Radiol 2007;10(2):88–101.

19. Loevner LA. Image-guided procedures of the head and neck: the radiologist's arsenal. Otolaryngol Clin North Am 2008;41(1):231–50, viii.

20. Mukherji SK, Turetsky D, Tart RP, et al. A technique for core biopsies of head and neck masses. AJNR Am J Neuroradiol 1994;15(3):518–20.

21. Sack MJ, Weber RS, Weinstein GS, et al. Image-guided fine-needle aspiration of the head and neck: five years' experience. Arch Otolaryngol Head Neck Surg 1998;124(10):1155–61.

Index

Note: Page numbers of article titles are in **boldface** type.

Neuroimag Clin N Am 23 (2013) 179–182
http://dx.doi.org/10.1016/S1052-5149(12)00188-8
1052-5149/13/$ – see front matter © 2013 Elsevier Inc. All rights reserved.

neuroimaging.theclinics.com

Moving?

Make sure your subscription moves with you!

To notify us of your new address, find your **Clinics Account Number** (located on your mailing label above your name), and contact customer service at:

Email: journalscustomerservice-usa@elsevier.com

800-654-2452 (subscribers in the U.S. & Canada)
314-447-8871 (subscribers outside of the U.S. & Canada)

Fax number: 314-447-8029

**Elsevier Health Sciences Division
Subscription Customer Service
3251 Riverport Lane
Maryland Heights, MO 63043**

*To ensure uninterrupted delivery of your subscription, please notify us at least 4 weeks in advance of move.

Printed and bound by CPI Group (UK) Ltd, Croydon, CR0 4YY

03/10/2024

01040347-0016